Multiple Sclerosis

The Questions You Have—
The Answers You Need

Second Edition

Edited by Rosalind C. Kalb, Ph.D.

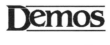

Demos

New York

Demos Medical Publishing, Inc., 386 Park Avenue South,
New York, New York 10016

Library of Congress Cataloging-in-Publication Data

Multiple sclerosis : the questions you have, the answers you need /
edited by Rosalind C. Kalb.—2nd ed.
     p.   cm.
  Includes bibliographical references and index.
  ISBN 1-888799-43-9
  1. Multiple sclerosis—Popular works. 2. Multiple
sclerosis—-Miscellanea. I. Kalb, Rosalind
  RC377.M564 2000   00-035857
  616.8′34—dc21

Printed in Canada

Dedication

To all those individuals and families living with multiple
sclerosis who continue to look for answers
And to my family—Nick, Johanna, and Alex

Frequent updates to this book can be downloaded from our Web site: demosmedpub.com. This site also contains information about Demos's other publications on multiple sclerosis.

Contents

Foreword

Randall R. Schapiro, M.D.

It is with pleasure and honor that I write this foreword to the new edition of *Multiple Sclerosis: The Questions You Have—The Answers You Need.* In the first edition of the book Rosalind Kalb, Ph.D., proved that it was possible to compile the commonly asked questions about a very complicated disease and deliver answers in a manner that was easily understood by all. However, new questions are asked, there is always new information for old questions, and sometimes even the old answers change! Thus this is a never-ending task. That is how it should be until the final answer to the mystery of MS is found. Once again Dr. Kalb has obtained consultation from the most experienced clinicians and researchers who tackle the issues associated with MS. None of these are simple, and simple answers do not always satisfy the thirst for knowledge, but this is a start.

The book—like life—represents teamwork. Surprisingly, it is not easy to compile answers to questions in a form that educates the naive and the well-informed at the same time. This is especially true when the topics range from toileting to immune modulation. The answers to such diverse questions often come from very diverse experts. To make the book flow and yet thoroughly answer the diversity of inquiries is truly a noble feat.

This was accomplished in the first edition and once again in this edition.

The issues surrounding MS are many. A day does not go by in my practice during which I am asked any number of the questions answered here. That is an indication of the practicality of this endeavor. There is no doubt in my mind that education empowers individuals to fight for a better quality of life. We all educate ourselves differently, but we all want quick answers to our questions. There are a number of sources for answers. They range from the medical community, to the voluntary health agencies, to people on the Internet expressing opinions without fact. It is incumbent upon us all to seek out the best information with the most factual basis. In the information-oriented society it is often hard to know who to trust. This book is trustworthy! It is factual! It is honest! However, it is no substitute for talking with your health professional about your problems. It is a jumping-off point to learning more about MS and with that knowledge developing new and better coping skills to deal with the ups and downs of the mysteries of MS. You may be disappointed that there are no easy answers to curing MS, but you should come away from reading this book understanding that while there are still gaps in our knowledge, much is now known and even more is being studied.

I personally am privileged to be a part of the "questions" team and look forward to discussing MS with each of you as you read on.

Acknowledgments

The teamwork continues. This new edition reflects the ongoing commitment of a multidisciplinary group of health care professionals to provide accurate and up-to-date information for individuals and families living with MS. In addition to the authors, I would particularly like to thank the following people: Stephen Reingold, Ph.D., of the National Multiple Sclerosis Society for his thoughtful and comprehensive review; Shirley Brown, M.A., CCC-SLP and Sandé Grant Goldman for their valuable comments and suggestions; Faith Seidman, C.S.W., for pointing me toward useful resources; Alex Kalb for his assistance in reviewing and updating the resource section; Christina Lipka and Ann Palmer of the Information Resource Center and Nancy Holland, Ed.D., of the Clinical Programs Department at the National MS Society for assisting me to find answers and stay current with information and resources; Nicholas LaRocca, Ph.D., for his ongoing help and support with the content and the process; and Diana Schneider, Ph.D., and Joan Wolk of Demos Medical Publishing for their enthusiasm and hard work in support of this project.

1

What Should I Know About This Book?

Nancy J. Holland, Ed.D.

Is this book for me?

Multiple Sclerosis: The Questions You Have—The Answers You Need was written primarily for people with multiple sclerosis. However, if you love someone with MS, work with a person who has MS, or are just curious about the disease, you will find this book helpful and informative. It covers a wide range of topics in a format that is familiar, accessible, and easily understood. The question and answer format was selected for several reasons. First, it reflects the collaborative relationship between individuals with MS and their health care professionals. The authors of each chapter answer the questions that they have been asked repeatedly in the course of their work with MS. Second, the questions included here provide a model and a vocabulary for those who are not certain what questions to ask or how to ask them. Third, the question and answer format makes it possible for readers to zero in on particular topics, and even particular questions, without having to wade through material that may be irrelevant to their individual needs.

What is the purpose of this book?

It is important for someone with a chronic illness to understand its potentially far-reaching impact and to know what positive actions can be taken to manage this unexpected intrusion into daily life. An open dialogue with the physician and other professionals on the health care team is an important part of the adjustment process. This book answers specific questions about living with MS and can help prepare you to interact with health professionals as an informed and active participant in your health promotion plan. Factors such as the symptoms you are experiencing, the course of your MS, and career and family plans all need to be considered in a thoughtful manner. This book provides one tool to help in that process. Concerned professionals will also assist and support you through the difficult aspects of adjusting to MS.

How were people selected to answer the questions in this book?

Recognized experts in the field of multiple sclerosis were invited to participate. Most of the authors are affiliated with a comprehensive MS care center and/or the National Multiple Sclerosis Society and have extensive experience in assisting people to deal with MS-related problems. Others work in related fields that target the medical, psychosocial, and economic challenges faced by those with chronic illness.

How were the questions selected for inclusion?

For the first edition of the book, each of the contributing authors was asked to provide a list of questions, related to his or her area of expertise, that are commonly asked by individuals with MS and their family members. Authors were also asked to include questions that they thought people should be encouraged to ask even if they were not routinely doing so. Additionally, the Information Resource Center at the National Multiple Sclerosis Society provided a computerized listing of topics most frequently asked about on the telephone information line. The proposed questions for each chapter were then reviewed by a number of people with MS, family members, caregivers, and health professionals in an attempt to ensure that the list of questions was both comprehensive and meaningful. The questions and topics that have been added to the second edition of the book were suggested by people with MS and their family members, professionals in the field, and other interested readers.

How should I use this book?

There are a few factors to consider before deciding how to use this book. First, the course of MS and its related symptom picture can vary significantly from one individual to the next, as can the individual's response to treatment. People also vary in the individual characteristics they bring to the situation—their age, sex, family composition, social support network, and occupation, to name a few. Personality characteristics can also influence how a person will deal with MS and how he or she will choose to use this book. For example, some people want to know *everything* about MS, regardless of immediate or long-term relevance to their own medical situation. For most people, however, this is not the case. They want to know answers to specific questions that are pertinent to decisions that they need to make now and in the immediate future. You can use this book in any way that best suits your needs and your style of dealing with information.

The book attempts to answer questions for everyone living with MS—those who have the disease and those who share life with someone who has it. Although many people with MS do not have serious or debilitating symptoms, others have a rougher time. Since all of the information in this book will not pertain to everyone, some material may be upsetting to those not experiencing the more disabling problems. We recommend that you be selective in your reading and not see this as a book you must read from cover to cover. No one person will face all of the problems addressed here, and the full range of circumstances can be overwhelming if not dealt with selectively. Each chapter has a short introduction to the particular topic, a series of questions and answers relating to the topic, and a listing of recommended readings for people who wish to pursue the topic in greater depth. Where applicable, the authors have also provided a list of available resources, including organizations, agencies, product manufacturers, and other potential sources of relevant information or goods and services.

The best strategy is probably to use this book for reference purposes, reading it now for background information and answers to your immediate questions, and in the future as other problems or questions arise. The "Neurology" and "Treatment" chapters provide a useful overview of the disease and its management. The "Employment," "Insurance," and "Life Planning" chapters will alert you to important issues that you need to be thinking about now in order to safeguard yourself and your family down the road. The chapter "Psychosocial Issues" addresses the ways in which people with MS and their family members react to the intrusion of MS and learn to cope with the changes that a chronic illness can impose on their lives. The introductions to the other chapters will help identify additional areas you might want to pursue in more detail. The Appendixes provide specific reference materials:

◇ **Glossary.** Medical words and phrases that are in bold type in the text are explained in the alphabetized glossary in Appendix A. Also included in the glossary are terms that you might encounter in other MS-related reading materials or in discussions with your health care providers. Multiple sclerosis is surrounded by a new and unfamiliar vocabulary of neurologic terms, anatomic parts, and rehabilitation language. Learning the meaning of these terms will increase your understanding of the complex information and facilitate your efforts to communicate with your health care providers.

◇ **Medication Information Sheets.** Many medications are used to deal with the variety of MS symptoms. A particular medication will likely be of interest only if your physician has recommended it or if you read or hear about it as a suggested therapy for a symptom you are experiencing. Each sheet in Appendix B describes how the particular drug is used in MS and provides important information that you need to know about any drug you are taking, including potential side effects and drug interactions. While the information sheets are designed to help you be a more informed participant in your own care, your physician should always be your primary source of information about the medications that he or she is prescribing for you.

◇ **Recommended Reading List.** Included in this list in Appendix C are books and other publications relating specifically to multiple sclerosis or to chronic illness.

◇ **National Multiple Sclerosis Society Consensus Statement.** Appendix C contains a statement, published in 1998, regarding early intervention and access to therapy for people with relapsing-remitting MS.

◇ **Resource List**. Your particular needs at any given time will direct your use of the Resource List in Appendix E. Included in this list are government and private agencies and organizations that provide information and/or services to deal with MS-related problems. Since many resources vary according to the state or community in which you live, the Resource List can also guide your efforts to identify local sources of information and assistance. Resources that are specifically relevant to the area covered in a particular chapter are listed at the end of that chapter.

◇ **List of Authors**. Brief professional biographies of the authors are included in Appendix F.

What if I have only recently been diagnosed with MS?

In general, it will not be helpful for someone with a recent diagnosis to read the entire book. If you were only recently diagnosed, you probably have a relatively short history of MS symptoms to look back on and limited experience with the impact of these symptoms on your daily life. People differ in their responses to both the diagnosis and the challenges it poses. Additionally, there is considerable variation in disease course and symptoms in MS. Therefore, much of the material in this book will not be pertinent for you now and may or may not be pertinent for you in the future. If your MS follows a mild or moderate course, some of this information will never be relevant to your situation.

What if some of the answers (and even the questions) upset me?

Multiple sclerosis is an unwelcome and distressing intruder for everyone involved. One way to reduce the discomfort is to have accurate information about what to expect and what can be done. Some people with MS have an easier time than others, but this book attempts to deal with the full range of possible problems, even the very difficult ones. Remember to focus on the topics that relate to your particular and unique situation, and try not to become preoccupied with questions and problems that are unrelated to your own. If you continue to have questions or concerns about the information provided here, be sure to contact a member of your health team for further discussion.

How can I get additional information about topics addressed in this book?

Each chapter includes a list of recommended readings for people who wish to pursue more detailed information about a particular topic. Most of the recommended readings are for lay audiences. Articles from professional journals have been included in some lists, particularly in those areas in which little has been written for nonprofessionals (e.g., speech and swallowing disorders, cognition). Information about professional articles pertaining to multiple sclerosis can be obtained from the Information Resource Center of the National Multiple Sclerosis Society; publications may be available at your public library, through the library's interlibrary loan service, or from an online computer service.

More general readings are listed in the Recommended Reading List in Appendix C. You can also contact a member of your health care team for additional recommendations. Your local chapter of the National Multiple Sclerosis Society (reachable by calling 1-800-FIGHT MS) is another valuable source of up-to-date information about MS. Staff will answer questions and send you reading materials on a wide variety of MS-related topics. Obviously, no single book can include every possible question. Each individual is different and will experience MS in his or her own way. You will probably have questions of your own that do not appear in this book. The goal of this book is to help you ask important questions—and find accurate, meaningful answers—so that you can manage life with MS in the way that best meets your needs.

2

Neurology

Charles R. Smith, M.D.
Randall T. Schapiro, M.D.

Multiple sclerosis (MS) is a **chronic** neurologic disease that is diagnosed most commonly in young adults. Although 90 percent of those diagnosed are between the ages of 16 and 60, MS has been known to make its first appearance in early childhood or long after age 60. The currently estimated **prevalence** of MS in the United States is 250,000–350,000 individuals, which means that more than one in a thousand people have the diagnosis at any given time. While an **incidence** rate of 10,000 new cases per year has been estimated in the United States, the availability of more effective diagnostic tools is gradually resulting in a higher rate of accurate diagnosis than was previously possible. Multiple sclerosis is more common in women than in men, by a ratio of approximately 2–3:1. It appears more frequently in whites than in Hispanics or African Americans and is relatively rare among Asians and certain other groups.

Multiple sclerosis is more common in temperate areas of the world and is relatively unusual in the tropics. The disease is seen more frequently in individuals from Great Britain, Scandinavia, and Northern Germany than from areas around the Mediterranean Sea; Canadians and individuals from the northern part of the United States develop MS more frequently than those living in the southern part of the continent. Multiple sclerosis is extremely rare among the Black peoples of Africa.

Although not directly inherited, the disease seems to appear in genetically predisposed individuals who are apparently more reactive or susceptible to whatever stimulus or agent causes the disease to become active. The general conclusion is that people of northern and central European ancestry, as well as those whose ancestry has become mingled with this group, seem to have some genetic predisposition to the disease. While we do not know as yet what factors within the environment cause MS to make its appearance in some of these individuals and not others, most researchers continue to believe that some unidentified infectious agent (e.g., viral or bacterial) is the likely culprit.

MS is thought to be an **autoimmune disease** in which the body's immune system attacks an apparently normal tissue or organ of the body. The immune attack involves inflammation directed against the **myelin** of the **central nervous system (CNS)** (see Fig. 2-1), in a process called **demyelination. Neurons**, or nerve cells, in the central nervous system are made up of the cell body, **axons** (the processes or extensions of nerve cells that conduct nervous impulses away from the cell body), and dendrites. Myelin is the insulation or coating that surrounds the axons and speeds nerve conduction. Demyelination results in **plaques** or lesions along the myelin sheath that interfere with nerve conduction. The symptoms that occur in MS result from this inflammatory process, as well as from inflammatory damage to the axons themselves. These symptoms can include loss of vision, double vision, stiffness, weakness, imbalance, numbness, pain, problems with bladder and bowel control, fatigue, sexual changes, speech and swallowing difficulties, emotional changes, and intellectual impairment. The type and number of symptoms vary tremendously from one individual to the next, depending on where in the CNS the myelin and axonal damage occurs. At this time, we do not know why the damage occurs or why some people get more or different symptoms than others.

As is clear from this description of MS, there is much that we do not know about its causes or its pattern of symptoms. This uncertainty has been largely responsible for the frustrations faced by scientists searching for a cure. We do know that the disease tends to appear during the early adult years, when career and family growth are at their peak. Fortunately, although MS is a

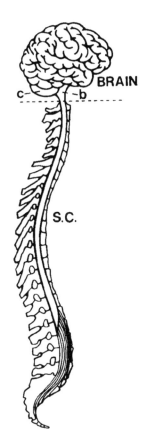

BRAIN

c—   —b

S.C.

Figure 2-1   Central nervous system. The brain and spinal cord (S.C.) are the principal components of the central nervous system and are separated by a broken line in this schematic diagram. The cerebellum (**c**) and brainstem (**b**) are regions of the brain often affected by multiple sclerosis.

chronic illness, it is not always a progressive one. Many people with MS are able to lead healthy and productive lives. For them, the symptoms of MS are more of an episodic discomfort or annoyance than a hindrance to their life's ambitions. For those whose MS is more severe and debilitating, we now have a variety of management strategies available that may help to keep the various neurologic **impairments** that can be caused by the disease from compromising a person's daily *activities* or interfering with their active *participation* in society. These categories of **disablement**, recently identified by the World Health Organization, are important to keep in mind as you read the questions and answers in this and other chapters. At the present time, we have almost no control over the neurologic changes (impairments) that occur in MS. Nevertheless, we can do a great deal to reduce the impact of those impairments on a person's ability to carry out specific tasks at home or at work (activities), and reduce or eliminate any societal barriers that prevent a person from being an active and productive member of society (participation).

Much can be done to improve quality of life after the diagnosis. Developing a positive attitude and getting educated are half the battle. Finding a health care team that understands and accommodates your needs is an important step. With their help, you can feel more in control and take on the challenges of life with MS with confidence. The following questions and answers highlight the primary concerns of people who are trying to understand this puzzling and unpredictable disease.

The Disease: Its Diagnosis, Course, and Prognosis

What goes wrong when a person has MS?

The body's actions and reactions to outside stimuli involve a lightning-quick and complicated process in which the body receives those stimuli through the various senses (vision or touch, for example), sends a report to the brain, and then responds to instructions from the brain about what to do next (see Fig. 2-2).

This ongoing process depends on the coordinated transmission of nerve impulses from one nerve cell to the next. Nerve impulses pass along nerve fibers, which connect at synapses. A fatty substance called myelin, which forms a sheath around the nerve fibers in the CNS (which is made up of the brain, optic nerves, and spinal cord) helps to speed this conduction of nerve impulses (see Fig. 2-3). The myelin, which is made and maintained by cells called **oligodendrocytes**, has a whitish appearance, leading to the identification of MS as primarily a **white matter** disease of the CNS.

Any damage to the myelin sheath results in some disruption of the impulse or message that is being transmitted, much as would occur in a damaged telephone wire. In MS, overactive, misguided cells of the immune system enter the CNS, causing inflammation in the brain and spinal cord. This inflammation causes damage to the myelin. Wherever myelin is destroyed, a **plaque** (lesion) forms, with a gradual buildup of hardened scar tissue (**sclerosis**) at the site. These sclerotic sites occur in varied locations throughout the CNS, giving rise to the name *multiple sclerosis*. While many of these scars may be "silent," causing no

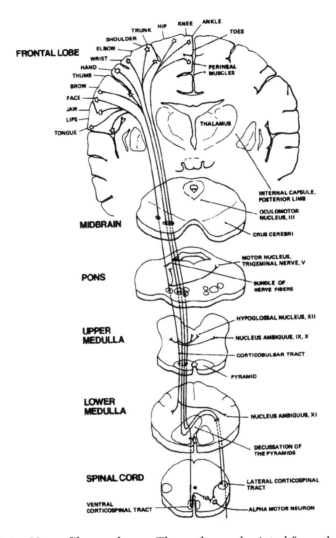

Figure 2-2   Nerve fiber pathway. The pathway depicted from the brain to the spinal cord involves fibers responsible for control of movements. (Adapted with permission from Gilman S, Newman SW: *Manter and Gatz's Essentials of Clinical Neuroanatomy and Neurophysiology*, 8th edition. Philadelphia: F.A. Davis, 1992:77.)

apparent symptoms, others can interfere with sensation or function. Additionally, demyelination may disrupt communication between different parts of the brain, even if the parts themselves remain intact.

While the name "multiple sclerosis" comes from the multiple sclerotic sites caused by demyelination, the disease can also

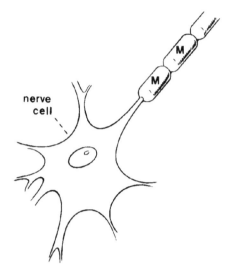

Figure 2-3   Myelin sheath.
Cuffs of myelin (M) insulate
fibers from the nerve cell that
carries electrical signals.

cause irreversible damage to the nerve fibers themselves. Recent
studies of brain tissue (on autopsy) have revealed the presence
of damaged nerve fibers (axons) in people with MS, even in the
very earliest stages of the illness.

Why is the diagnosis of MS so difficult?

At the present time, there are no specific blood tests, imaging
techniques (e.g., **magnetic resonance imaging (MRI)** or **computerized axial tomography (CAT) scan**), tests of immune function, or genetic tests that can, by themselves, determine if a person has MS or is likely to have it in the future. The diagnosis is
a clinical one, made on the basis of a person's medical history,
an assessment of the **symptoms** experienced and reported by the
person, and the existence of **signs** detected by the physician (but
not necessarily noticed by the person) during the neurologic
examination. Both symptoms and signs are necessary because
symptoms are subjective complaints that can vary tremendously
from one individual to another, while signs are more measurable, objective observations. Examples of symptoms that are
commonly reported by people with MS include problems with
vision, walking, bladder control, fatigue, and uncomfortable sensations such as numbness or "pins and needles." Common signs
that can be detected by the doctor during a physical examination, even if the person has never noticed or been troubled by
these changes, include altered eye movements and abnormal

responses of the pupils, subtle changes in speech patterns, altered reflex responses, impaired **coordination**, sensory distur- bances, and evidence of **spasticity** and/or weakness in the limbs.

In order to make a definite diagnosis of MS, the physician must find the following:

◇ plaques or lesions in at least two distinct areas of the CNS white matter;

◇ evidence that the plaques have occurred at different points in time; and, perhaps most importantly,

◇ that these plaques in the white matter have no other rea- sonable explanation.

In other words, MS is a diagnosis that can be made only after every other possible explanation of the signs and symptoms has been ruled out.

How will the doctor try to determine if I have MS?

The physician will first take a very careful history, including any past and present complaints that you have, any pertinent family history of disease, the places you have lived and visited, sub- stance use (alcohol, drug, and smoking habits), and any medica- tions that you are taking. Through detailed questioning, the doc- tor can determine whether you have ever experienced other symptoms—no matter how slight or transient—that might be indicative of MS-related disease activity.

The physician will do a neurologic examination to check for signs that can explain the symptoms you are experiencing or point to disease activity of which you may have been totally unaware. An eye examination with an **ophthalmoscope** may reveal the presence of damage to the optic nerve. A pale optic nerve in MS is often indicative of earlier damage even if the per- son reports no past or current visual symptoms. The doctor will also test visual acuity and look for evidence of double vision or incoordination of eye movements.

The physician will test for evidence of weakness by asking you to resist efforts to pull or push your arms and legs. You may also be asked to squeeze his or her hand. Your coordination will be tested in a variety of ways, including the **finger-to-nose test,** in which you are asked to bring the tip of your index finger to your nose rapidly, with your eyes open and then closed, and the *heel-knee-shin test*, in which you are asked to move one heel up and down the shin of the other leg. The physician will evaluate your balance by asking you to perform a variety of tasks, including walking on your heels and then on your toes, performing a *tandem gait* (placing the heel of one foot directly against the toe of the other foot in an alternating fashion), and standing still with your eyes closed.

Sensory changes will also be tested in a variety of ways. Your physician will determine if you can tell, with your eyes closed, where your body parts (e.g., fingers and toes) are in space (*position sense*). *Vibration sense* will be tested with a vibrating tuning fork placed against various points on your body. The physician may also use a (gentle) pinprick to test for changes in skin sensitivity. Unfortunately, many of the sensory changes experienced by people with MS, such as numbness, pain, or tingling, cannot be seen or objectively measured on examination, with the result that some physicians have tended to ignore or dismiss these uncomfortable symptoms as unimportant.

The physician will test the reflexes in various parts of your body. Inequality of reflexes on the two sides of your body is indicative of an abnormal reflex. Absent reflexes, particularly in the abdomen, are also common in MS, although they can have other explanations such as obesity or multiple pregnancies. The *Babinski reflex*, a frequent finding in MS, is clearly indicative of disturbances in major nervous pathways. This neurologic sign is elicited when the physician draws a bluntly pointed object along the outer edge of the sole of the foot from the heel to the little toe. Instead of the normal downward flexion of the toes, it results in an abnormal response in which the big toe extends upward and the other toes fan outward.

For some people, no tests beyond this history and neurologic exam are necessary to make the diagnosis. If the doctor is able to find evidence of multiple lesions in the CNS that have occurred at different points in time and have no other reasonable explanation, the diagnosis can be made without any other testing being done. However, most physicians will not rely entirely on this type of evaluation and will do at least one other test to confirm the diagnosis. This is especially true if the history and examination have not been able to provide conclusive evidence of more than one lesion in the brain or spinal cord. The most commonly done test is MRI (*magnetic resonance imaging*) of the brain, which is abnormal in about 90 percent of people with definite MS.

MRI of the spinal cord can also be useful but is not as frequently positive as MRI of the brain. Prior to the development of MRI, a specialized X-ray technique known as the CAT scan (*computerized axial tomography*) was used to demonstrate the presence of lesions. However, MRI, which is safer and more accurate than any X-ray technique, provides clear evidence of white matter lesions in the CNS.

Other good tests to help confirm a diagnosis of MS include the *visual evoked potential (VEP)* and the *somatosensory evoked potential (SSEP)*. These tests, which look at the speed and efficiency of myelin conduction, are frequently abnormal in definite MS. VEPs, for example, are abnormal in about 90 percent of people with MS. Evoked potentials are particularly useful in confirming the diagnosis because they can demonstrate a completely asymptomatic lesion that would otherwise go unnoticed. Like MRI, these evoked responses tests are noninvasive and painless.

In some instances, a person will be advised to have a *lumbar puncture* (spinal tap). In this test, *cerebrospinal fluid* (fluid that bathes the spinal cord and brain) is collected for chemical analysis. In performing this test, the physician is looking for (1) elevations in IgG (immunoglobulin G, a protein fraction of gamma globulin), and other proteins which are indicative of some abnormality in the immune system; and (2) the presence of a specific IgG that appears in the spinal fluid as *oligoclonal bands*. Neither of these is specific to MS, making a lumbar puncture primarily useful for confirming the diagnosis of MS when there is other suggestive evidence. Because this test is somewhat uncomfortable, it is not done as frequently as MRI or evoked potentials. However, one of the most important reasons for doing diagnostic tests is to make sure that some other disease is not masquerading as MS, and a lumbar puncture is an effective means of ruling out other diagnoses.

Thus, a variety of diagnostic procedures may be used to help *confirm* the diagnosis of MS if the physician believes that one or more are necessary. Keep in mind that the diagnosis cannot be made solely on the basis of these tests because MS is only one of several conditions that can cause them to be positive. Your medical history and the symptoms and signs of CNS demyelination that you and the doctor are able to piece together are the clear-est evidence for the diagnosis of MS.

Why did I get MS? Did I do something to make this happen to me?

Because the cause of MS is unknown, why any one person gets the disease remains a mystery. Nothing that you had any control over could in any way have caused your MS. Multiple sclerosis is believed to be an autoimmune disease caused by some infectious agent in the environment. It is also believed that the disease occurs in a person who is genetically predisposed to its development.

What does this mean? Most doctors believe that MS is an autoimmune disease because the plaques or scars in the myelin that are caused by MS have all the signs of an immune-mediat-ed process. For example, immune cells such as *lymphocytes*, *plasma cells* (white blood cells that make antibodies), and *macrophages* (cells that destroy myelin) can be found at sites being actively damaged. Many plaques start around a small vein, suggesting that these immune cells escape from the blood, pass through the *blood-brain barrier*, and enter the brain and spinal cord to do damage. There is a good animal model for MS, called *experimental allergic encephalomyelitis (EAE)*, which we know is an autoimmune disease. We can cause this disease to occur by injecting animal myelin into laboratory animals, mak-ing it an extremely valuable tool in the research efforts to find the cause and treatment of MS (see Chapter 3).

Although no one has yet identified what in the environment causes MS, the fact that the disease is definitely more common in certain parts of the world seems to point to some kind of envi-ronmental agent. Additionally, some studies have shown that the chances of getting MS seem to depend in part on where a person lives before the onset of adolescence. There are also some report-ed "epidemics" of MS, which would tend to support the notion of an environmental agent as the cause of the disease. However, no virus or toxin has ever been proven to cause the disease.

Are there different types of MS?

The basic types of MS are now defined in the following way:

◇ *Relapsing-remitting MS* is characterized by clearly defined acute attacks that last from days to weeks, with either full recovery or residual deficit(s). Whether or not there are deficits remaining after the attacks, the periods between attacks are characterized by stability and absence of disease progression. One subtype of this category is commonly referred to as "benign sensory" MS. Individuals with this type of MS have attacks of numbness or tingling in various parts of the body or visual blurring (caused by optic neuritis) as their only symptoms.

◇ *Primary progressive MS* is characterized by progression of disability from onset, without any obvious plateaus or remissions, or with only occasional plateaus and temporary, minor improvements.

◇ *Secondary progressive MS* begins initially with a relapsing-remitting course, which later becomes a more consistently progressive course. A physician cannot predict who will remain relapsing-remitting and who might in the future become secondary progressive. This is the reason why it is difficult to give any person a firm *prognosis*.

◇ *Progressive-relapsing MS* shows clear progression in disability level from the onset of the disease, but with clear, *acute* relapses that may or may not have some recovery following the acute episode.

These definitions clearly convey that multiple sclerosis is an unpredictable disease that can change course along the way. Research indicates that the vast majority of people (85 percent) have relapsing-remitting disease at the time of diagnosis, while only 15 percent initially have progressive disease. Within a period of ten years, more than half of those whose disease was initially relapsing-remitting will have developed progressive disease. After a period of 25 years, approximately 90 percent will have changed from relapsing-remitting to progressive disease.

I have a neighbor with MS and her symptoms are completely different from mine. How can the same illness cause such different symptoms in people?

Just as there are different courses of MS, there are different kinds of symptoms, even among people of the same sex and age who have had the illness for the same length of time. This results from the fact that the plaques of MS are scattered throughout the white matter of the brain and spinal cord. Although there are areas where the plaques are more likely to occur, the distribution is random. Therefore, one person might experience loss of vision and another might have problems controlling urination. All MS symptoms are caused by damage to the myelin sheath (demyelination) or axons in the central nervous system; however, the particular areas that become damaged vary from person to person.

How is an exacerbation different from a pseudo-exacerbation and what causes each to happen?

An *exacerbation* or "attack" of MS is caused by a new plaque of demyelination or the reactivation of an old plaque. For a symptom to qualify as an exacerbation it must, by definition, last for at least twenty-four hours and be separated from the previous attack by one month. Although these limits are somewhat arbitrary, it is important that they be considered so that symptoms will not be misinterpreted.

A *pseudo-exacerbation* is unrelated to new disease activity. It results from some other problem, such as a fever or pain, which aggravates the neurologic effects of the preexisting plaques. For example, people with MS who develop a fever often feel—and appear—much worse as long as their temperature remains elevated. Once their temperature drops to normal, they return to their baseline neurologic function. Similarly, people with *spasticity* in their lower limbs notice more spasms and stiffness when they have a bladder infection. Once the bladder infection is cured with antibiotics, the spasms and stiffness return to their previous level.

Although there are many identifiable causes for pseudo-exacerbations, nobody knows the cause of true MS exacerbations. There is no convincing evidence for the commonly held belief that stress or trauma can produce exacerbations (see Chapter 11). Some studies have indicated that viral infections such as the common cold or flu can trigger a true exacerbation. This may happen because viral infections trigger the body's immune response.

Is there anything I can do to prevent an exacerbation?

There is no proven way to prevent MS attacks. We know of no medical treatment that always works to prevent an exacerbation or every person with MS would be taking it. There is no convincing evidence that a person can prevent an exacerbation by avoiding or controlling life stresses. However, we now have three medications—Betaseron® (interferon beta-1b), Avonex® (interferon beta-1a), and Copaxone® (glatiramer acetate)—that have been approved in the United States and Canada for the treatment of relapsing-remitting MS. Betaseron® has been shown to reduce the frequency and severity of MS attacks. Avonex® has been shown to reduce the frequency of disease attacks and slow disease progression. Copaxone® has been shown to reduce the frequency of attacks. All three drugs have been shown to reduce new and active lesions in the brain as shown on MRI. Betaseron® has also demonstrated positive results in secondary progressive MS (see Chapter 3 and Appendix B). A fourth drug, Rebif® (also beta interferon beta-1a), has been approved in Europe and Canada for the treatment of relapsing-remitting MS.

Because many scientists believe that some infectious agent (either viral or bacterial) might trigger an exacerbation, it also makes sense to employ good personal hygiene to reduce the possibility of getting such an infection. For example, washing your hands is known to reduce the chance of getting many contagious viral illnesses such as the common cold.

Is there anything I can do to prolong a remission?

There are medical treatments that may help to prolong remission for some people. For example, Betaseron®, Avonex®, Copaxone®, and Rebif® have been shown to reduce the frequency of attacks in some individuals with relapsing-remitting MS (and secondary-progressive MS, in the case of Betaseron®). Although doctors frequently use **corticosteroids** to treat MS flare-ups, there is no proof that these medications prolong remission or prevent exacerbations. Once an exacerbation has begun, however, corticosteroids seem to make it resolve more quickly than if no treatment were given.

How will my MS affect me in the future? Will I end up in a wheelchair or bedridden?

It is not possible for the physician to predict with complete accuracy what the future holds for any particular person with MS because it is such an unpredictable disease. However, many physicians will hazard a guess based on such factors as the frequency of attacks and the types of symptoms that the person has experienced. Individuals who have frequent attacks, especially during the first few years of illness, seem to do less well than those who have infrequent attacks. People whose attacks last for a long time, especially if these attacks are characterized by weakness or incoordination, tend to do less well than those who have brief attacks consisting primarily of numbness or visual loss. Those individuals who have prominent weakness or incoordination that does not go away with time tend to have a worse prognosis, as do males and those people who are diagnosed at a later age.

Can a person die from MS?

Like everyone else, most people with MS die from "natural causes" that include heart attacks, strokes, or cancer. Death caused directly by the plaques of MS is highly unusual. Sometimes a plaque occurs in the part of the brain that regulates breathing and consciousness, in which case death could result if adequate medical care is not provided. In very rare instances, large areas of demyelination could cause swelling of the brain that puts pressure on the life-supporting systems, ultimately causing respiratory failure and death.

People sometimes die because of complications of their disease. These complications include choking because of swallowing difficulties, serious kidney or blood infections, or aspiration pneumonia (see Chapter 8). Because most physicians who care for people with MS are aware of these potential complications, they are able to provide the kind of preventive health care that minimizes the risk of their occurrence. The relatively recent availability of a wide range of antibiotic medications has also greatly reduced the numbers of deaths from infection.

Another notable cause of death in MS is suicide. Although the rate of suicide in MS is somewhat higher than the rate in the general population, we still do not have a clear understanding of why this is so. These suicides may be the result of severe depression, the outcome of a person's decision to terminate life in the face of severe and incapacitating disability, or the result of some other factor(s) of which we are still unaware (see Chapter 11 for a more complete discussion of emotional issues in MS).

I know a family in which the mother and son both have MS. No one else in my family has MS. Is it hereditary?

Although MS is not inherited, we pass on to our children the genes that determine all of their characteristics, including the way their immune systems behave. It seems that a certain genetic pattern may make a person more likely to get MS than if those genetic characteristics were not present.

A good way to study how genes influence the likelihood of getting disease is to study twins. Identical twins have the same genetic makeup, whereas nonidentical (fraternal) twins have different genes and are similar to other non-twin siblings. If one identical twin has MS, the chance of the second twin having MS is about 30 percent. For fraternal twins, the chance is 2 percent, about the same as for any non-twin siblings. If MS was inherited in the same simple and direct way as eye color, the chance of identical twins both having MS would be 100 percent. Therefore, the twin studies support the theory that there is genetic involvement in MS, but also demonstrate that other factors must be involved. The current thinking is that MS: is the result of an immune-mediated attack against myelin; is triggered by some factor in the environment; and occurs in those individuals with some genetic predisposition for producing this particular immune response.

What does this mean for a person with MS who is concerned about having children? The risk of MS in the general population is approximately 1/1000. In a family in which one person has MS, the risk for other family members (except identical twins) is approximately 2–5/100. This means that the probability that one of the children will get MS is 20–50 times greater than it is for people in the general population. While this certainly represents an increased risk, it is important to keep in mind that the risk to these children is still only 2–5 percent. Most MS physicians today will encourage prospective parents with MS to proceed with their family plans based on their feelings about parenting and children, and their personal assessment of their ability to raise their children in a loving and secure environment, rather than on this low risk (see Chapter 13).

To date, there is no test available (e.g., tissue typing) to determine whether a relative of someone with MS is genetically-susceptible to the disease.

Am I susceptible to other autoimmune diseases because I have MS?

There are no clear associations between other autoimmune disorders and MS. There is not, for example, an increased chance of having psoriasis or rheumatoid arthritis because one has MS.

What type of physician should I see for help with my MS? What are the differences between going to an MS center and seeing a private practice neurologist?

You should get treatment from a doctor with whom you feel comfortable and who gives you sound advice. Of course, it is not always possible for someone to know when advice is sound or not. Look for a physician who listens carefully to your problems and concerns and offers suggestions on how to remedy them. A good physician will explain what is known about your disease and its symptoms and what treatment options are available. A physician who merely answers all your questions with "That's caused by MS and there's nothing that can be done . . . go home and learn to live with it" is not giving you the best possible service.

Generally, **neurologists** are best equipped to answer your questions and give you the guidance you need. Obviously, physicians who see many people with MS, and work at an MS center, are more likely to have a broad base of experience. They also tend to work within a multidisciplinary team of professionals (including, for example, nurses, physical therapists, occupational therapists, psychologists, social workers) who are knowledgeable about specialized aspects of MS care. The variable and complex symptoms of MS have the potential to affect many different aspects of a person's physical, emotional, and social functioning. The members of a multidisciplinary MS team have the expertise to diagnose and treat the varied problems potentially associated with the disease. Additionally, the team approach ensures that a person's care is coordinated rather than spread out among several specialists who are working independently without communicating with one another.

What is a physiatrist?

A **physiatrist** is a physician whose speciality is rehabilitation medicine. Although these physicians prescribe medication, their primary emphasis is on physical treatments (e.g., **orthotics**, mobility aids, and exercise) designed to ease or improve important functions such as walking. While some physiatrists treat MS patients, and manage the full range of symptoms, others see MS patients who are referred to them specifically for **rehabilitation** purposes.

The neurologist in my managed care program does not specialize in MS. How will I know if I am getting appropriate or up-to-date medical care?

While it is not always easy to tell if you are getting the most up-to-date treatment and advice, there are several ways that you can educate yourself about current treatment strategies in MS. The National Multiple Sclerosis Society publishes pamphlets and brochures describing the symptoms of MS and their management, as well as information about what can be done to control the disease. The Society also makes this information available on its website (www.nmss.org). Most local chapters sponsor open lecture and discussion meetings throughout the year as well as support groups. Support groups may be particularly helpful because you can listen to what other people with MS have to say about their experiences. If you have a computer and modem, there are several Internet forums you can access to raise questions and discuss topics of interest with other individuals who have MS (see Appendix E).

If you learn about a treatment, medication, or management strategy that you think might be beneficial for you, ask your doctor about it and see what kind of response you get. If you always seem to know more than your doctor, it may be time to consider a change.

How often do I need to get an MRI done?

You may never need an MRI. If your history and physical examination confirm the diagnosis of MS, no additional testing is needed. However, most physicians recommend MRI of the brain at the time of diagnosis to help confirm that the problem is indeed MS rather than some other condition. Since MRI does not reliably predict the course of the disease, there really is no reason why the test should be regularly repeated. However, it might be useful to repeat the test if there is some question about whether or not the disease is progressing, and if a particular treatment is being considered based on the answer to this question. In other words, the MRI should be done when there is a specific question to be answered or a treatment decision to be made. A chemical compound called ***gadolinium*** can be administered during the MRI to help distinguish between new—or active—lesions and old ones. The MRI is best repeated with the same MRI machine used on the first study so that reasonable comparisons can be made.

How do allergies affect MS?

There is no evidence that allergies, such as those to food, animal dander, or pollen, cause MS or lead to MS attacks. However, it is possible that an allergic reaction could trigger a **pseudoexacerbation**. Unfortunately, some individuals have deliberately popularized the notion that allergies are the cause of MS so that they can recommend useless and expensive treatment to "desensitize" the person with MS.

Does owning a pet cause MS?

Some years ago, it was suggested that the cause of MS was an infection carried by dogs, possibly canine distemper virus. A report suggested that owning a small dog was associated with a greater risk of getting MS. A national study was undertaken, which showed this was definitely not the case. However, ideas such as this one often seem to linger even though they have been disproved.

What is the EDSS?

Neurologists who see many people with MS need some basis of comparison so that they can communicate findings and conclusions about them in an effective and consistent way. Although the neurologic examination gives a great deal of useful information, it takes a long time to describe the different parts of the examination.

The Expanded Disability Status Scale (EDSS), which is part of the *Minimal Record of Disability*, summarizes the neurologic examination and provides a measure of overall disability—at least as it relates to the ability to walk. It is a 20-point scale, ranging from 0 ("normal examination") to 10 ("death due to MS"). A person with a score of 4.5 can walk three blocks without stopping; a score of 6.0 means that a cane or a leg brace is needed to walk one block; a score over 7.5 indicates that a person cannot take more than a few steps, even with crutches or help from another person. The EDSS is used for many reasons, including deciding future medical treatment, establishing rehabilitation goals, and choosing subjects for participation in clinical trials. The major drawback of the scale is that its emphasis on gait impairment ignores disability that results from other impairments such as upper limb problems or memory loss. However, no other scale for MS is as widely used in clinical trials as this one.

Symptom Management

If there is no cure for MS, why do I need to bother seeing a doctor at all?

A close look at medical practice today reveals that relatively few chronic diseases can actually be cured. Most must be treated on an ongoing basis to allow the individuals who have them to function at their best—comfortably and productively. This is particularly true of MS, which can be so varied and unpredictable in its symptoms and associated problems. Periodic medical follow-up will help you manage the symptoms you have in order to increase your mobility, enhance day-to-day functioning, improve your comfort and, most importantly, help you avoid needless complications. Additionally, these visits with your physician will help to ensure that you have up-to-date, accurate information about available medications and treatments so that you can be an active participant in the management of your MS. You may also be able to learn about upcoming *clinical trials* in which you might be eligible to participate (see Chapter 3 for further discussion of clinical trials).

How often do I need to be seen by the doctor?

How frequently you should be seen and how long a visit should take will be determined by the types of problems you are experiencing. A person with relatively "benign" MS who has very few symptoms can probably do well with just a thorough yearly visit. The person who has more complicated symptoms that require ongoing medical management and a rehabilitative regimen will need more frequent visits. Because the symptoms of MS can come and go over time, you may find that you need to see your physician more frequently at some times than at others. Of greatest importance is that your questions be answered and that a workable treatment and management strategy be understood and agreed upon by you and your physician.

Why do some symptoms come and go while others seem to stay for a long time?

Symptoms of MS initially appear because of inflammation within the brain and spinal cord. The inflammation results in swelling (edema), which can cause symptoms. The symptoms start to go away as the swelling gradually subsides. Sometimes the inflammation in a particular area is severe enough to cause demyelination and axonal damage. Once the myelin and axons have been severely damaged, the symptoms are likely to remain.

Symptoms of MS can also worsen temporarily for reasons unrelated to the disease process itself. Temporary elevations in body temperature, such as those caused by infection or over-exertion, can cause a person's symptoms to flare until the body temperature returns to normal. Similarly, symptoms may temporarily worsen during periods of intense fatigue and subside following a period of rest. These episodes are called pseudo-exacerbations because they do not reflect an actual change or progression in the disease.

To me, every new symptom feels like an emergency. How do I know when it's important to call the doctor?

A disease such as MS, with its varied symptom picture and unpredictability, tends to make a person very aware of day-to-day changes in the way his or her body feels. Each new symptom or sensation feels strange and perhaps somewhat frightening. In general, if you are experiencing a symptom that is puzzling or bothersome, a telephone call to your doctor is appropriate. As you become more familiar with your MS and the patterns your symptoms tend to follow, you may find that you are comfortable waiting a few days to see if the problem goes away before making the call. Keep track of the changes so that when you do call your physician you are able to describe how and when the problem started. Keep in mind that very few MS-related symptoms are medical emergencies and that most can be handled safely and effectively during normal working hours.

My symptoms are so varied and unpredictable that it's hard for me to know which are caused by MS and which might be due to some other medical problem. How do I know which doctor to call for a new problem or symptom?

The symptoms of MS can be quite varied, appearing in many different parts of your body. It is important for you to be educated about MS and the types of symptoms it tends to cause so that you can make reasonable judgments about what is MS-related and what is not. In general, any symptom that seems to be neurologic, and is not otherwise easily explained by some other common illness, should be reported to the doctor who is treating your MS. Symptoms that are not common in MS, such as chest pain, shortness of breath, stomach pain, and so on, should be discussed with your family physician. Since the neurologist functions as the principal physician for some people with MS, he or she will make an appropriate referral if the problem you are having is unrelated to your MS.

What causes the stiffness in my arms and legs and what is the best treatment for this problem?

Muscle stiffness associated with MS is "spasticity"—an increase in **muscle tone** that can interfere with normal movement of the affected limb even though the strength of that limb might be normal. This increased muscle tone is caused by a dysregulation of nerve impulses in the spinal cord, resulting in too much stimulation in some muscles and too little in others. Spasticity tends to occur most frequently in postural muscles (those that enable us to stand upright), including muscles in the calf, thigh, groin, buttock, and occasionally the back. Spasticity can also occur in the arms. Very mild spasticity can sometimes be managed with appropriate stretching and range of motion exercises (see Chapter 5).

If exercises alone are too uncomfortable or do not provide adequate relief and mobility, antispasticity medications may be used. A variety of medications are available for this purpose, including baclofen (Lioresal®), tizanidine (Zanaflex®), clonazepam (Klonopin®), diazepam (Valium®), and dantrolene (Dantrium®). Your physician will select the particular medication best suited for your needs; baclofen is the drug most commonly used (see Appendix B). The correct dosage of baclofen will differ from one individual to another. The goal of treatment is to find the dosage level that provides adequate muscle relaxation without producing excessive fatigue or weakness. Tizanidine has been shown to relieve spasticity without causing muscle weakness but is often sedating.

Occasionally, people with MS-related spasticity develop *flexor* or *extensor spasms*. These spasms, which typically last two or three seconds, are disinhibited (hyperactive) spinal reflexes that can occur in response to the slightest of noxious stimuli (e.g., the rubbing of bed sheets against the foot during sleep). Flexor spasms cause both legs to pull upward into a clenched position, while extensor spasms cause the legs to straighten into the stiff, extended position. These uncontrolled spasms can be sufficiently intense and sudden to propel the person out of his or her chair. Baclofen (Lioresal®), gabapentin (Neurontin®), diazepam (Valium®), clonazepam (Klonopin®), and tizanidine (Zanaflex®) are the medications of choice for the management of this problem (see Appendix B).

In the case of severe spasticity that cannot be managed comfortably or effectively with oral baclofen (tablets), a pump can be surgically implanted in the abdomen to automatically administer low doses of liquid baclofen directly into the spinal cord. The pump's usefulness stems from its ability to reduce spasticity with a much lower dose of medication, thus eliminating the side effects (e.g., severe drowsiness, dizziness, weakness, or nausea) that can occur with higher doses of baclofen.

In some instances of spasticity, Botox (made from botulinum toxin) may be used to block a nerve's function. The Botox is injected into the affected muscle at the point where the nerve enters the muscle, and prevents the nerve from exciting the muscle to contract. Botox, which can be administered by the neurologist, may require repetitive injections to achieve sustained blockage of the nerve. It is best used for focal spasticity in small muscles like those of the upper limbs.

Severe spasticity that does not respond to medications, or for which Botox is not suitable, may also be treated with a procedure called a **nerve block** or **motor point block**. An injection of phenol into the affected nerve chemically damages the nerve and interferes with its function for up to three months. This temporary destruction of the nerve prevents the affected muscle from contracting and allows the person to feel more comfortable. The nerve block may also improve gait and mobility. The injections of phenol are usually given by a **physiatrist** or anesthesiologist using an **EMG** to pinpoint the location of the nerve.

On rare occasions, surgery is required to cut one particular nerve to the affected muscle without endangering other nerves that are in close proximity. This surgical procedure is permanent and irreversible. Fortunately, the recent availability of the baclofen pump has greatly reduced the need for nerve blocks or surgery to reduce spasticity.

My doctor has told me that I may be a suitable candidate for a baclofen pump. How does the pump work and how will I know if it is the right treatment for me?

Your physician may recommend the baclofen pump if your spasticity is not adequately controlled by oral spasticity medication or if you are experiencing intolerable side effects such as drowsiness, dizziness, weakness, or nausea. The pump is a surgically-implanted device that is programmed to deliver the prescribed dose of liquid baclofen (Lioresal® Intrathecal), on a continuous basis, directly into the area surrounding your spinal cord (*intrathecal space*). Because the drug is administered in this way, it is possible to obtain positive results using a lower dose with fewer side effects.

Before implanting the baclofen pump, your doctor will inject a test dose of liquid baclofen into the intrathecal space of your lower back to see how you respond to the medication. The test dose is given in the hospital so that you can be observed for changes in rigidity and spasms and for any side effects you might experience. If the test dose proves to be comfortable and effective, you and your physician will decide whether to proceed with the baclofen pump.

In order to receive liquid baclofen on a regular, long-term basis, it is necessary to implant a pump and catheter into your body. The pump (a round metal disk weighing about six ounces) is placed under the skin of the abdomen during a surgical procedure. A catheter connects the pump to the intrathecal space in your back. The pump is refilled at periodic intervals by injecting the baclofen through your skin into the pump's drug reservoir.

The pump has been shown to be a safe and effective treatment for the management of severe spasticity. Its potential to reduce the discomforts and possible complications associated with spasticity makes it a valuable treatment option for you and your physician to consider. The, pump is, however, an invasive and expensive intervention, and should be reserved for those who have not responded to other treatments.

What are contractures and how are they treated?

Contractures are an abnormal, sometimes permanent flexion (bending) of a joint that can occur if significant spasticity goes untreated. When spasticity prevents a limb from moving freely about the joint, some of the muscles and tendons around the joint become shortened. This shortening further constricts movement of the joint. Without treatment, the joint may freeze and become immobilized. Contractures can usually be prevented with a careful regimen of antispasticity medication and physical therapy techniques designed to maintain joint flexibility, mobility, and full range of motion.

Severe contractures may require more drastic treatment measures in order to reduce the intractable pain, positioning problems, and possible skin complications that can result. For example, surgery may be performed to sever the affected tendon, thus allowing the contracted limb to be straightened. This irreversible procedure is used only in individuals whose prolonged spasticity has resulted in permanent paralysis of the contracted limbs. By far the best treatment of contractures is to prevent them from occurring in the first place. With the advent of the baclofen pump, this type of unmanageable spasticity should be seen less frequently.

At night I experience painful spasms in my legs that make it very hard for me to sleep. Is there anything I can do about this problem?

These painful flexor spasms are involuntary muscle contractions that result from spasticity or increased muscle tone. They seem to occur in response to such stimuli as sheets being rubbed over the skin of the lower limbs. Stretching exercises before bedtime may be helpful, but medication is often necessary. Baclofen (Lioresal®), diazepam (Valium®), clonazepam (Klonopin®), gabapentin (neurontin®), L-dopa/carbidopa (Sinemet®), and tizanidine (Zanaflex®) are the medications most commonly used to treat these spasms. Diazepam and clonazepam are somewhat sedating, making them particularly useful for the management of nighttime spasticity. Both of these drugs can be habit-forming, however, and must therefore be prescribed and used with some caution (see Appendix B). Some people find that the over-the-counter medications threonine and quinine are also helpful with this problem. Be sure to discuss the situation with your physician before beginning any treatment.

My hands and feet often get numb or feel like "pins and needles." Are there any medications for this problem?

"Pins and needles" are one example of sensory symptoms in MS. Sensory symptoms are those that a person can feel but for which the physician cannot see objective evidence during the neurologic exam. Other examples include numbness, tingling, decreased or blurred vision, dizziness, or pain. These symptoms occur because of demyelination in the sensory pathways of the spinal cord or brain. Although they can be quite uncomfortable, sensory symptoms are generally considered relatively benign because they tend to come and go without severely restricting a person's ability to function. Although there is no specific medication for most sensory symptoms, antiseizure medications such as gabapentin (Neurontin®), carbamazepine (Tegretol®), and valproic acid (Depakene®) may decrease their intensity. A tricyclic antidepressant medication such as amitriptyline (Elavil®) can provide some relief, particularly if the symptoms are painful (see Appendix B). In the meantime, remember that these symptoms tend to go away on their own and seldom signal significant impairment.

What causes tremor in MS and are there any treatments available for it?

Tremor is an involuntary, relatively rhythmic movement of the arms, legs, or head. While several types of tremor can occur in MS, the most common one results from demyelination in the pathways leading to or from the balance center of the brain (*cerebellum*). Damage in this area of the brain causes an *intention tremor*, a relatively slow, oscillating (back and forth) movement of a limb engaged in purposeful movement. For example, a person with an intention tremor finds it difficult to perform the finger-to-nose test on the neurologic exam because the intentional movement of the finger toward the nose triggers a tremor in that arm.

Tremor is one of the most difficult symptoms to treat and can be among the most disabling. There are balance and coordination exercises (see Chapter 5) that can help a person to develop compensatory techniques, but the results are far from satisfying. Weights can be placed on the affected limbs to lessen the oscillations somewhat, or weighted utensils can be used for such activities as eating, dressing, and writing (see Chapter 6).

No medication has been developed specifically for tremor. However, some medications designed to treat other conditions have secondary antitremor properties. These include the beta-blocker propranolol (Inderal®), clonazepam (Klonopin®), primidone (Mysoline®), isoniazid (Laniazid®—United States; Isotamine®—Canada), and buspirone (Buspar®). A medication used for nausea resulting from cancer treatment, ondansetron (Zofran®), may be helpful but is prohibitively expensive on a long-term basis. While these medications are not usually effective with MS-related tremor, it is impossible to predict who will respond to one or another of the medications and who will not. Therefore, it is worthwhile to try them singly or in combination in an effort to control the tremor.

I take a lot of different medications now—some prescribed by my neurologist and others by my family doctor. Do I need to be concerned about the interactions of all of these drugs?

Everyone needs to be concerned about the actions and interactions of the drugs they take. Each physician involved in your care must know all of the prescription and nonprescription medications that you are taking. Keep a list of all your medications and ask that a copy of that list be included in your medical chart. When the doctor prescribes a new medication for you, feel free to ask about its possible interactions with the others you are taking. Usually there is not an interaction problem, but it makes good sense to ask.

Refer to the Medication Information Sheets in Appendix B for information about the drugs commonly used in MS. You can also ask your pharmacist to give you the "package insert" that comes with each medication, read about your medication(s) in one of the standard drug references, or get information from one of the on-line computer services.

Is there any treatment for my balance problems? People who see me on the street think I'm drunk.

Balance problems in MS, like tremor, are usually caused by damage in the cerebellum. Balance and coordination exercises may offer some compensatory strategies, but there is no effective treatment at this time for damage to the cerebellum. Assistive devices such as a cane, crutches, or a walker will offer you varying degrees of stability and, just as importantly, tell the world that you are not drunk (see Chapter 5). Many people initially take the emotional plunge of using an assistive device for this reason; they would rather be identified as having a physical impairment than as having had too much to drink.

I have always gotten a lot of exercise and been in pretty good shape. Now I feel weakness in my legs in spite of the exercise. What is causing this weakness and is there anything I can do about it?

Weakness in MS is caused by faulty transmission of impulses from the brain through the spinal cord to the muscle. *The problem is not due to a bad or weak muscle.* Weakness from poor nerve transmission will not be altered by exercise and, in fact, can be worsened by aggressive exercise that produces fatigue. At the same time, however, inadequate use of the muscle will produce its own kind of "weakness" that is really a result of deconditioning. Therefore, an effective exercise program for weakness must include exercises to strengthen the muscles that have adequate nerve conduction, as well as useful movements for the weakened muscles that lack adequate nerve conduction (see Chapter 5). There is currently no medication to treat weakness in MS; researchers are working to identify medications that might improve nerve conduction in demyelinated nerves.

Fatigue has become my most disabling symptom. Sometimes I even feel it right after I wake up in the morning. Is there any treatment for this problem?

Fatigue is one of the most common symptoms in MS. There are several distinct types of fatigue, each with its own management strategy.

◇ *Normal fatigue* results from physical, mental, and emotional exertion. This type of fatigue is managed with rest, just as it is in people without MS.

◇ The most common fatigue seen in MS is also referred to as "*lassitude.*" This fatigue is described as an overwhelming tiredness that seems unrelated to activity level or even time of day. While most people report this type of fatigue in the late afternoon or early evening, it can also occur in the morning. While some people find that a brief rest alleviates this fatigue to some degree, others report that it is unaffected by sleep or relaxation. Lassitude of this type often responds to neurochemical medications (see Appendix B) such as amantadine, pemoline (Cylert®), and fluoxetine

(Prozac®), as well as to a personalized regimen of aerobic exercise.

◇ *Muscle fatigue* can occur in an arm or leg following repetitive movements. After walking some distance, for example, you might find that one leg begins to drag and feel very weak. This type of fatigue is caused by a temporary blocking in the nerve and is best managed by stopping the walk long enough to allow nerve conduction to restart. Cooling strategies may also be beneficial.

◇ *Deconditioning fatigue* results when muscles are under-utilized. People with MS who experience weakness, heat sensitivity, and fatigue tend to become less active. This inactivity, in turn, leads to greater fatigue and weakness. Therefore, it is important to engage in some form of regular exercise to increase your stamina. Your doctor or physical therapist can help you design an exercise regimen that is suited to your needs and abilities.

◇ *Disability-related fatigue* results from the impact of MS on muscle control, coordination, and strength, and the increased effort and energy needed to accomplish routine tasks. This kind of fatigue is best managed with assistive technology (e.g., tools and devices to simplify everyday activities and mobility aids to ease ambulation problems).

◇ *Depression-related fatigue* is very common in anyone who is experiencing significant depression. This type of fatigue is best managed by addressing the depression itself with a regimen of psychotherapy and, if needed, antidepressant medication.

◇ *Medication-induced fatigue* can be an unfortunate side-effect of some of the medications used in MS. Obviously, the best strategy is to identify the medication that provides the greatest amount of symptom relief with the least amount of associated fatigue. When it is necessary to use a medication that causes significant fatigue, it can be helpful to start with a very low dose, building up gradually to allow your body to become adjusted to it.

◇ *Fatigue from sleep disturbances* is usually managed by addressing the symptoms or problems that interfere with sound sleep.

I don't seem to sleep as well as I used to. Could this have anything to do with my MS?

Many people with MS report problems with their sleep. For most, "not sleeping well" means that the time spent in bed *trying* to sleep is substantially greater than the total time they *actually* sleep. This kind of reduced sleep efficiency often results from an increase in the number of awakenings during the night.

There are many reasons why a person's sleep might be interrupted. We know that periodic limb movements (PLMs) are more common in people with MS than in the general population. Although PLMs are often very slight movements (a flexion of the big toe, for example), they alter the *quality* of the person's sleep. Therefore, people with MS can have PLMs that interrupt or disturb sleep without even being aware of them. In addition, people with MS are often awakened by spasms in their limbs or the need to urinate. Finally, stress and depression, both of which are quite common in MS, can result in insomnia. There are several kinds of insomnia, including trouble falling asleep, trouble staying asleep, and early morning awakening.

A variety of medications and behavioral strategies are available to manage sleep disturbances. In order to determine which interventions would be most helpful for you, it is necessary to identify the source(s) of your sleep problems. Talk to your doctor, being as specific as possible about your sleep schedule and habits. Your sleep partner may also be able to provide valuable information about limb movements or spasms that occur during the night. The doctor may refer you to a sleep specialist (usually a physician or psychologist with specific training in this area) if the specific causes of your sleep disturbance are not readily apparent. The sleep specialist will use a variety of techniques to identify the source(s) of your problems and recommend a treatment regimen. It is important to address any sleep problems you are having because they can contribute significantly to your day-to-day fatigue.

My MS seems to get worse every summer. I feel so weak and tired when it's hot that I can hardly move. Why does this happen and is there any solution to this problem?

For many people, heat temporarily worsens MS symptoms. This can occur with as little as a one-degree elevation in body temperature. There is no evidence that heat actually makes the disease worse. Instead, heat alters nerve conduction (the passage of nerve impulses) and causes a feeling of weakness in the limbs. This same phenomenon often occurs when a person becomes overheated following strenuous exercise or develops an elevated body temperature due to a viral or bacterial infection. In fact, the "hot bath test" for MS was used (before current imaging techniques made it unnecessary) to capitalize on this heat sensitivity; a person suspected of having the disease was put in a bathtub of hot water to see if MS symptoms could be elicited. Thus, it is not surprising that the heat and humidity of summer make your symptoms feel worse.

Keeping your body cool helps to alleviate this problem and is certainly the best management strategy for the heat of summer and of a fever. Avoid unnecessary heat—hot showers and sunbathing, for example, are not good activities for someone with MS—and make use of air conditioning, cold drinks, or a body cooling system like the ones designed for laborers in heat-intensive occupations (see Appendix E). Body cooling systems come in two basic types and seem to be most helpful for those individuals who are sensitive to the heat rather than the humidity of summer. The simplest cooling system is a vest designed to hold frozen gel packs in front and back compartments (e.g., Steele Vest®). A person can wear this type of vest for driving in a warm car, engaging in outdoor activities, cooking over a hot stove, or just staying cool in a warm house. A somewhat more complex cooling system electronically pumps a cold liquid through a specially designed garment (e.g., the cooling suits made by Life Enhancement Technologies, LLC). Research is currently underway to determine the effectiveness of these types of cooling apparatuses for people with MS.

What types of pain can be caused by MS? What are the best treatments for the different types of pain?

Pain in MS can take different forms. The most common is called **dysesthesia**, referring to a burning sensation caused by abnormalities in the sensory pathways in the brain and spinal cord. Demyelination in the sensory pathways can result in pain, numbness, tingling, itching, or other abnormal sensations. Sometimes the pain is quite severe or sharp, most commonly in the trigeminal nerve of the face. **Trigeminal neuralgia** is often described as a stabbing or shock-like pain along the side of the face. These types of pain do not respond to ordinary pain medications. The preferred treatment is to try to alter the faulty nerve conduction with other types of medications, including antiepileptic drugs such as gabapentin (Neurontin®), carbamazepine (Tegretol®), phenytoin (Dilantin®), and valproic acid (Depakene®). Antidepressant medications such as amitriptyline (Elavil®) may also relieve the pain (see Appendix B). Some people find that acupuncture and meditation are effective for dysesthesias.

Unusually severe cases of trigeminal neuralgia that do not respond to any of these interventions can also be treated with an outpatient surgical procedure called a **percutaneous rhizotomy**. Under local anesthesia, the surgeon makes a tiny incision in the side of the face and blocks the function of the trigeminal nerve using one of several possible techniques, including laser surgery, cryosurgery (freezing), and cauterization.

A second, relatively common type of pain or discomfort in MS results from the symptom of spasticity—increased muscle tone and muscle spasms can be quite uncomfortable. Antispasticity medications are the most effective treatment for this type of discomfort.

In addition to these more common types of pain in MS, secondary orthopedic pain can result from changes in a person's posture or gait. If a person begins to walk or stand differently because of weakness or spasticity, for example, these changes can in turn cause pain in the knees, back, or hips. It is important to identify the causes of this type of secondary pain so that an appropriate treatment regimen of physical therapy, gait training, seating assessment (for someone in a wheelchair), exercise, and pain relief can be implemented.

My eye doctor says he can't give me glasses to correct the vision problems caused by MS. What is causing my visual problems and why can't they be corrected?

Visual symptoms are quite common in MS. They can result from damage to the optic nerve or from an incoordination in the eye muscles, neither of which is correctable with eyeglasses. The optic nerve connects the eye to the brain. Inflammation or demyelination in the optic nerve causes **optic neuritis**, which is experienced as a temporary loss or disturbance in vision and possibly pain behind the affected eye. Typically, vision returns partially or fully within a few weeks. While it is quite rare for a person with MS to become totally blind, it is not at all uncommon for an individual to have recurrent episodes of optic neuritis over the course of the disease, usually in one eye at a time. Damage to the optic nerve can result in a blurring of vision, which may or may not totally resolve over time. This blurring of vision is not correctable with eyeglasses because it is the result of nerve damage rather than changes in the shape of the eye. Color vision requires a great many nerve fibers from the eye for accurate transmission and is particularly susceptible to changes from demyelination.

Although episodes of optic neuritis typically resolve spontaneously, acute loss of vision used to be treated fairly routinely with low doses of oral cortisone in order to end the episode more quickly. Recent research has demonstrated that high-dose corticosteroids such as methylprednisolone (Solu-Medrol®) or dexamethasone (Decadron®) are more effective in the treatment of optic neuritis. If visual loss is relatively mild and manageable, the best alternative is probably to wait for the episode to remit on its own. However, a course of high-dose corticosteroids may be prescribed if everyday functioning becomes too impaired.

Optic neuritis can cause a large, noticeable "blind spot" in the center of the visual field, and the person experiences a visual image with a dark, blank area in the middle. This is called a central **scotoma** and is not correctable with either eyeglasses or medication, although steroids may be helpful in the early, acute phase.

Diplopia (double vision), the experience of seeing two of everything, is caused by weakening or incoordination of eye muscles. This symptom is typically treated with a short course of steroids. Patching one eye while trying to drive or read will stop the double image; however, permanent patching of the eye will slow the brain's remarkable ability to accommodate to the weakness and produce a single image in spite of the weakened muscles. Some physicians are prescribing eyeglasses with special prisms that help to minimize double vision.

Upon examination, the physician may detect a rhythmic jerkiness or bounce in one or both eyes. This relatively common visual finding in MS is **nystagmus**. Nystagmus does not always cause symptoms of which the person is aware. In the event that

it does become troublesome, clonazepam (Klonopin®) is sometimes effective in reducing this annoying but painless problem.

**I have developed a lot of problems with my memory and think-
ing in the last few years. Is there any medication I can take to
help with these problems?**

Some degree of measurable cognitive change occurs in 50 percent to 60 percent of people with MS. Fortunately, the majority
of these changes progress quite slowly and are relatively mild.
For a complete discussion of cognition in MS, please refer to
Chapter 9. The answer to your specific question is that no medication has been shown to treat or manage these changes successfully. You and your doctor should be alert to any signs of
depression, which can sometimes mimic changes in cognition
and is far more amenable to treatment. Research is currently
underway to determine whether Aricept®, a drug recently
approved for use in Alzheimer's disease, is effective in treating
cognitive symptoms in MS. Research is also being done with the
neurostimulant pemoline (Cylert®).

**Sometimes the treatment I get for one symptom makes another
problem worse (e.g., my bladder medications make my mouth
uncomfortably dry, the antidepressant I took interfered with my
sex life, the medication I took for pain made me constipated).
How can I learn more about these side effects so that I can make
reasonable decisions about what is best for me?**

Side effects are very common with certain medications and
should be discussed with your physician. The MS health care
team is quite knowledgeable about frequently used medications
and has a great deal of experience with people's reactions to
them. Using the information you give them about your symptoms, as well as feedback about the beneficial and not so beneficial responses you are having to the medications, your health
care team can help you maximize the positive treatment effects
while minimizing side effects. They will usually be able to
reduce any unpleasant side effects to a manageable level with
minor adjustments in level and timing of dosages. For additional information about medication side effects, you can refer to the
Medication Information Sheets in Appendix B, read the "package insert" available at your pharmacy, or consult a drug reference book or on-line computer service for information about a

particular medication that has been prescribed for you (see Appendix E).

I've read that people who aren't very mobile are at greater risk for osteoporosis. I am now in a wheelchair most of the time. How can I prevent osteoporosis and what is the treatment for it?

Osteoporosis, defined as a gradual loss of calcium from the bones, which causes them to be fragile and easily broken, is caused by a combination of factors. Hormones, vitamins, genetic predisposition, and level of physical activity all play a role. In fact, the National Multiple Sclerosis Society is currently sponsoring a clinical study of vitamin D and osteoporosis. Any person who has decreased mobility, particularly a loss of weight-bearing activity (as would be true of a person using a wheelchair most of the time) needs to be concerned about osteoporosis. Additionally, excessive or prolonged use of steroids can lead to osteoporosis. Talk to your physician about your risk for osteoporosis and the advisability of a baseline evaluation to determine the health of your bones. You may be referred to a physical therapist for a regimen of weight-bearing exercises to enhance bone strength. Vitamin D, calcium, and appropriate hormone treatment may also be recommended to you. Do not begin any exercise program or medication regimen without first consulting your physician.

Recommended Readings

Holland, N. & Halper, J. *Multiple Sclerosis: A Self-Care Guide to Wellness.* Washington, D.C.: Paralyzed Veterans of America, 1998.

Kraft, G. & Catanzaro, M. *Living with Multiple Sclerosis: A Wellness Approach (2nd edition).* New York: Demos Medical Publishing, 2000.

Lechtenberg R. *Multiple Sclerosis Fact Book (2nd edition).* Philadelphia: F.A. Davis, 1995.

Schapiro R. *Symptom Management in Multiple Sclerosis (3rd edition).* New York: Demos, 1998.

Selected booklets available from your local chapter of the National Multiple Sclerosis Society (800-FIGHT-MS; 800-344-4867):

◇ *Living with MS* (ES 0087)
◇ *What Everyone Should Know About Multiple Sclerosis* (ER 100)
◇ *Things I Wish Someone Had Told Me: Practical Thoughts for People Newly Diagnosed with Multiple Sclerosis* (ES 6028)
◇ *Managing MS Through Rehabilitation* (ECS 6022)

Facts and Issues (reprints of articles from the National Multiple Sclerosis Society magazine, *Inside MS*):

◇ *Diagnosis: The Whole Story*
◇ *Genes and MS Susceptibility*
◇ *Digging for Clues to Fatigue*
◇ *Pain: A Certain Four-Letter Word*

Knowledge is Power—a series of articles written for people newly diagnosed with MS
Living Well with MS—a series of workbooks written for, and by, people who have been living with MS for some time.

Reprint available from the Canadian Multiple Sclerosis Society (416-922-6065):

◇ *Coping with Fatigue in MS Takes Understanding and Planning*—Alexander Burnfield, M.D., M.R.C. Psych.

3

Treatment Issues

Aaron E. Miller, M.D.
Robert M. Herndon, M.D.

Any discussion of treatments for multiple sclerosis must start with a careful look at what we mean by the word *treatment*. To most people, being "treated" for an illness means that they report their symptoms to a physician, are prescribed a medication (an antibiotic, for example), the symptoms go away, and they are cured. In another familiar scenario, the person gets the flu or some other viral infection, goes to the doctor or the pharmacy for some medications to relieve discomfort, and waits patiently for the virus to run its course and go away. In the case of physical injury, the treatment may be even more direct and clear-cut. The person who temporarily cannot walk because of a broken leg is treated for the injury, and walking ability is restored. Of course, the best strategy of all is a vaccine to prevent the disease in the first place.

At the present time, none of these familiar notions of treatment applies in MS. We are unable to prevent the illness from occurring, we do not know how to cure it, we have not found a way to restore damaged *myelin, axons*, or lost functions, and the disease is a chronic one that refuses to run its course and go away. While efforts continue in the scientific community to find a cure for MS and restore damaged myelin, the primary focus of day-to-day medical care in MS is symptom management (see Chapter 2) and efforts to stabilize the disease course. These efforts to stabilize the disease are the main focus of this chapter.

In order to understand why efforts to find an effective treatment for MS have been so frustrating, it is important to review some of the characteristics of the disease. Although we believe MS to be an **autoimmune disease** that is triggered in genetically susceptible individuals by some infectious agent in the environment (see Chapter 2), we do not yet have any definitive answers. Not knowing the cause of a disease makes looking for its cure significantly more challenging. Additionally, the disease tends to progress quite slowly, with a symptom picture that is highly variable from one person to the next. These characteristics make it difficult for researchers to know how to evaluate the efficacy of any particular treatment. If the disease manifests itself differently from one person to the next, what symptom or other aspect of the disease should be looked at to determine if a treatment is working?

Furthermore, although a review of treatments used in MS over the 15-year period from 1935 to 1950 indicated that 66 percent of the patients improved, none of these interventions has been shown *over time* to be any more effective than no treatment at all. Other studies have demonstrated that 70 percent of individuals treated for a recent worsening of their disease will improve, at least temporarily, with a **placebo**, or inactive, medication. Thus, treatment of a recent **exacerbation** in MS can only be considered effective if it leads to long-lasting improvement in significantly more than 70 percent of people who are given it.

This brings us back to the question of measuring the outcomes obtained when evaluating experimental treatments. Recent research efforts have targeted the number of exacerbations, length of exacerbations, length of time between exacerbations, severity of exacerbations, and the total area or volume of lesions shown on **MRI** as reasonable indicators of treatment impact in **relapsing-remitting** multiple sclerosis. In 1981, at the first international conference on therapeutic trials in MS, it was clear that there had been only one successful treatment trial in MS that met the scientific standards of its time. In that trial of **adrenocorticotropic hormone**

(ACTH), it was demonstrated that ACTH could shorten attacks even though it had no effect on the ultimate degree of recovery or long-term disability.

Since that time, there have been several high-quality drug trials in MS. There currently are more trials in progress in North America and Europe than at any time in the history of the disease. These include small-scale (fewer than 20 patients) and large-scale (several hundred patients) trials, targeting acute relapses, as well as *exacerbating-remitting, secondary progressive*, and *primary progressive* MS. They involve experimental therapies designed to affect immune function, fight infectious agents, restore myelin, and improve symptoms. The trials are evaluating new drugs, old drugs, and drugs used in various combinations. In addition, treatments that have already been approved for use in MS are beginning to be compared to one another.

Based on data from recently completed European trials of mitoxantrone, an advisory panel for the *Food and Drug Administration* (FDA) recommended that the FDA approve Novantrone® (mitoxantrone for injection concentrate) to slow worsening of neurologic disability in secondary progressive and relapsing-remitting forms of MS. In recently completed trials of oral myelin, cladribine, and sulfasalazine, these agents were found not to be of benefit. Roquinimex (linomide) proved to be toxic so the trial was stopped. *As the results from new or ongoing trials become available, the information will be incorporated into periodic updates available from the publisher.*

This is an exciting time for both individuals with MS and their health care providers. Interferon beta-1b (Betaseron®), the first drug approved by the FDA for treatment of MS, became available for relapsing-remitting MS in the fall of 1993. Betaseron® has had a noticeable impact on the frequency and severity of attacks in many of those receiving the drug. In 1994, reports were made of successful trials of interferon beta-1a (Avonex® and Rebif®) and glatiramer acetate (Copaxone® formerly known as copolymer 1) for exacerbating-remitting MS. Avonex® and Copaxone® are now approved and in wide use. In February of 2000, Biogen, Inc. announced the early termination of its clinical trial of Avonex® for individuals with initial signs of demyelinating disease who are at risk for developing clinically definite MS. When used at the standard dose of 30 micrograms in once-weekly intramuscular injections, Avonex® (in comparison to a placebo treatment) significantly delayed development of a second objective sign that would signal clinically definite MS. [Publication of these data, and their review by the FDA had not yet occurred when this book went to print.] Rebif® has already been approved in Canada and Europe, and is expected to become available in the United States within the next few years. While these offer neither a cure nor any restoration of lost function, they do represent a significant advance in our efforts to stabilize the disease process.

What makes it so difficult for scientists to find a cure for multiple sclerosis?

Physicians and researchers have found it difficult to find a cure for MS because the underlying cause of the illness is not known. Current thinking is that some "environmental" trigger (a viral infection, for example) initiates a process in which the individual's **immune system** inappropriately attacks the myelin in his or her own **central nervous system**. This process probably occurs more readily in people born with a genetic predisposition to the disease. Since we do not know the exact triggers for the initial and ongoing immunological assault, it is difficult to devise specific treatments to prevent it.

The ultimate result of the immunologic process in MS is damage to the myelin and destruction of nerve fibers or **axons**. While myelin has the potential to regenerate to some degree, and does so early in the course of the disease, damaged axons do not regenerate. Once this damage has proceeded beyond a certain point, there are insufficient nerve fibers left to carry out normal functions, and permanent weakness, numbness, or visual loss begins to occur. Thus, much of the function lost during acute attacks early in the disease tends to be recovered, with the remaining fibers compensating for those that are lost. As the disease progresses, cumulative damage to myelin and nerve fibers leads to increasing, persistent neurologic dysfunction. Research has also demonstrated that some degree of brain atrophy, or shrinkage, occurs in MS, even in the early years of the illness. However, the cause or causes of this atrophy remain to be determined. At present, we do not know how to repair or restore myelin and are, therefore, unable to reverse the neurologic symptoms, i.e., cure the disease. One hopeful sign is that we have recently come to realize that mammals, including humans, do have the capacity for spontaneous repair of central nervous system myelin and there is experimental evidence that this process can be favorably influenced.

When I have an exacerbation my doctor prescribes *intravenous* steroids (e.g., Solu-Medrol®). Why are steroids prescribed and what is the difference between steroids taken orally and those taken intravenously?

Steroids are a group of chemicals, some of which are naturally occurring hormones. They have many important hormonal functions but they have various additional effects when administered as medications (usually in synthetic preparations). Their utility in MS stems from their ability to decrease inflammation in the central nervous system, at least in part by closing the damaged ***blood-brain barrier.*** The steroids used in MS should not be confused with the anabolic steroids used by athletes to build muscle; the corticosteroids used in MS suppress inflammation.

Under normal circumstances, many potentially damaging substances are prevented by the blood-brain barrier from passing out of the blood stream into the brain and spinal cord. During attacks of MS, this barrier can break down and begin to allow damaging chemicals and cells to leak into the central nervous system. Inflammation then ensues, resulting in both ***acute*** neurologic injury—sometimes with accompanying symptoms—and ***chronic*** damage to myelin and axons. Steroids appear to decrease this inflammation.

Most neurologists caring for MS patients believe that steroids work best when given directly into the veins in high doses. We do not know whether equivalently high doses given orally would be equally effective, but some MS centers are taking this approach. In the past, it has been more common to prescribe lower doses of steroids orally. However, recent studies in patients with **optic neuritis**, a condition that is often the first sign of MS, suggest that this strategy is less effective than high doses given intravenously.

Do steroids have any long-term benefits? I feel much stronger while I'm taking steroids but my doctor says they should not be used frequently or for very long periods. Why not?

Continuous administration of steroids has never been shown to provide long-term benefits for people with MS. There is some suggestion that short courses of high-dose intravenous steroids may have a longer-term benefit in delaying further disease activity. Many people feel better while taking steroids, in part because these drugs can have a mood-elevating effect. However, the chronic use of steroids is fraught with many potentially dangerous side effects and is currently thought to be unwise in the treatment of MS. Their long-term use can be associated with such side effects as hypertension, diabetes, bone loss (*osteoporosis*), cataracts, and ulcers. These potential detrimental effects outweigh the possible benefits when steroids are used on an extended basis.

When I take steroids I get very emotional and have intense mood swings. I also feel very down or depressed toward the end of the treatment. Why does this happen and is there anything to do about it?

Short courses of steroids, even in very high doses, are usually well-tolerated. Many people, however, do have some minor mood changes, both highs and lows. Others may have difficulty sleeping. A much smaller group of individuals may have more severe disturbances in mood or behavior. Lithium, a medication often prescribed for people with bipolar disorder (formerly called manic-depressive disorder), is sometimes used to prevent or manage these mood swings. Carbamazepine (Tegretol®) and divalproex (Depakote®) have also been shown to be very effective. On occasion, antidepressant medications may be prescribed, but they are seldom needed because the "blues" associated with a short course of steroids usually disappear spontaneously before the antidepressants would begin to take effect (usually a few weeks).

Once a promising new treatment has been identified, why does it take such a long time for it to be available for patients?

Unfortunately, the process of new drug development is very slow, particularly for a chronic disease like MS. The typical sequence initially begins with animal studies (see Fig. 3-1). This is a crucial first step because an experimental model for MS, *experimental allergic encephalomyelitis (EAE)*, exists in laboratory rodents (as well as other species). This allows a quick

Figure 3-1. Summary table of steps involved in the development of a new drug

◇ Preclinical Phase	Animal studies
◇ Phase I	Preliminary human clinical trials
	✚ small, unblinded, open label trials (for safety)
◇ Phase II	✚ small, often double-blind, for additional safety and efficacy information
◇ Phase III	Multicenter, randomized, double-blind, placebo-controlled trials needed for FDA approval
◇ Data Analysis	
◇ Application for approval of drug by the FDA	
◇ Pharmaceutical company brings drug to market	

assessment of the possible benefits of a treatment, as well as the preliminary evaluation of its safety. A promising agent then moves into human clinical trials.

Human clinical trials begin with very small "open label" (unblinded) trials in which the physicians *and* subjects know what drug is being taken. Initially, these are usually done in normal individuals without known disease. An unblinded trial is aimed at demonstrating the safety of a treatment and may be followed by an open trial in a few patients with known disease. These trials are typically of much shorter duration than later studies, but still take many months to a year or longer because of the variable nature of MS. The open label trials are then followed by relatively small, usually ***double-blind***, pilot trials designed to give stronger evidence suggesting that a new treatment may be effective as well as safe. "Double-blind" means that neither the subject nor the investigators know which subjects are receiving the real medication and which are getting the placebo (an inactive substance). This procedure is followed in order to prevent hopes and expectations on the part of researchers or subjects from affecting the course or evaluation of the treatment.

If the drug still appears promising, testing will move into Phase III, involving large, multicenter, randomized, placebo-controlled, double-blind trials. In this stage of drug development, typically hundreds of subjects are entered into a study in which some are randomly assigned to receive the medication and others to get placebo. Because MS is a chronic disease in which changes occur relatively slowly in most people, these

Phase III trials typically last for several years in order to obtain enough information on which to base fair and statistically valid conclusions. These trials are expensive, costing many millions of dollars that are essentially wasted if the drug does not work. This accounts, in large part, for the high cost of new drugs.

Following the completion of the trial, another six months may be necessary to analyze the large quantity of data and prepare submission of documents to the Food and Drug Administration (FDA). The FDA, which is ultimately responsible for the approval of new drugs, carefully reviews both the data and the methodology of the trial. This agency must be convinced of both the *effectiveness* and *safety* of the treatment before giving its approval. The review process typically takes another six to twelve months. Finally, after approval of a drug, the pharmaceutical company typically needs a few more months to get the drug to market.

Thus, the process is extremely long and arduous, as well as very frustrating for people with MS and their families. However, it is a process designed to assure that everyone receives safe treatments and that no one misses out on the opportunity to take other, potentially useful treatments while taking something that is ineffective. The problem with many of the publicly acclaimed "treatments" that receive so much attention in the press (e.g., snake venom and the removal of tooth amalgams) is that they have not been through this process. In other words, they have not been proven to be safe or effective in a clinical trial and can sometimes be quite harmful.

What is the "placebo effect?"

A placebo is a non-active substance that is designed to look just like the drug that is being evaluated in a research protocol. Investigators repeatedly find that a substantial proportion of patients with a variety of diseases experience some benefit even when they are treated with a placebo. This phenomenon is known as the **placebo effect**. Although this effect may occur in part through unconscious psychological mechanisms, some studies have also demonstrated the production of certain chemicals in such individuals that may contribute to this improvement. Even though the benefits are not usually sustained, this short-lived effect confounds the study of new drugs. Randomized, placebo-controlled, double-blind trials are used in order to determine the advantage (if any) that the new drug shows over placebo effects. Thus, to demonstrate the value of a new treatment, it must be proven to have a benefit *superior* to that offered by a placebo.

It is important to remember that being treated with a placebo is not the same as receiving *no* treatment. Taking the placebo fosters certain expectations for improvement that are not present when no treatment is given. That is why new drugs are always compared with a placebo rather than with no treatment at all. The drug must demonstrate a specific benefit beyond the placebo effect or the improvement that might occur spontaneously with no treatment, or with an existing treatment. Now, with the availability of several treatments for relapsing-remitting MS, many future trials will probably compare a new drug with an existing drug rather than with placebo.

If alternative treatments like bee stings and cobra venom work well for some people, why aren't they more widely prescribed?

Alternative treatments for MS such as bee stings are often touted as helping people with MS. The problem is that these reports are always "anecdotal"; they consist mostly of individual *claims* of success, without any scientific study. It is well-known that MS often undergoes spontaneous improvement or remission. Furthermore, as discussed previously, virtually every study of MS indicates a significant placebo effect, whereby people taking placebo (non-active substance) do better than they would with no treatment. Therefore, claims of success with any therapy, including alternative treatments, must be regarded with considerable skepticism unless controlled clinical trials are done. Additionally, some of these treatments, such as bee stings, carry potentially severe risks. Specifically, fatal allergic reactions can occur in some individuals receiving bee stings. These comments are not to suggest that there might not be merit to some alternative treatments, but rather to emphasize the importance of proper scientific investigation under controlled and *safe* conditions.

Who designs clinical trials and decides when and where they will take place, and who can participate?

Clinical trials may originate from several different sources. Early trials are often initiated by investigators interested in MS, whereas more definitive trials of promising new treatments are generally undertaken by pharmaceutical companies interested in marketing a product. Although these companies often have physicians and basic scientists in their direct employment, they usually recruit outside investigators to help plan a clinical trial. Then, depending on the size of the study, additional investigators are invited to participate in the trial in order to enter the required number of subjects as quickly as possible. The lead investigators design the protocol or format for the trial, deciding how the trial will be carried out and who will be eligible to participate. The design of the trial is then submitted to the Food and Drug Administration for approval before the trial is begun.

How can I get into a clinical trial?

Various sources of information about clinical trials are available. The best place to start is with your own physician, who will often be able to direct you to a particular trial. The National Multiple Sclerosis Society can also provide information about the sites participating in particular clinical trials. Some of the local chapters of the National Multiple Sclerosis Society publish newsletters in which they announce trials in their area. Many of the member centers of the Consortium of Multiple Sclerosis Centers (see Appendix E, Resources) participate in one or more clinical trials. It is important to remember that each trial has a very specific protocol that details the types of patients who are eligible to participate. For some trials, the eligibility criteria are quite restrictive; for others, the criteria are more liberal. Your willingness to participate in a clinical trial is greatly appreciated by investigators because successful completion of such studies is the only way that we will definitively identify effective new treatments. Do not be discouraged if you do not meet the entrance criteria for a particular trial. Keep informed—the next one might be right for you.

Why should I participate in a clinical trial if I have a significant chance of getting the placebo instead of the real drug?

There are several reasons to participate in clinical trials.

◇ It has been demonstrated repeatedly in MS trials that even those subjects who receive the placebo usually do better than they would have done without any intervention. The quality of medical care in trials tends to be very high, and is provided without cost to the participants.

◇ Clinical trials are the best mechanism currently available to identify effective treatments; therefore, your participation ultimately helps investigators answer important questions.

◇ Standard, accepted treatments continue to be allowed under the research protocols of most placebo-controlled trials. For example, acute exacerbations could be treated with steroids in the interferon beta-1b (Betaseron®) and interferon beta-1a (Avonex®) trials.

◇ With Betaseron®, Avonex®, and Copaxone® currently available in the United States, Rebif® available in Canada and Europe, and Novantrone® recommended for approval by the FDA, it is likely that we will shift away from placebo-controlled trials to drug comparison trials in which a proposed new drug will be compared with the most effective available drug. Thus, any proposed new drug would have to demonstrate its superiority over those that have already been approved for use. Participants in this type of drug comparison trial would therefore be randomly assigned to either the proposed drug or one that has already been shown to be effective in treating MS.

Why do so many clinical trials require that participants be able to walk?

The entrance criteria for particular trials are very specific. Many of the trials require that subjects be able to walk, sometimes without the use of aids. This requirement is made because it is often more difficult to detect changes in disease activity in individuals whose illness is more advanced, and the inclusion of people with more advanced disease might cause investigators to discard potentially useful treatments because they erroneously failed to detect a benefit.

Why were the disease-modifying agents (Betaseron®, Avonex®, Copaxone®, and Rebif® [not available in U.S.]) originally tested on people with relapsing-remitting disease?

These agents (see Appendix B) were originally tested on people with relapsing-remitting MS because investigators thought those with milder disease would be more likely to show a benefit from the treatment. Also, previous studies had shown that it might be easier to demonstrate an effect by measuring a reduction in attack rate than by showing a reduction in disease progression.

How does Copaxone® differ from the interferon medications, Betaseron®, Avonex®, and Rebif® [not available in U.S]?

Betaseron®, Avonex®, and Rebif® are interferons, a group of immune system proteins, produced and released by cells infected by a virus, which inhibit viral multiplication and modify the body's immune response. Copaxone® is unrelated to the interferons. It is a synthetic polypeptide (like a protein) that may act by fooling the immune system, and by suppressing the immune attack on myelin that is believed to occur in MS.

Copaxone® is administered by daily subcutaneous (under the skin) injection. Unlike Betaseron®, Avonex®, and Rebif®, it does not cause flu-like reactions. Injection-site reactions are generally minor. Depression, which has been associated with all interferons administered in high doses for human disease, does not occur with Copaxone®. However, people who are taking Copaxone® should be aware of one peculiar reaction that, although infrequent, can be quite alarming. On rare occasions (perhaps once in 800 to 1,000 injections), a person taking Copaxone® may experience an immediate post-injection reaction involving sensations of tightness in the chest and flushing of the face, perhaps accompanied by palpitations, shortness of breath, or anxiety. This reaction passes within 15 to 30 minutes and has never proved to be serious.

Table 3-1 compares the four drugs currently approved for the treatment of relapsing-remitting MS. *Note: Betaseron®, Avonex®, and Copaxone® have been approved in the United States and Canada. Betaseron® is approved in Canada and Europe for both relapsing-remitting and secondary-progressive MS. To date, Rebif® has been approved only in Canada and Europe.*

At a recent MS educational meeting, sponsored by my local chapter of the National Multiple Sclerosis Society, I heard about a drug named Rebif®. What is it, and why isn't it available in the United States?

Rebif®, like Avonex®, is beta interferon-1a. In a multicenter trial in Canada, Europe, and Australia, for relapsing-remitting disease, Rebif® was found to reduce the number and frequency of MS attacks, slow the progression of disability, and reduce the number of brain lesions as measured by magnetic resonance imaging (MRI). It also reduced the number of hospitalizations and steroid use. The drug was tested in two dose strengths, administered subcutaneously three times per week. In this study, amounts of interferon beta-1a were higher on a weekly basis (by weight) at each dose than the weekly amount of Avonex® that has been approved by the FDA for use in relapsing forms of MS. In addition, people with a broader range of disabilities were studied, and shown to benefit.

In a separate, three-year, controlled clinical trial of (Rebif®) for secondary progressive MS, two doses of the drug were compared to placebo. Compared to placebo, neither dose of Rebif® delayed progression of disability (the primary goal of the study). However, both treated groups had significantly fewer and less severe relapses, fewer hospitalizations, reduced use of steroids, and fewer total lesions and new lesions in the brain as detected by MRI. The manufacturer of the drug has suggested that the failure to delay progression of disability in these secondary-progressive patients (in contrast to their positive findings in relapsing-remitting disease) may be due to the fact that the patients in this study started with higher levels of disability and had had the disease longer than the patients in previous studies.

Rebif® is now available for use in some countries. The trial sponsor, Ares Serono, has applied to the FDA for approval to market Rebif® in the United States as a treatment for relapsing-remitting MS. The FDA ruled that Rebif® was not sufficiently different from Avonex® to be marketed in the United States at this time. Under the provisions of the U.S. Orphan Drug Act, which provides financial incentives to the developers of drugs for rare diseases, Rebif® may not be allowed to compete with Avonex® on the U.S. market until 2003 unless Rebif® can be shown to be clinically superior to other products currently on the market. This ruling was made to allow the manufacturers of Avonex® time to recoup some of their costs. While this is frustrating for people with MS in the United States, the importance of the Orphan Drug Act should not be underestimated. Without the protections provided by this law, pharmaceutical companies would be unable, and unwilling, to undertake the development of new drugs for diseases like MS that affect relatively small numbers of people.

Table 3-1

	Betaseron® Interferon beta-1b	Avonex® Interferon beta-1a	Copaxone® Glatiramer acetate	Rebif® Interferon beta-1a
BRAND AND GENERIC NAME				
MANUFACTURER/DISTRIBUTOR	Berlex	Biogen	TevaMarion Partners	Serono Laboratories (U.S.), Serono Canada
APPROVAL	1993 U.S. 1995 Canada (R-R) 1999 Canada (S-P)	1996 U.S. 1998 Canada	1996 U.S. 1997 Canada	1998 Canada
FREQUENCY/ROUTE OF DELIVERY	Every other day; subcutaneous injection	Weekly; intramuscular injection	Daily; subcutaneous injection	Three times per week; subcutaneous injection
COMMON SIDE EFFECTS	Flu symptoms following injection, which lessen over time for many people; injection site reactions, about 5% of which need medical attention. Rarer: elevated liver enzymes, low white blood cell counts.	Flu symptoms following injection, which lessen over time for many people. Rarer: mild anemia, elevated liver enzymes.	Injection site reactions. Rarer: a reaction immediately after injection which includes anxiety, chest tightness, shortness of breath, and flushing. This lasts 15–30 minutes and has no known long-term effects.	Flu symptoms following injection, which lessen over time for many people; injection site reactions; Rarer: elevated liver enzymes, low white blood cell counts.

RETAIL COST, APPROXIMATE
(SOURCE: WWW.DRUGSTORE.COM)

$10,800/year* (U.S.)	$11,000/year (U.S.)	$10,000/year (U.S.)	$17,000/year (Canada)-lower dose
$17,000/year (Canada)	$16,970/year (Canada)	$12,300/year (Canada)	$21,000/year (Canada)-higher dose

PATIENT INFORMATION AND FINANCIAL
SUPPORT PROGRAMS

"Pathways"	"Avonex Alliance"	"Shared Solutions"	"Multiple Support Service":
1-800-788-1467;	1-800-456-2255	1-800-887-8100	1-888-MS-REBIF
1-800-948-5777	www.biogen.com	www.tevamarionpartners.com	www.ms-network.com
(financial issues)			
www.betaseron.com			

Once I start taking one of the disease-modifying drugs (Betaseron®, Avonex®, Copaxone®, or Rebif® [not available in the United States]), how long will I need to take the medication?

No one knows how long a person "needs" to take these medications. Since none of these medications completely prevents disease activity, the occurrence of an occasional attack in someone taking one of these medications does not necessarily mean drug failure. Data from the original three-year trial of Betaseron® indicated that, compared to the group receiving a placebo, the group treated with high-dose Betaseron® (the same dose that is currently prescribed for patients) had about a 30 percent reduction in annual exacerbation rate and showed no increase in total amount of lesion area in the CNS as detected with MRI. Follow-up data from the original group of 372 individuals with ambulatory, relapsing-remitting MS in the interferon beta-1b trial indicate the continued benefit and safety of Betaseron® for up to 10 years.

Additional clinical data on the safety and efficacy of glatiramer acetate (Copaxone®) were reported in 1998. Data for up to 35 months of treatment showed that the beneficial effects of daily subcutaneous injection of the drug persist for at least three years, and the benefit tends to improve as time progresses. These benefits, which include a further reduction in the relapse rate and extended time to first relapse, also suggest a slowing of the progression of disability. Safety continues to be acceptable, and the drug continues to be well tolerated. Experience with Avonex® now extends to at least five years and suggests continued efficacy and safety as well.

After a year or longer on Betaseron®, there is some evidence that approximately 38 percent of individuals develop substances in the blood called antibodies—proteins of the immune system that protect the body from foreign substances such as viruses and bacteria. The development of neutralizing antibodies was originally thought to be associated with a reduction in treatment benefits in some individuals. Follow-up data from the Betaseron® trial initially indicated that the exacerbation rate of the subgroup of treated individuals who developed the antibodies was significantly higher than the exacerbation rate for those who did not develop antibodies; in fact, it did not differ from the exacerbation rate for the group receiving a placebo. More recent data, however, indicate that the antibody level declines again, so that after a number of years they are no longer found. This means that there is no simple way for a person to determine his or her likelihood of developing antibodies to Betaseron®, or the impact that these antibodies are likely to have. Although similar neutralizing antibodies were reported in some of the patients in the Avonex® trial, data from the extension study show only about 5% of individuals developing antibodies. In the Rebif® trial, the relapse rate of those who developed neutralizing antibodies in the two treatment groups did not differ from the relapse rate of those who did not develop antibodies.

In general, people taking these medications should remain on the medication unless they are clearly having frequent attacks, significant disease progression, or severe side effects. Of course, the availability of newer effective treatments will require continual reassessment of an individual's situation.

I have been taking one of the disease-modifying agents for more than two years and I still don't feel better. Does this mean that the drug isn't working for me?

In the clinical trials of interferon beta-1b (Betaseron®), interferon beta-1a (Avonex® and Rebif®), and glatiramer acetate (Copaxone®), there was no evidence that the drugs made the treatment groups "feel better." Betaseron® was found to reduce the frequency and severity of exacerbations in relapsing-remitting MS. Avonex® reduced the frequency of relapses and slowed disease progression. Copaxone® reduced the frequency of exacerbations. Rebif® was found to reduce attack frequency and slow progression of disability. And all four drugs showed a reduction in new or active lesions on MRI. Although a significant effort has been made to inform people about the possible benefits and limitations of these treatments, it is clear that many people harbor a hope that they will feel better as a result of taking one of these treatments. This is not particularly surprising since most people's life experience with medical treatment in general, and medication in particular, is that it is designed to make a person feel better.

In a study of 100 individuals eligible for Betaseron® (funded by the National Multiple Sclerosis Society at the University of California, San Francisco), a significant proportion of those surveyed had misconceptions about the drug's potential effects. More than 80 percent expected that the drug would reduce their level of physical discomfort and improve their overall quality of life. Unfortunately, misconceptions such as these may cause people to become disappointed or dissatisfied with the effects of the drug they are taking and stop it prematurely, even if the drug is working for them in ways they cannot readily see or feel.

Since it is not possible to evaluate the extent to which any of these drugs is working for any one individual at any particular point in time, it is advisable for you to remain on the drug unless you are having frequent attacks, rapid disease progression, or severe side effects.

Why do all of these medications have to be taken by injection?

Injection is the only route of administration that has been shown to be effective at the present time. Betaseron®, Avonex®, and Rebif® are proteins, and proteins are degraded in the stomach and intestinal tract. The degradation products may not have the same effects in modulating the immune system that the intact molecule has. Copaxone® is a synthetic polypeptide (like a protein) that is unrelated to the interferons. An oral form of Copaxone® has been tested very successfully in EAE, the animal model of multiple sclerosis, and a major trial in MS is being launched. Oral and inhaled forms of interferons are also in development.

What will happen if I lose track of the date and forget to give myself a shot of Betaseron®, Avonex®, Copaxone®, or Rebif®?

Missing an occasional Betaseron® or Rebif® injection is not thought to be harmful. If that should happen, just give yourself the injection at the next most appropriate opportunity and continue the every-other-day routine from that point. The same holds true for Copaxone®. If you miss an injection, simply continue with your daily routine as soon as you remember. Do not, however, take two injections in one day. If you miss a dose of Avonex®, take it as soon as you remember and continue on a weekly schedule. Do not, however, take two doses within two days of each other.

Why are the disease-modifying medications so expensive and will the cost of these drugs ever come down?

These drugs are expensive for several reasons. First, the technology to develop and produce them is highly specialized.

Interferon beta-1b and interferon beta-1a are not naturally occurring substances. They are produced in the laboratory— grown in, and harvested from, bacteria and mammalian cells respectively. Glatiramer acetate is synthesized in a complex process that is difficult to standardize and requires precise control to maintain standardization. Manufacturing is thus complex and costly. More importantly, however, the costs of developing the products are extremely high and are passed along to the consumer. It is important to realize that for every drug that does reach the marketplace, dozens of others have failed to achieve that goal. The costs of testing those unsuccessful drugs must also be recouped through sales of the drugs that are successful.

Unfortunately for the public, pharmaceutical companies, like all other businesses, have a fiduciary obligation to their stockholders to try to maximize profits. Therefore, new drugs are generally quite expensive, especially those without similar competitive medications. With the approval of additional treatments, many people expect that competition may bring down the cost of these drugs.

I have recently been diagnosed with MS and have no apparent symptoms at this time. Should I start taking Betaseron®, Avonex®, Copaxone®, or Rebif® [not available in U.S.] right away?

The decision to begin one of these medications should be made with your physician, taking into account your history, current symptoms, exacerbation rate, and any evidence on MRI of new lesion development. In general, the person whose disease shows signs of relatively recent activity is the likeliest candidate to benefit from the treatment. Although people who are feeling and doing relatively well may see little reason to begin one of these medications, the fact is that multiple sclerosis is a very unpredictable disease. These medications are designed to reduce the number and severity of attacks in the hope that they will slow disease progression *over the long term*. Particularly in light of the new data indicating irreversible axonal damage, and possible brain atrophy even in the early stages of the disease, it is important to consider these medications carefully. Most MS experts now believe that one of the medications should be started early in the course of the disease, before significant, permanent damage occurs. Thus, if there are clear signs on clinical examination or on MRI that the disease process is active, *even if you are not currently experiencing significant symptoms*, most experts would favor initiating treatment. The National Multiple Sclerosis Society has recently published a Consensus Statement of the Medical Advisory Board advocating early and sustained treatment with one of these medications for individuals with relapsing forms of MS (see Appendix C).

Recently there have been reports about axonal damage and brain atrophy that can occur even in the early stages of MS. Can you tell me what these terms mean?

It is generally believed that the inflammatory process in MS causes damage primarily to the myelin sheath surrounding the nerve fibers in the central nervous system. Since the earliest descriptions of MS pathology, however, it has been known that the nerve fibers (axons) themselves also sustain damage. While inflammation is probably responsible for this phenomenon as well, the details of how axonal damage occurs remain unclear. Recent research has confirmed that nerve fibers can be affected or even severed in MS, and that this damage can occur very early in the disease. There is some speculation that this damage to the axons may be responsible for the permanent symptoms or impairments that can occur in MS.

Damage to nerve fibers and their loss may be partly responsible for the recently confirmed "atrophy" or brain shrinkage that occurs in MS. Loss of myelin and changes in brain fluids are also likely contributors. While myelin has the potential capacity to regrow, at least early in the disease, the regrowth of nerve fibers is much more problematic.

Perhaps the greatest significance of these findings lies in the fact that these irrevocable changes can occur early in the disease. It is in part because of these findings that MS experts are advocating early treatment, with one of the disease-modifying agents, for anyone with a confirmed diagnosis of relapsing-remitting MS. The goal is to slow the progression of the disease and prevent as much of this early, irreversible damage as possible.

What are the long-term side effects of taking the interferons (Betaseron®, Avonex®, and Rebif®) or glatiramer acetate (Copaxone®)? Will I get cancer because of these drugs?

No severe, long-term side effects have as yet been recognized with the use of these treatments. However, it is important to realize that only very small numbers of people have taken the drug for more than a few years. There is nothing at present to suggest an increased risk of cancer in people taking Betaseron®, Avonex®, Copaxone®, or Rebif®.

Follow-up data from the original group of 372 individuals with ambulatory relapsing-remitting MS in the interferon beta-1b trial showed a significant drop over time in the numbers of people experiencing flu-like symptoms and injection-site reactions. While 76 percent of the high-dose treatment group experienced flu-like symptoms during the initial months of the clinical trial, only 3 percent to 8 percent of this group reported these symptoms through the next five years. Similarly, the injection-site reactions experienced by 80 percent of the high-dose group in the early months of the trial were reported by 44 percent to 50 percent of this group in years four and five. Thus, most people taking Betaseron® over an extended period of time seem to be doing so with relatively little problem or discomfort.

In the Avonex® trial, 4 percent of patients discontinued the drug due to adverse effects. Modest side effects, including flu-like symptoms, muscle aches, fever, chills, and weakness, diminished with continued treatment. Four percent of patients experienced mild injection-site reactions.

During the two-year Rebif® trial, 3 percent of patients discontinued the drug due to adverse effects. The flulike symptoms and injection-site reactions tended to diminish with time. No long-term follow-up data on these subjects are yet available.

There are no long-term adverse effects known for Copaxone®.

If I have an exacerbation while I'm taking Betaseron®, Avonex®, Copaxone®, or Rebif®, can I still be given intravenous steroids?

Individuals taking any of these medications can still be treated with intravenous steroids in the same manner as those not on the medication.

I read on the Internet that some people with MS are being prescribed double doses of their injectable medication. Are double doses more effective that single doses, and will the insurance companies pay for them?

At the present time, little information is available to permit a reliable decision about what is the most effective, well-tolerated dose of the currently available injectable medications for MS. The recommended dose of Betaseron® was based on a very small pilot trial, which suggested that this was the maximum dose that was reasonably well tolerated. Nonetheless, recent trials of the drug in patients with secondary progressive MS have included some individuals who received slightly higher doses, based on their body weight.

It is difficult to compare doses of Betaseron® and Avonex®. Although both are interferon beta preparations, the drugs are chemically slightly different. In addition, their different routes of delivery (subcutaneous vs. intramuscular, respectively) can affect dose response. However, some experts do believe that the currently FDA-approved dose of Avonex® may not be maximally effective. Higher doses are likely to be tolerated, and are currently being tested in the Avonex® trial for secondary-progressive disease and in a dose-response study in Europe for relapsing-remitting MS. Rebif® (also interferon beta-1a) was recently tested successfully in Europe using three injections per week, thus providing a much larger, weekly dose of medication.

Despite the possibility that higher doses of the interferons may ultimately prove better, at the present time there remains insufficient information to justify their routine administration. Furthermore, it is extremely unlikely that insurance companies will be willing to pay for the higher doses unless and until there is more conclusive evidence of their effectiveness.

Very little is known about the optimal dose of Copaxone®. The current dose of 20 mg daily was rather arbitrarily chosen for the clinical trials. In one small trial in progressive MS, 30 mg was administered daily in two divided doses. This higher dose was well tolerated, but the trial did not show any convincing benefit for progressive disease.

My MS used to be relapsing-remitting. Now that it seems to be secondary progressive, would Betaseron®, Avonex®, Copaxone®, or Rebif® still be appropriate treatment for me?

In the United States, Betaseron®, Avonex®, and Copaxone® have been approved by the FDA solely for the treatment of relapsing-remitting MS. In Canada, Betaseron®, Avonex®, Copaxone®, and Rebif® are approved for relapsing-remitting MS. Following a recent European trial that demonstrated the effectiveness of Betaseron® in secondary-progressive MS, the drug was also approved in Canada and Europe for secondary-progressive disease. A similar trial of Betaseron® in secondary-progressive MS is still underway in North America. The FDA is awaiting results of the North American trial before deciding whether to approve Betaseron® for use in secondary progressive MS. The Rebif® trial in secondary progressive MS did not show an effect on progression and its approval for the treatment of secondary progressive MS in Canada is still in question.

A study is currently underway with Avonex® to investigate its effectiveness in secondary progressive MS. One small trial of Copaxone® in progressive MS, done in the late 1980s, failed to show a statistically significant benefit, but the trial was too small to be conclusive. Currently, Copaxone® is being tested in a larger primary progressive trial.

From a theoretical standpoint, it is reasonable to believe that these agents may all be effective for secondary-progressive MS. Difficulty may be encountered in obtaining insurance coverage in the United States for treatment of secondary progressive MS with these drugs since the drugs have either not been tested or are not yet approved by the FDA for progressive disease. At the moment, the only choice available in Canada for those with secondary, progressive disease is Betaseron®.

I have progressive MS and I'm wondering what treatments are available for me.

The answer to your question depends, in part, on what you mean by "progressive MS." There are two recognized types of progression in MS: *Primary progressive MS* refers to a disease course that is characterized by progression of disability from the outset, without an early phase of acute attacks and remissions. This course is seen in only 15 percent or so of people with MS. *Secondary progressive MS* refers to a disease course that is initially relapsing-remitting but subsequently becomes more consistently progressive. Of the 85 percent of people with MS who start out with relapsing-remitting disease, more than half will develop secondary progressive within a period of 10 years, and 90 percent within 25 years.

Of the treatments that have already been approved by the FDA for relapsing-remitting MS, Copaxone® (glatiramer acetate) and

Avonex® (interferon beta-1a) are currently being studied in people with primary progressive disease. However, the results from these studies will not be available for a few years.

Avonex® is currently being studied in secondary progressive MS. A European trial of Betaseron® (interferon beta-1b) in secondary progressive MS was terminated prematurely due to overwhelmingly positive results, and the drug is now approved for this use in Europe and Canada. The results of a similar study in the United States are not yet available. The FDA's decision about the use of Betaseron® in secondary progressive MS is awaiting these results. A study of Rebif® (interferon beta-1a; not available in the United States) for secondary progressive MS showed no benefit on slowing progression of disease, although a positive effect on relapses was seen.

One immunosuppressive agent is likely to have an increasing role in the treatment of progressive MS. Novantrone® (mitoxantrone for injection concentrate) is a potent immunosuppressing agent that is approved by the FDA for use in adult myeloid leukemia and for pain associated with certain types of prostate cancer. Its modes of action include inhibition of cell division, suppression of immune system B cells and helper T cells, and modulation of other immune cells and substances.

In a large, multicenter, controlled clinical trial, 194 individuals with secondary progressive MS (*with or without relapses*) and mild to moderate disability were randomly assigned to a low-dose, high-dose, or placebo group. Treatment was delivered by intravenous infusion once every three months over 24 months. After two years of treatment, the high-dose group was significantly less likely than the placebo group to demonstrate increased disability on the EDSS rating scale. The high-dose group also experienced significantly fewer relapses requiring corticosteroid treatment. The beneficial effects of treatment continued through one year of post-treatment follow-up.

A second study, focusing on MRI findings in individuals with highly active MS, compared monthly infusions of Novantrone® plus intravenous steroids with intravenous steroids given alone, over a six-month period. Compared with those treated only with steroids, the subjects treated with Novantron® plus steroids demonstrated significantly lower numbers of active inflammatory lesions in the brain, slower progression of disability, and reduced relapse rate.

The most common side effects in these two trials were nausea, hair loss, urinary and upper respiratory tract infections, and menstrual disorders. Cardiac toxicity has previously been reported, primarily in cancer patients exceeding a certain *cumulative* dosage level (i.e., accumulated level in the body over time). No cardiac toxicity was evident in the MS trials because none of the participants reached an equally high cumulative dose during the two years of the study.

Based on all of these findings, an advisory panel for the FDA recommended in January 2000 that the FDA approve Novantrone® to slow worsening of neurologic disability in people *with normal cardiac function* who have secondary progressive and relapsing-remitting forms of MS. Because of the dose-related toxicity that has been reported, its use will require cardiac monitoring above a certain cumulative dose and termination once the maximum cumulative dose is reached. Thus, Novantrone® will likely be prescribed to treat aggressive disease for a time-limited period, followed by one of the other available therapies. In fact, a trial is under way in Europe in which Novantrone® is being given in combination with methylprednisolone for six months, followed by interferon beta-1b for 27 months.

Although the FDA is not required to follow the advisory panel's recommendations, it usually does so. A final decision is expected in the near future. At the time of approval, the FDA will issue specific recommendations for the dosing and monitoring of Novantrone®.

Various other immunosuppressive agents (e.g., Imuran® (azathiaprine), Cytoxan® (cyclophosphamide), and methotrexate) have been used by some MS physicians to treat progressive disease; however, the clinical trials of these chemotherapeutic agents have not conclusively demonstrated their value for a broad spectrum of secondary progressive MS. A trial of cladribine failed to show benefit in progressive disease.

Thus, there is no simple answer to your question. Novantrone® is likely to be approved for the treatment of secondary-progressive disease very soon. While there are no currently approved treatments for primary progressive disease, there is reason to be optimistic that some will become available in the not-too-distant future.

What is immunosuppressive therapy and will it make my MS better?

Immunosuppressive therapy utilizes treatment agents that dampen the body's natural immune response, which is designed to protect it from foreign substances. In MS, we believe the immune system mistakenly attacks the person's own myelin as if it were foreign. By suppressing the immune system, such therapy may reduce the severity of the attack and thus reduce further damage to the myelin in the nervous system.

Immunosuppressive drugs such as mitoxantrone, cyclophosphamide, methotrexate, and azathioprine have been shown to slow the progression of MS. An advisory panel to the FDA has recently recommended that mitoxantrone (Novantrone®) be approved by the FDA for use in secondary progressive and relapsing-remitting forms of MS to slow worsening of neurologic disability. Cyclophosphamide proved too toxic for widespread acceptance by physicians or their patients. Methotrexate has been used in cancer treatment, for immunosuppression in organ transplantation, and for the treatment of rheumatoid arthritis. In relatively low doses, it has been shown to slow the rate of progression in MS. However, methotrexate is potentially toxic to the liver, and treatment with this drug must be carefully monitored. It is not compatible with nonsteroidal antiinflammatory drugs (e.g., aspirin or ibuprofen) or with alcohol, so that the use of methotrexate involves a number of restrictions. It is currently being used in some individuals with progressive MS. There is some evidence that azathioprine may slow progression in MS, but the effect, if it exists, is small and somewhat controversial.

All treatments currently available or in advanced stages of testing are aimed to reduce further damage. Of course, individuals with MS often improve spontaneously. However, the longer symptoms of MS have been present, the lower the likelihood that this spontaneous improvement will occur.

Now that there are several disease-modifying treatments available, how will I know whether to continue with my current treatment or try one of the others?

This is a question to be answered by you and your physician. The three therapies currently available in the United States have similar effectiveness but somewhat different side effect profiles. If side effects are causing significant problems, one of the other medications may be better tolerated. If you are doing well on what you are taking, however, you probably should not change since there is a certain period of time required for any treatment to take effect in your body.

While the mode of action of interferon beta-1b (Betaseron®) and interferon beta-1a (Avonex® and Rebif®) are probably identical, the third drug, glatiramer acetate (Copaxone®), is completely unrelated to the interferons. It is believed to "fool" the immune system in some way and interfere with its ability to damage myelin.

We currently have no data comparing the relative effectiveness of the three drugs. Many MS specialists believe that the dose of Avonex® may be sub-optimal, and that some people will require higher doses of interferon. This conclusion is derived principally from studies of Rebif®, an identical interferon to Avonex®, produced by another pharmaceutical company. Clinical trials with this agent showed substantially better responses, both clinically and on MRI, when the drug was administered three times a week rather than once. A study funded by Serono (the makers of Rebif®) is currently under way to compare the relative efficacy of Avonex® and Rebif®.

My friend's doctor recently started him on a combination of Copaxone® and Avonex®. Does combining these drugs provide more protection than either one of them alone?

Many people with MS, as well as MS investigators, would like to see results of a trial combining one of the interferons with glatiramer acetate (Copaxone®). Although this pairing might be beneficial, it is also possible that the combination could pose unexpected hazards (as seen in animal studies using this combination) or be less effective than either drug used alone. A current small pilot trial is examining the safety of Copaxone® and Avonex® used together in humans with MS, by evaluating their effect on MRI scans over a six-month period. If this trial does not lead to disease worsening or other unforeseen problems, it is probably that a full-scale trial of the two drugs together will be undertaken. In the meantime, there does not appear to be sufficient safety and efficacy information available to warrant use of two agents simultaneously, making it highly unlikely that insurance companies will be willing to pay for two drugs at the same time.

My family is worried about my using Betaseron® because of the reported suicides. What is the risk of depression and/or suicide with this drug?

Depression is very common in people with MS. Fortunately, however, it is usually not severe and generally responds well to a combination of psychotherapy and medication. Nevertheless, suicide occurs more frequently among people with MS than among comparable groups of people without the disease. In the Betaseron® definitive trial, four suicide attempts and one completed suicide occurred. Because of the frequency of depression and suicide in the MS population (see Chapter 11) and the small number of events in the trial, one cannot conclude that these episodes of depression were caused by the drug. It is known, however, that very high doses of interferon, such as those used in cancer treatment, do cause depression. As a result of concerns about interferons and depression, the emotional state of patients receiving these drugs has been followed carefully since marketing. In addition, the subjects in the Rebif® trial, who were receiving higher doses of interferon than subjects in previous interferon trials, were carefully monitored for depression. Rates of depression and suicide did not differ between the two treatment groups (high and low dose) and the group receiving a placebo. Now that more experience with these agents has been gained, severe depression and suicide seem to occur among individuals taking interferons at the same rate as they occur in the general MS population.

The best recommendation is that people with a previous history of severe affective disorder (depression or bipolar [manic-depressive] illness), or previous suicide attempts, should probably not take either interferon beta-1b (Betaseron®) or interferon beta-1a (Avonex®). Individuals with milder forms of depression can probably safely take Betaseron® or Avonex® under close supervision. Family members, other loved ones, and caregivers should be advised to be alert to any changes in mood and report them promptly to the physician. Sometimes the physician will wish to consult with a psychiatrist before starting a person on interferon beta-1b or interferon beta-1a, even though no suicide attempts or serious depression occurred in individuals in the Avonex® trial.

My doctor has recommended that I begin taking one of the interferons (Betaseron® or Avonex®). I've been reading about them on the Internet and hearing about the side effects people experience with these drugs. I'm reluctant to start an interferon because I don't want to feel worse than I already do.

The Internet has been a useful forum for people to exchange views and information about MS. It is probably a fact of life, however, that people tend to report side effects and problems more commonly than they "go on record" with positive feelings. Certainly, side effects do occur with Betaseron® and Avonex®. Most common are flulike symptoms that occur primarily in the first few months of treatment. For the majority of people, these are relatively mild and can be managed by taking injections at night and using minor analgesics (pain relievers), such as ibuprofen or acetaminophen. People taking Betaseron® also experience local injection-site reactions. Most typically these are confined to the appearance of red blotches and, perhaps, minor pain. Only infrequently do more severe reactions occur that may necessitate stopping the medication. We now have experience with many thousands of people taking Betaseron® or Avonex®. In general, with proper education and support from physicians and nurses, the medications are well tolerated and people can readily continue taking them. Overall, perhaps about 15 percent of people need to discontinue treatment for one reason or another and, certainly, not all of these are because of side effects.

One of the people in my MS support group is getting a treatment called IVIg. What can you tell me about it?

Intravenous immunoglobulin (IVIg) is a treatment that has been used in other autoimmune disorders, including neurologic diseases such as myasthenia gravis and Guillain-Barré syndrome, although the mechanism of action in any of these disorders is not known. IVIg, which consists of the antibody-containing portion of blood collected and fractionated from pools of donors, requires periodic intravenous administration. Several different treatment schedules have been employed, but most have involved monthly infusions.

Several reports have now indicated a beneficial effect in MS. All of these studies have evaluated the treatment with relapsing disease. No data have yet been reported for individuals with progressive forms of MS. Direct comparisons of the effectiveness of this treatment with those approved by the FDA—Betaseron®, Avonex®, and Copaxone®—are not available.

The treatment is generally well tolerated, although kidney problems may occur, and there is some concern about potential liver damage. Because IVIg is derived from natural blood products, there can be inconsistencies between batches and a potential risk from blood-borne viruses. For these reasons, IVIg is not considered by many North American experts in the field to be the treatment of choice for MS.

Insurance companies are likely to vary in their willingness to pay for the treatment, the costs of which tend to be higher than those for the other injectable medications.

I recently heard a news report about plasma exchange as a treatment for MS. I was just diagnosed and would like to know where I can get this treatment.

Although a recent study of ***plasma exchange*** (also called plasmapheresis) suggested a significant potential benefit for certain individuals with MS, its use is not appropriate for everyone. The study included 12 people with MS and 10 people with other disorders involving myelin destruction in the brain and spinal cord. *All subjects in the study were experiencing acute, severe attacks that had failed to respond to standard treatment with high-dose steroids.*

Before the plasma exchange, neurologists selected for each study participant one or two neurologic deficits or disabilities, resulting from the acute attack, that were to be the target of treatment. After plasma exchange, four of the 12 study participants with MS showed improvement in at least one of their targeted deficits and were considered treatment successes. For these individuals, plasma exchange was a major treatment intervention, resulting in a degree of recovery that would otherwise have been impossible

The investigators concluded that plasma exchange might contribute to recovery from an acute attack in people with MS or other inflammatory demyelinating diseases who have not responded to standard steroid treatment. They recommend, therefore, that this treatment *only be considered for individuals experiencing a severe, acute attack that is not responding to high-dose steroids.* Since the vast majority (approximately 90 percent) of people experiencing acute attacks respond well to the standard steroid treatment, plasma exchange would be considered a treatment alternative only for the 10 percent or so who do not. For those 10 percent, however, plasma exchange may offer an important and beneficial treatment option.

The plasma exchange procedure can be performed at most major medical centers without hospitalization. It involves seven treatments over a 14-day period, and costs approximately $18,000. Because this treatment is considered experimental for MS, the cost is not likely to be covered by most insurance carriers. The procedure also carries with it certain risks, including anemia and infection.

What new drugs are currently being tested for MS and how do they differ?

The following is a partial list of current and planned drug trials, divided by the type of MS being studied. Because this list is an ever-changing one, it is provided here merely to give an idea of the range of potential treatments currently under evaluation.

Acute Attacks: gamma globulin; monoclonal antibodies

Relapsing Forms of MS: glatiramer acetate (in oral form; in children with MS); interferon alpha (oral); interferon beta-1a + glatiramer acetate; monoclonal antibodies; peptide therapy; T cell vaccination; valacyclovir; vitamin D

Progressive Forms of MS (including all forms of progressive disease, separately or in combination): bone marrow transplantation; glatiramer acetate; interferon beta-1a; interferon beta-1b; mitoxantrone; T cell vaccination; valacyclovir

Combined Relapsing and Progressive Forms of MS: aspirin; gancyclovir; estriol

Is it possible to replace or repair the myelin that has been destroyed by MS?

It is not currently possible to enhance or improve myelin repair in MS. However, recent animal and laboratory investigations have shown that myelin repair occurs spontaneously in mammals and that this repair can be enhanced in animals. Some myelin repair occurs naturally in MS, particularly early in the disease, and this may be an important aspect of recovery from attacks. Further study is underway to try to find ways to enhance myelin repair in humans.

I have a friend who is taking 4-AP for his MS. What is 4-AP and is it likely to help me?

4-AP, which stands for 4-aminopyridine, is a chemical that acts on the channels in nerve fibers that control the passage of potassium. In so doing, it appears able to improve temporarily the transmission of impulses through these fibers. Some individuals with MS have experienced improvement in neurologic symptoms when taking 4-AP orally. In particular, it seemed to help some people whose MS was heat-sensitive. Although 4-AP has never had FDA approval, a physician could legally write a prescription for the chemical to be made up for a patient by a compounding pharmacy that would put the substance into a medicinal form.

Recently, however, the FDA recommended that pharmacies no longer be allowed to compound this substance because of significant safety problems and problems with inconsistency in products made by compounding pharmacies. 4-AP has a number of potentially serious side effects, most noteworthy of which are seizures. Furthermore, it has a low toxic-therapeutic index, meaning that the dose that may cause problems is not very much higher than that which may be beneficial. Because compounding pharmacies may not have the same high level of standardization controls that exist for prescription drugs marketed by regulated pharmaceutical companies, a lack of precision about dosage may pose significant risks to people who obtain the substance from compounding pharmacies.

Oral myelin is sold at my local health food store. Will this product help my MS symptoms?

Oral myelin did not produce detectable benefit in a recent therapeutic trial so it is unlikely that the product sold in your local health food store will be helpful. Unfortunately, preparations touted as containing oral myelin are presently being sold at

many health food stores. Such products are essentially unregu-
lated. The amounts of oral myelin that they contain are
unknown, but usually much smaller than that which was tested.
Furthermore, the source of the product is generally not indicated. Certain herds of cattle, though not those in the United States,
have harbored a fatal, transmissible disease that may pose risks
to humans. Extreme precautions were taken to eliminate any risk
to subjects in the FDA-approved trial of Myloral®, but the same
cannot be said for these uncontrolled products distributed
through health food stores.

**One of my friends recommended that I try marijuana to relieve
my MS symptoms. Is marijuana an effective treatment for MS?**

Smoking marijuana has been reported by some individuals to
benefit some of their symptoms, particularly spasticity. However, small clinical trials of orally-administered tetra-hydro-
cannabinol (THC), the active chemical in marijuana, have had
mixed results. While some treated individuals reported feeling
"looser" and less stiff, objective evaluations by physicians could
not always confirm any change. Effects lasted less than three
hours, and side effects included weakness, dry mouth, dizziness, mental clouding, short-term memory impairment, space-
time distortions, and incoordination.

In March 1999, the National Academy of Sciences/Institute of
Medicine released their White House-commissioned report on
medical uses of marijuana. The report stated that the medical
benefits of marijuana are modest, and that for most symptoms,
more effective medicines are already available. The report did
recommend, however, continued research on the biological
effects of cannabinoids, the active compounds in marijuana, to
determine if it is possible to derive their benefits without their
detrimental side effects. In the meantime, the use of marijuana is
not legal for the treatment of MS.

**My friends and relatives are always pushing me to try different
diets and vitamins. Does diet have any effect on this disease?**

Many diets have been touted as being useful for MS, but none
has ever demonstrated its efficacy in a controlled trial. While
some of these (e.g., the popular Swank diet) are generally health-
ful if extremely demanding, others are inconvenient, and some

are possibly harmful. The same is true for vitamins and other supplements, none of which has been shown to help MS. It is clear, however, that maintenance of good health and physical condition is valuable and may help a person with MS cope better with the physical and emotional challenges of the neurologic disease. Thus, a diet such as the American Heart Association diet—which resembles the Swank diet but is a little less rigid—may be worthwhile if a person with MS wants to follow a nutritional regimen.

Recommended Readings

Giffels JJ. *Clinical Trials: What You Should Know Before Volunteering to Be a Research Subject.* New York: Demos Vermande, 1996.
Sibley WA. *Therapeutic Claims in Multiple Sclerosis (4th edition).* New York: Demos Vermande, 1996.

Selected booklets available from the National Multiple Sclerosis Society (800-344-4867):

◇ *Research Directions in Multiple Sclerosis* (ES 6017)

◇ *Clear Thinking About Alternative Therapies* (ECS 6038)

References in this area become outdated very quickly. The most accurate, up-to-date information about treatments and drug trials is available through the National Multiple Sclerosis Society Society (800-FIGHT-MS; www.nmss.org).

Recommended Resources

Avonex®: "Avonex Support Line" (800-456-2255); www.bio-gen.com

Betaseron®: "Multiple Sclerosis Pathways" (800-788-1467); www.betaseron.com

Copaxone®: "Shared Solutions" (800-887-8100); www.tevamarionpartners.com

Rebif®: "Multiple Support Program" (888-MS-REBIF); www.ms-network.com

National Multiple Sclerosis Society (800-FIGHT MS); www.nmss.org

4

Nursing Care
to Enhance Wellness

June Halper, MSN, RN.CS., ANP

Multiple sclerosis can affect many aspects of a person's functioning over its long and unpredictable course. Some of the problems caused by the illness, such as weakness, imbalance, optic neuritis, or bladder and bowel symptoms, are a direct result of *plaque* formation in the *central nervous system.* Others, including skin breakdown or *osteoporosis*, can result from the lack of mobility caused by the illness. Much has been learned in recent years about successful management of these primary and secondary problems in MS. With education and support provided by the health care team, people can learn to manage their symptoms and avoid unnecessary problems and complications.

The nurse can be a helpful ally in these management efforts, whether as a member of an MS center's health care team, in the community's Visiting Nurse Service, on a hospital inpatient service, in a rehabilitation facility, or in the home. A primary goal of nursing care in MS is to help people learn effective, preventive self-care in order to manage minor problems before they become major ones. This chapter has as its focus three areas in which nursing plays a key role—bladder function, bowel management, and skin care. The chapter also addresses important wellness strategies for maintaining an optimal level of health and well-being in spite of a chronic illness.

Bladder Function

The neurologic changes in MS sometimes interfere with bladder function. These changes can be distressing and occasionally disabling, but they are manageable with effective interventions including education, thorough diagnostic testing, medications, and self-care activities.

The urinary system (see Fig. 4-1) includes:

◇ kidneys, which filter impurities from the bloodstream and excrete them in the urine
◇ ureters, the small tubes that transport urine from the kidneys to the bladder
◇ urinary bladder, which stores urine until it is time to void (urinate)
◇ urethra, which transports the urine out of the body

In order for normal urination to occur, the detrusor or bladder muscle must contract to expel urine at the same time that the

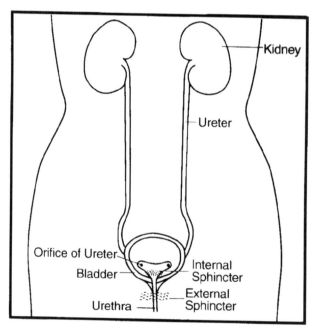

Figure 4-1. Diagram of the urinary system.

internal and external sphincters are relaxed to allow the urine to pass freely out of the body. In normal function, the urine is collected slowly, causing the bladder to expand. When approximately six to eight ounces (180–240 ml) of urine have accumulated, nerve endings in the bladder send a message to the voiding reflex area of the spinal cord which, in turn, sends a message to the brain signaling the need to urinate. The brain then sends a message back to the spinal cord that signals the voiding reflex to contract the **detrusor muscle** and relax the urethral sphincter. Thus, a functional urinary system depends on an intact nervous system.

In multiple sclerosis, the excretion or elimination of urine can be altered in the following ways:

◇ **Failure to store** urine, usually seen in a small, spastic bladder, results from **demyelination** of the pathways between the spinal cord and the brain. The bladder fills quickly and sends messages to the spinal cord, which, because of demyelination, is unable to forward the message to the brain. As a result, voluntary control of urination is interrupted and voiding becomes a reflex response to repeated signals from the spinal cord. Failure to store can result in symptoms of **urinary urgency** (having to get to the bathroom quickly), **urinary frequency** (feeling the urge to urinate even when urination has occurred very recently), dribbling, **incontinence** (wetting oneself), and **nocturia** (being awakened at night by the need to urinate).

◇ **Failure to empty** urine occurs when there is demyelination in the voiding reflex area of the spinal cord. Even though the bladder fills with large amounts of urine, the spinal cord is unable to send the necessary messages—either to the brain that the bladder is full or to the bladder and sphincter. The resulting absence of either voluntary or reflexive voiding causes the bladder to overfill. Failure to empty results in a large, **flaccid** (atonic) bladder and symptoms of urgency, dribbling, hesitancy, and incontinence.

◇ **Combined dysfunction** can result from a failure to store/failure to empty combination called **detrusor-external sphincter dyssynergia (DESD)**. Combined dysfunction involves a lack of coordination between muscle groups, whereby the detrusor and external sphincter contract simultaneously, trapping urine within the bladder. Both urgency and hesitancy may occur, as well as dribbling or incontinence.

It is important to remember that a particular symptom does not point to a particular type of bladder failure. In fact, each of the primary urinary symptoms—urgency, frequency, hesitancy, incontinence, and nocturia—can be caused by any of the functional abnormalities that have been described. Careful evaluation is needed in order to identify the cause of the problem and select appropriate treatment measures.

I have just been diagnosed with MS. What are the chances that I will develop problems controlling my bladder or bowel?

Multiple sclerosis can affect the motor and sensory pathways from the brain and spinal cord that control both bladder and bowel function. Over the course of the disease, as many as 80–90 percent of people develop transient or persistent urinary symptoms. Bladder symptoms can occur at the onset of the illness or at any time thereafter. They can usually be controlled with medications, self-care activities, and some possible modifications in lifestyle. Bowel problems occur somewhat less frequently but are still common enough that everyone with MS needs to be aware of their relationship to the disease and familiar with effective prevention and management strategies.

The most important thing to remember about bladder and bowel symptoms in MS is that they can be helped. The MS health care team is familiar with these problems and their management. Although you may initially find it difficult or uncomfortable to discuss bladder and bowel questions with your doctor or nurse, the more open you are about any problems you are having, the more quickly and easily you can learn effective management techniques and avoid unnecessary complications and discomfort.

I have recently begun having trouble controlling my urine. All of a sudden, without any warning, I have to get to the bathroom immediately or risk wetting myself. What is the treatment for this problem?

The sudden sensation of having to urinate quickly is called urinary urgency. It usually results from the bladder's failure to store urine properly or from a failure to store/failure to empty combination (bladder detrusor-external sphincter dyssynergia— DESD). A careful evaluation is needed in order to determine the cause of the urgency. Urgency resulting from a failure to store can be managed with an **anticholinergic** medication, such as oxybutynin chloride (Ditropan® or Ditropan XL®), that controls spasms in the bladder and other smooth muscles of the body by inhibiting transmission of parasympathetic nerve impulses (see Appendix B). While Ditropan® is taken three to four times daily, Ditropan XL® is an extended-release formula that needs to be taken only once a day. Tolterodine tartrate (Detrol®) is an anti- spasmodic agent that reduces urinary urgency by reducing spasms of the detrusor muscle of the bladder. Certain tricyclic antidepressants, most notably imipramine (Tofranil®), share these anticholinergic properties and have been found to be use- ful in controlling urinary muscle contractions (see Appendix B). Feelings of urgency resulting from the bladder's failure to empty or from DESD are best managed with a treatment regimen that includes anticholinergic medication and **intermittent self- catheterization (ISC)**.

What is intermittent self-catheterization?

If the bladder fails to empty properly or the bladder and sphinc- ters do not work together in the proper rhythm, your physician may suggest that you do intermittent self-catheterization (ISC) on a scheduled basis—from one to five times a day. ISC can be thought of as physical therapy for your bladder because it pro- motes regular filling and emptying (expanding and contracting) of the bladder muscle and may help restore normal function. You begin by emptying your bladder as thoroughly as you can. Then you drain the residual or remaining urine by passing a **catheter** (a very thin, hollow, plastic tube that resembles a straw) into your bladder through the urethra. The catheter stays in your bladder until the urine stops draining—no more than a minute or two—and is then removed. With a little practice, the procedure is easy, quick, and painless. ISC can be done while sitting on the toilet, lying on the bed, or even in the public restroom of your favorite restaurant. Your doctor or nurse can instruct you in the appropriate use, care, and cleaning of the urinary catheter. If you are unable to self-catheterize, the proce- dure may be carried out by your spouse, partner, or a visiting nurse. Typically, the nurse will stay involved only long enough to ensure that you or your spouse/partner have mastered the technique.

What kinds of tests will the doctor do to find out why I am having problems urinating?

A number of tests are used to diagnose urinary problems. Your physician will first determine whether a urinary tract infection (UTI) is causing your urinary symptoms. Infections in one or more of the structures of the urinary tract are caused by bacteria and can be detected by microscopic examination of a urine specimen. A test called a **urine culture and sensitivity (C&S)** will be used to identify the particular bacteria that is present and the antibiotic to which it is sensitive. The bacteria from a midstream urine sample is allowed to grow for three days in a special laboratory medium and then tested for sensitivity to a variety of antibiotics. This allows your physician to prescribe the antibiotic most likely to kill the bacteria. An antibiotic that commonly cures UTI may be prescribed until the results of the C&S are known.

In order to determine whether your urinary symptoms are caused by the bladder's failure to empty, failure to store, or combined dysfunction, the doctor can evaluate your **post-void residual (PVR)**. You will be asked to drink ample fluids for a day or two before the test and two glasses just prior to the PVR. As soon as you feel the need to urinate, you will do so and the amount of urine will be measured. After you have urinated, the nurse will pass a catheter into the bladder to drain and measure the urine remaining in the bladder. A completely noninvasive way of measuring residual urine that is now being used by many MS centers and urologists involves a bladder scanner. This scanner uses an external "wand" and a computer to determine the amount of urine remaining in your bladder after voiding. It is important to determine if urine is being retained in the bladder because urine that is not voided can cause a urinary tract infection. Depending on the amount of urine that is found in your bladder after voiding, your doctor may suggest a program of self-catheterization and/or an anticholinergic medication to manage your symptoms.

In most instances, the results of either kind of post-void residual assessment, in combination with your body's response to the prescribed treatment regimen, will provide ample information about the source of your urinary symptoms. Further testing may be required if the physician is still unable to diagnose the problem. In an intravenous pyelogram (IVP), dye is injected into your vein so that sequential X-ray pictures can be taken of the kidneys, ureters, and bladder. Ultrasound technology (utilizing sound waves) can also be used to determine the presence of stones or other abnormalities in your bladder. A somewhat more invasive test, a urinary **cystoscopy**, which can be done in a urologist's office or in the hospital, allows the physician to examine the inside of the bladder.

Sometimes when I feel that I have to urinate I find that I have trouble getting started. I feel the pressure to empty my bladder but nothing comes out. Is there anything I can do about this?

The inability to initiate urination in spite of the sensation of a full bladder is called **urinary hesitancy** and usually results from the bladder's failure to empty properly. Patience almost always pays off; people find that the urinary stream usually starts within a minute or two. You can try running water in the sink to help relax the urinary sphincter. "Tickling" the opening to the urethra (the opening behind a woman's vagina or the tip of a man's penis) with a moist tissue may also promote relaxation. If these techniques do not produce results, you may tap lightly on the lower part of your abdomen. Do not press or hit yourself too forcefully as this might worsen the problem.

Speak to your physician if you are unable to manage the hesitancy. A medication such as baclofen (Lioresal®) will relax the sphincter to allow the bladder to empty more effectively (see Appendix B).

After I finish urinating I sometimes feel that my bladder is still full. Nothing more comes out but I'm afraid to leave the bathroom in case of an accident. How can I tell if there is more urine left in my bladder?

The sensation of a full bladder after voiding can be caused by the bladder's failure either to empty or store properly. A PVR can be done to determine if you are retaining urine in your bladder and what treatment would be most beneficial. As indicated, it is important that you be able to empty your bladder fully, using whatever combination of medication and/or ISC is appropriate, both to maintain your personal comfort and to reduce your risk of bladder infections. Some individuals with multiple sclerosis find relief from this problem by "double-voiding"—urinating once, waiting a minute or more, and then voiding again.

I'm so worried I'll have a bladder accident that I hardly drink anything any more. My doctor says that I need to drink fluids so that I won't get bladder infections. What can I do to handle this problem?

Urine, which consists of solid and liquid waste substances that are not needed by your body, is manufactured continuously by the kidneys. It is important for urine to be diluted with water because urine that contains more solid particles than liquid will increase your risk of infection. Many people who experience urinary urgency or frequency restrict their intake of fluids in the hope of relieving their symptoms and freeing themselves from the bathroom. As a result, their urine becomes too highly concentrated with solid particles (resulting in a dark brownish appearance) and therefore more susceptible to infection. You should drink between six and eight glasses of fluid per day, early in the day if you prefer in order to avoid having to go to the bathroom at night. You can also get fluids in such foods as soup, Jell-O®, fruits, puddings, and compotes. In addition to reducing your risk of bladder infections, adequate fluid intake will help you to maintain satisfactory bowel function.

Identifying the cause of your bladder accidents will make it possible for your physician to design a bladder management program, possibly including medication and scheduled voiding, in an effort to "train" your bladder and help reduce the risk of accidents.

Sometimes I wet myself without even knowing that it is happening—I can't feel either the urge to urinate or the urine itself. Why is this happening and is there anything I can do about it?

Spontaneous voiding (urinary incontinence) can occur in MS for a number of reasons. Because uninhibited bladder spasms and a weakened bladder muscle can both cause urine to pass out of the bladder before the urge to urinate is felt, post-void residual testing is required to determine the cause of the problem. Diminished sensations in the genital area will reduce a person's awareness of the urge to void and perhaps even of the sensation of being wet. Usually a treatment regimen consisting of ISC and/or a trial of anticholinergic medication will be sufficient to

control the incontinence. If the bladder dysfunction that is causing the incontinence does not respond to this type of treatment
regimen, your neurologist will probably refer you to a urologist
for more extensive bladder studies to determine if some other
problem is contributing to your symptoms.

**I seem to be getting up three or four times during the night to
urinate. This is very unusual for me. Is there anything I can do
about this problem?**

The first step in dealing with *nocturia*, as this problem is called,
is to make sure that you do not have a urinary tract infection.
Then your physician or nurse will do a PVR to determine the
probable cause of the problem. Nocturia is most commonly
caused by spasms in the bladder muscles that result in the bladder's failure to store urine properly. It can usually be treated very
effectively with a bedtime dose of either imipramine (Tofranil®)
or desmopressin (DDAVP Nasal Spray®) (see Appendix B).

**I think I have memorized the location of every bathroom in the
city. Is there anything I can do when I'm going out so that I
don't constantly have to be near a toilet?**

The urinary symptoms of urgency and frequency, which sometimes make people feel as though their lives are controlled by
the location of the nearest bathroom, can usually be treated and
managed once they are properly diagnosed. Your health care
team can diagnose the source of these symptoms and prescribe a
course of medication and/or ISC that will allow you to regain
control of your bladder.

Once this sense of control is regained, you will feel more confident about venturing farther from the bathroom. Most people
still find that they feel more comfortable if, upon arriving at
their destination, they check out the location of the bathroom so
that they can get there without having to search for it. Some
people choose to wear some protective pad (e.g., Serenity® or
Depends®) so that they do not have to panic about possible leakage. If you know that you have trouble controlling your bladder
for long periods of time and that you are going to be in a situation in which getting to a bathroom quickly is impossible (a
football game, a wedding, or a long bus ride, for example), you
can discuss with your doctor the occasional use of a drug such

as desmopressin (DDAVP Nasal Spray®) or imipramine (Tofranil®).

What are the symptoms of a urinary tract infection and what are the treatments for it?

Urinary tract infections can sometimes occur without any apparent symptoms or discomfort. More often, however, an infection causes symptoms such as urinary urgency and frequency, a burning sensation, abdominal pain, an elevated body temperature, increased spasticity, and possibly foul-smelling, dark-colored urine. Urinary tract infections most commonly occur in the bladder and are usually treatable with oral antibiotics. An infection in the upper portion of the urinary tract, including the kidneys and ureters, is more serious and potentially more debilitating. Kidney infections are usually accompanied by a high fever and may require intravenous treatment with antibiotics. Both types of infection are treated by increased fluid intake and rest, as well as close medical monitoring.

Individuals who are particularly prone to urinary tract infections may be prescribed an antiseptic, such as methenamine (Hiprex® or Mandelamine®), to use on a routine basis to "cleanse" the urine and reduce the number of bacteria (see Appendix B). Additionally, maintaining an acid urine will help in the prevention of urinary tract infections because the organisms that cause infections do not grow as easily in an acidic environment. You can make your urine more acid by following certain dietary guidelines. *Increase* your daily intake of: (1) protein, such as that found in meat, fish, fowl, eggs, and gelatin; and (2) cranberries (and their juice), plums, and prunes. The cranberry juice, which provides a replacement for the vitamin C found in citrus fruits, should be taken at frequent intervals throughout the day because vitamin C is processed and excreted very rapidly by the body. *Decrease* your intake of: (1) citrus fruits and juices (grapefruit, oranges, lemons, and tomatoes); (2) milk and milk products; (3) beverages or antacids containing sodium carbonate or sodium bicarbonate (use Gelusil® or any other aluminum-type antacid in their place); and (4) potatoes.

To treat chronic, recurrent UTIs, your physician may prescribe long-term, low-dose antibiotics such as sulfamethoxazole

(Septra® or Bactrim®) in an effort to suppress bacterial activity and reduce the risk of infection (see Appendix B).

I feel very weak when I have a bladder (urinary tract) infection even though I never seem to run a very high fever. Does this mean that the infection is making my MS worse?

Any type of infection is likely to cause a feeling of weakness and an apparent exacerbation of symptoms, especially one that causes an elevation in body temperature. This is referred to as a *pseudoexacerbation* because it is caused by the underlying infection and not by an actual progression of the disease. The important strategy when this occurs is to treat the infection promptly, thus removing the trigger for this temporary worsening of the symptoms. A pseudoexacerbation and accompanying weakness typically remit or disappear once the infection is brought under control.

Is a urinary tract infection ever life-threatening?

A urinary tract infection can be life-threatening if left untreated and allowed to spread into the kidneys. Since all blood is filtered through the kidneys, the infection can pass into the bloodstream and cause serious problems.

Are there different types of urinary catheters? How do I know what type of catheter is best for me?

The type of catheter used for intermittent self-catheterization resembles a straw and is called a straight catheter. One end is tapered and has a small hole called a port. This end is inserted into the bladder for urinary drainage. The other end has a larger opening that allows the urine to flow into the toilet or a collecting device.

A *Foley catheter* is an *indwelling catheter* that remains in the bladder for longer periods of time, allowing continuous drainage into a collection bag. The tapered end has a balloon that is inflated when the catheter is placed into the bladder. The balloon is filled with sterile water while in the bladder and emptied when the catheter is withdrawn, but cannot be felt by the person at any time. A Foley catheter is used for continuous drainage of urine when bladder function cannot be improved by the other means discussed in this chapter or if a person is experiencing skin breakdown (*decubitus* ulcer) because of chronic wetness that cannot be otherwise managed.

My doctor wants me to do intermittent self-catheterization. Why can't I just use a Foley catheter all the time so I don't have to be bothered?

ISC is a strategy to maintain and sometimes improve bladder tone and bladder function. It prevents infections, reduces symptoms, and prevents the long-term complications of chronic urinary tract infections. People may find that their bladder symptoms are more problematic some times than others; they may need to do ISC for a period of time and then find it unnecessary for a while. A Foley catheter is used by people who are unable to manage their bladder function with medications or self-care, either because their symptoms cannot be controlled or their other symptoms interfere with their ability to do ISC.

The urinary system is normally closed to the outside environment even when a person self-catheterizes. Once an indwelling catheter is inserted into the bladder, this closed system remains open at all times, making the person susceptible to ongoing infections, the development of bladder stones, and other complications of the urinary system. Foley catheters are now thought of as the last resort when other treatments are not viable.

Is it possible to use a Foley catheter for some situations and catheterize myself the rest of the time?

Some people who self-catheterize regularly can insert Foley catheters for situations when ISC is not possible. Airline flights or long car trips, for example, make ISC somewhat problematic. The Foley catheter is inserted prior to the journey and then removed. Because of the increased risk of infection with an indwelling catheter, it is very important to discuss the advisability of this strategy with your physician; it may be reasonable for some individuals but not others. Anyone using a Foley catheter needs to increase fluid intake to minimize the risk of infection. You can resume your normal ISC bladder routine once the Foley catheter is removed.

Will my bladder symptoms ever get better or go away?

This is not an easy question to answer. Many people report that their bladder symptoms improve or disappear, at least temporarily, with the appropriate use of medications and ISC. Others report that their bladder dysfunction waxes and wanes but never fully disappears. As with other symptoms of MS, bladder symptoms vary from person to person and from one period of time to another. The key to bladder management is accurate knowledge about what is causing the problem followed by appropriate action to minimize complaints and control symptoms.

Are there any surgical procedures that would take care of my bladder symptoms?

No surgical procedures can resolve bladder problems caused by neurologic changes. In certain rare instances, when none of the medications or self-care techniques have successfully relieved urinary symptoms, surgery (e.g., suprapubic *cystostomy*, *sphincterotomy*, *transurethral resection*) is performed to help bladder management.

Bowel Function

The gastrointestinal tract, which is responsible for the digestion and absorption of food and the elimination of waste, is composed of the following parts (see Fig. 4-2):

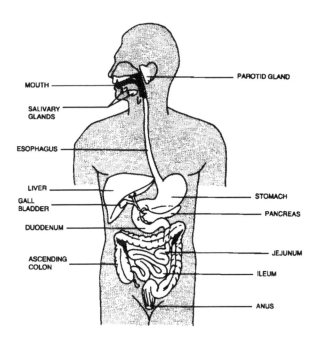

Figure 4-2.   The gastrointestinal tract.

◇ the mouth, in which digestion is initiated by the chewing process and the addition of saliva;

◇ the esophagus, which connects the mouth to the stomach;

◇ the stomach, which stores food and advances the digestive process;

◇ the small intestine, where the digestive process is continued;

◇ the large intestine, where stool is formed;

◇ the rectum, in which the stool is stored just prior to defecation; and

◇ the anal canal, which contains the internal and external sphincters that normally remain closed to prevent leakage.

Stool normally passes into the rectum just prior to a bowel movement. When the rectum becomes full, it sends nerve impulses to a critical area of the spinal cord. The stool then passes through the anal canal, where it encounters first the internal sphincter, which opens reflexively in response to signals from the spinal cord, and then the external sphincter, which responds to signals from both the spinal cord and brain. The external sphincter is under "voluntary control," which means that a person can consciously tighten it to prevent defecation until the time and place are convenient. As with the urinary system, a functional gastrointestinal system is dependent on a functional nervous system.

Changes in bowel function can be manifested as **constipation**, bowel urgency, or loss of bowel control (incontinence). People rarely complain about loose stools or diarrhea unless they have taken excessive amounts of laxatives or stool softeners. Constipation, by far the most frequent bowel complaint in MS, refers to infrequent, incomplete, or difficult bowel movements. The management of constipation in MS is important not only because of the abdominal discomfort it can cause, but also because of its potential for exacerbating other symptoms such as spasticity and urinary urgency and frequency.

Several factors conspire to produce MS-related constipation:

◇ Demyelination in the brain or spinal cord and reduced physical movement can each slow the passage of stool through the bowel. Because the body continuously draws moisture from the stool as it makes its way through the body, stool that remains in the intestine for extended periods of time becomes overly dry, hard, and difficult to pass.

◇ Dry, hardened stool can also result from decreased sensation in the rectal area. A person with decreased sensation may not experience the need to have a bowel movement, with the result that the stool remains in the rectum for an overly extended period of time.

◇ The same problem sometimes occurs because weakened abdominal muscles make it difficult to push the stool out of the rectum.

◇ A reduced fluid intake (usually in response to anxiety over bladder problems) will also cause the body to absorb more water from the stool.

◇ Certain medications slow bowel function and therefore contribute to the stool's loss of moisture.

Bowel changes in MS can be successfully managed with a self-care program that starts with a thorough evaluation of your dietary habits, medications, past and present bowel habits, and physical requirements for safe and comfortable toileting. If needed, an individualized bowel management program can be initiated with the help of the physician and nurse; successful bowel management then depends on the patience required to find the right combination of dietary changes, medications, and a consistent regimen. In general, a healthy bowel program consists of adequate fluid intake, a high fiber diet, adequate exercise, and a consistent, relaxed time for bowel evacuation, preferably thirty minutes after a meal when the **gastrocolic reflex** is at its strongest.

Are the bowel and bladder symptoms I have related? Some of my friends with MS have one or the other symptom but not both.

Bowel and bladder symptoms in MS may be related to one another, but they do not necessarily have to be. Spasms resulting from impaired neurologic function can cause symptoms of urgency and frequency in both the bladder and bowel systems. Weakened musculature can also interfere with the emptying process in either system. A full bowel can press on the bladder, causing symptoms of urinary urgency and frequency. Individual factors, such as diet, amount of exercise, and pre-illness patterns are more likely to affect a person's bowel regimen independently of what is occurring with the bladder.

My doctor says that drinking more fluids will help with my constipation, but when I drink I have difficulty controlling my urine. I can't decide which problem is worse!

Increasing your fluid intake is certainly one important method for improving bowel function. It is generally recommended that you drink two quarts of fluid every day. Be sure to discuss any problems you are having with urinary control with your physician or nurse so that they can recommend appropriate management techniques. The dilemma, of course, is that both problems are annoying and uncomfortable. Bladder problems need to be addressed first so that you can manage the high fluid intake needed for satisfactory bowel function. It may take some time and patience on your part to balance your bladder and bowel management, but it can be accomplished in ways that will reduce your symptoms, make you more comfortable, and avoid future complications.

Are there special diets that can help me with my bowel problems?

In addition to increased fluid intake, it is equally important to add fiber to your diet, usually in the form of bran, grains, fresh fruits and vegetables, prunes and prune juice. Fiber increases the moisture-retaining bulk of the stool, allowing it to pass more quickly and easily through the intestinal tract. Also be sure that you engage in some form of physical exercise each day to help promote regular bowel function.

What should I do if increasing my intake of fluids and fiber doesn't relieve the constipation?

In addition to the high fiber diet and increased intake of fluids, you can take a natural bulk supplement (made from the psyllium seed) such as Metamucil® on a daily basis, as well as a stool softener such as Colace®. These over-the-counter products will help to keep the stool soft enough to pass easily through your system. Regular adherence to this type of high fiber regimen will be sufficient for most people to control constipation. If the problem continues, your physician will probably recommend that you use a *mild* laxative such as Milk of Magnesia® every other night or so, and perhaps a glycerin suppository 30 minutes before you plan to move your bowels. Bisacodyl (Dulcolax®) suppositories can also be tried if the glycerin suppository is ineffective. Those who are unable to move their bowels even with these additional measures may require a Therevac Plus® or Fleet® enema to move the bowels. The Therevac Plus® is generally preferred because it is the size of a suppository and therefore much easier to use. As you can see, there are a variety of steps that can be taken to control constipation and create a comfortable bowel regimen. The goal is to maintain a consistent schedule of bowel evacuation using the mildest form of intervention that will encourage your body to function on a regular and comfortable basis.

Why can't I just use a laxative or enema whenever I need to move my bowels?

Laxatives and enemas should ideally be used only to help evacuate impacted stool that has remained in your bowel for a prolonged period. You might need a laxative or suppository to empty the bowel if you have not moved your bowels in more than four or five days and the stool has become too dry and difficult to pass. These products should be used only on an intermittent, as-needed basis because their chronic use can actually slow the bowel and increase constipation. As noted, the more effective technique for treating constipation is with a management regimen that prevents it in the first place.

If I'm so constipated most of the time, why do I sometimes seem to have diarrhea at the same time?

Occasionally, people who become severely constipated will find that looser stool from higher in the intestinal tract leaks around the impacted (dry and hard) stool. The solution to this problem is to remove the impacted stool with either a laxative or enema, and then begin a structured bowel program to retrain the bowel.

Sometimes I have bowel accidents even though my stomach is not upset and I don't have diarrhea. I lose control of my bowels without even realizing that it is going to happen. What is causing this and is there anything I can do about it?

Neurologic impairment in MS can cause spasms in the involuntary muscles of the bladder and bowel just as it does in the voluntary muscles of the legs and arms. These spasms can lead to involuntary loss of bowel control. Additionally, full or partial loss of sensation in the rectum allows it to fill with stool without your being aware of this fullness. The rectum stretches beyond normal capacity and then empties unexpectedly in response to an involuntary relaxation of the anal sphincter.

The most effective management of this infrequent but distressing problem is to retrain your bowel by establishing a bowel regimen. This regimen should include the dietary changes already discussed, as well as having a *consistent* time for moving your bowels. The frequency of evacuation matters less than the regularity of the interval and particular time of day that you choose. After breakfast every other day would be appropriate for one person; every day after lunch might be more comfortable for someone else—it does not matter as long as you stick with a consistent schedule. Whichever time you choose, make sure to allow yourself a quiet, relaxed period of time in the bathroom. Some people find that hot liquids such as coffee or tea help to stimulate the urge to defecate. If necessary, your physician may supplement this bowel regimen with an anticholinergic medication to relieve the spasms. Bowel retraining can take several weeks or even months, but it will help you to avoid bowel accidents and feel more in control of your body.

It has become increasingly difficult for me to move my bowels even with the use of laxatives and suppositories. I have not had a bowel movement in more than a week and don't know what to do.

A week is too long for most people to go without a bowel movement. In general, a person should take measures to have a bowel movement once three or four days have passed. You should notify your physician or nurse so that you can receive assistance emptying your bowel. In all likelihood, your bowel has become impacted with hardened stool that you will not be able to pass without help. Once your bowel has been emptied, the doctor or nurse will help you to establish a regimen to retrain your bowel and thus avoid the prolonged use of laxatives and/or laxative suppositories. Chronic use of these products results in "tolerance" to them so that the bowel will no longer respond to the medications in them.

Skin Care

The skin is the largest organ of the body. An intact skin protects the organs by maintaining body structure and preventing infections.

The risk of skin changes and skin breakdown is increased when people who are severely disabled with MS become less active, sitting or lying for longer periods. Continuous pressure on any area of skin decreases the flow of blood to that area. Without the flow of blood to bring oxygen and other nutrients, the skin can become damaged or die in a process referred to as ulceration. Pressure sores (also known as **decubitus** ulcers) occur most frequently in areas where the skin is thin and lies over protruding bones that cause pressure (the base of the spine and around the elbows, heels, and ankles) (see Fig. 4-3). Additionally, a person who has increased muscle tone and spasticity is at greater risk of skin breakdown because the skin has a tendency to rub against supporting surfaces and become irritated. Bowel and bladder inconti-

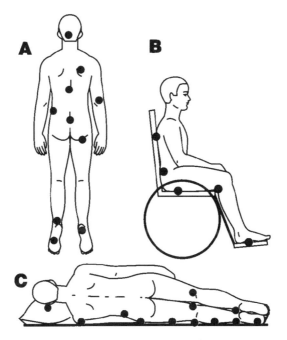

Figure 4-3. Dots show pressure points when lying on back (**A**), when sitting (**B**), and when lying on side (**C**).

nence can also increase the risk of skin breakdown because the accumulation of moisture can cause ulcers around the genital region.

Good skin care requires an adequate intake of nutritious foods and fluids as well as frequent changes of position, comfortable seating with even weight distribution, skin cleanliness and moisturizing, and frequent skin checks to identify current and potential problems. Once skin breakdown occurs, it requires prompt medical and nursing attention. Pressure sores are very slow to heal and the most effective treatment is prevention.

Now that I use a wheelchair much of the time, my doctor has ordered a special seat cushion. How is this cushion going to help my skin?

A good cushion for your wheelchair helps to distribute your weight evenly and prevent any single area of skin from being put under constant pressure. In addition to using this specially designed cushion, it is important for you to shift your weight regularly, either by yourself or with someone else's assistance. This will periodically relieve pressure on the skin of your lower back, buttocks, and thighs, and allow the blood to circulate freely. A physical therapist can teach you wheelchair activities that are specially designed to relieve pressure on the skin and prevent decubitus ulcers.

How can I tell if I am developing a problem with my skin?

The best way to determine if you are developing skin problems is to be on the lookout for changes in skin coloring. Since it is difficult for you to get a clear view of the areas that are most prone to irritation, you may want to use a mirror for self-examination of at-risk areas. It is also advisable for you to be given a fairly regular "once over" by a nurse or family member. This is particularly important if you have experienced any loss of sensation, since this loss would probably prevent you from becoming aware of the sore. The earliest sign of a pressure sore is usually a reddening of the skin, which gradually becomes blistered and then opens. Sometimes the first sign is a soft, blackened area under the skin. If the sore is allowed to progress, fluid will begin to ooze from the opening, which gradually becomes wider and deeper.

Since my most recent MS exacerbation I have spent many hours of the day in bed. Should I be using a special type of bed or mattress?

Anyone who spends many hours of the day in bed should be evaluated by a nurse familiar with skin care. The nurse will examine your skin, paying particular attention to the areas over bony projections (e.g., base of the spine, hips, heels), and evaluate your body alignment in bed. This type of examination will enable the nurse to identify current and potential skin problems and make any necessary recommendations about the use of special bedding, including a special air mattress, mattress overlay, or other products designed to prevent skin breakdown. In addition to appropriate bedding, it is important for you to turn and reposition yourself at least every two hours throughout the day and night.

Why is skin breakdown a serious problem for someone with MS?

Skin breakdown is a serious problem for anyone. A pressure sore can develop in a few hours but take several months to heal. Once a sore has formed, long periods of immobility are required to relieve pressure and provide adequate air to the affected area. Such periods of immobility can easily cause troublesome secondary problems. Untreated sores can lead to an infection of the underlying bone (osteomyelitis), which is difficult to treat. Since the skin protects the body from outside infections, its breakdown can allow the tissues underneath to become infected. This type of infection might ultimately lead to septicemia (blood poisoning), which can be life-threatening.

I recently developed a pressure sore on my buttocks. What is the treatment for this type of sore?

Any area of the skin that has become reddened should be massaged regularly with a skin lotion. You should change your position frequently so that the area has plenty of exposure to the air. Be sure to notify your doctor or nurse immediately if you have already developed a small opening in the skin. Your physician will start you on a treatment regimen that involves keeping the area clean (with a providone iodine solution such as Betadine®), dry, and pressure-free. If the sore has gone below the surface of the skin, the wound will be kept dry and open until the deeper area has healed. The nurse will monitor the status of the sore on a regular and frequent basis and keep your physician informed. Since the sore is on your buttocks, you will need to remain in bed and on your side or stomach for fairly long periods each day in order for it to heal. If the decubitus continues to grow deeper or wider, you will probably need to go into the hospital for further treatment involving antibiotics to prevent infection and immersion in a whirlpool-type bath for deep cleansing of the area. While in the hospital, you may also be given a special Clinitron® bed that promotes healing of the skin. A flotation effect, created by tiny, constantly moving, silicone balls, relieves pressure on your skin without your having to move or turn.

My doctor has said that I may need surgery for a pressure sore. Why would surgery be needed and how is the procedure done?

Occasionally, pressure sores do not respond to the measures already described. The blood circulation in the area of the sore may simply be too impaired for the healing process to proceed. If your decubitus has continued to worsen in spite of all treatment efforts, surgery may be required to close it. During surgery, any dead (necrotic) tissue in the area will be removed. A piece (flap) of skin from another area of your body that has better circulation may then be grafted onto the area of the sore. In the rare instances in which this type of surgery is required, healing of both the grafted skin and the area from which it was taken is generally quite successful.

Does my diet have anything to do with the condition of my skin? Are there any foods that will protect me from skin breakdown?

Skin integrity depends on activity and exercise, your general state of health, and adequate nutrition. While one factor alone is unlikely to cause skin breakdown, a combination of deficits in any of these areas can certainly lead to problems. No specific food or diet will protect your skin from breaking down. Your best strategy for avoiding skin breakdown is to keep your skin clean, free of urine and other irritants, and moisturized; learn the exercises you need to know in order to enhance circulation and relieve areas of pressure on your body; and maintain a healthy diet.

I know that lying constantly in one position can be harmful to my skin, but it is very difficult for me turn myself over. Is there anything I can do to make the turning easier so that I don't have to ask my husband (or aide) to help me turn?

Your physician can refer you to a physical or occupational therapist for a home evaluation of this problem. Depending on your physical abilities and the type of bed you have, these professionals can help you learn ways to maneuver yourself independently. Some people can make use of bars on the side of the bed to pull themselves over. There is also a bedsheet available that has fabric strips to allow people to turn and position themselves in bed.

Promoting General Wellness

What can I do to keep myself as healthy as possible in spite of my MS?*

This is a very important question because the evidence indicates that people with a chronic illness like MS often neglect their general healthcare needs. They begin to think of their neurologist (or other specialist) as their primary doctor, forgoing visits to their internist or general medical doctor. The result is that medical checkups and preventive health screening measures tend to go by the wayside.

The strategies for protecting and enhancing your overall health and well-being, whether or not you have MS, include:

maintaining a healthy diet that:

◇ contains a variety of foods, as shown in the food guide pyramid of the USDA
◇ is high in fiber (grain products, vegetables, and fruits)
◇ is low in fat, saturated fat, and cholesterol
◇ is moderate in salt

protecting your heart by:

◇ not smoking

*Adapted from K. Birk, General Health and Well-Being. In R. Kalb (ed.), *Multiple Sclerosis: A Guide for Families.* New York: Demos Medical Publishing, 1998.

◇ maintaining a healthy cholesterol level (less than 200 for
  the total and above 45 for the HDL [good cholesterol])
◇ engaging in some form of aerobic exercise (as recommended by your physician) for 30 minutes, 3-5 times a week
◇ following your doctor's recommended schedule for regular
  health screenings

obtaining periodic health appraisals and screening tests,
including:

◇ a general physical (20–40 years old—every 5 years; 40–50
  years old—every 3 years; 50–65 years old—every two
  years; over age 65—yearly). The evaluation should include
  a history, physical examination, blood and urine laboratory tests, and a chest X-ray and electrocardiogram, depending on age and history. Women should have pelvic and
  breast examinations on an annual basis.
◇ annual cancer screening, depending on the person's age
  (breast or testicular examination by the healthcare
  provider; Pap smear for women of reproductive age; mammogram for women over 40 years of age; rectal examination
  for men and women after 40 years of age; stool blood testing and other color cancer testing for men and women after
  age 50)

learning to manage stress by:

◇ examining your priorities
◇ eliminating the unnecessary stresses in your life while
  identifying more effective ways to manage those that are
  unavoidable
◇ finding activities that provide you with regular periods of
  relaxation, enjoyment, and "down-time" (e.g., deep-mus-
  cle relaxation exercises, meditation, listening to music,
  socializing with friends, watching television, yoga)
◇ consulting with a psychotherapist, if you feel the need, for
  help in identifying the sources of stress in your life and
  developing effective stress management strategies.

Recommended Readings

Carroll D, Dorman J. *Living Well with MS*. New York: Harper-Collins, 1993.

Holland, N. & Halper, J. (eds.) *Multiple Sclerosis: A Self-Care Guide to Wellness*. Washington, D.C.: Paralyzed Veterans of America, 1998.

Kraft, G. & Catanzaro, M. *Living Well with Multiple Sclerosis (2nd edition)*. New York: Demos Medical Publishing, 2000.

Lechtenberg R. *Multiple Sclerosis Fact Book (2nd edition)*. Philadelphia: F.A. Davis, 1995.

Maloney F, Burks J, Ringel S. *Interdisciplinary Rehabilitation of Multiple Sclerosis and Neuromuscular Disorders*. New York: J.B. Lippincott, 1985.

Rosner L, Ross S. *Multiple Sclerosis. New Hope and Practical Advice for People with MS and their Families*. New York: Simon and Schuster, 1992.

Schapiro R. *Symptom Management in Multiple Sclerosis (3rd edition)*. New York: Demos Medical Publishing, 1998.

Selected materials available from your local chapter of the National Multiple Sclerosis Society (800-FIGHT-MS):

◇ *Controlling Bladder Problems in MS* (ES 0039)

◇ *Understanding Bowel Problems in MS* (ECS 6036)

◇ *Food for Thought; MS and Nutrition* (ES 6020)

◇ *Facts and Issues* (reprints of articles from the National Multiple Sclerosis Society magazine, *Inside MS*).

◇ *MS and Wellness*—Janie Brunette, R.N., M.S.N., and Diane Reaves, B.S. One in a series of workbooks entitled *Living Well with MS*, written for, and by, people who have been living with MS for some time.

5

Physical Therapy

Angela Chan, B.P.T., M.H.Sc.

The **physical therapist** is a healthcare professional trained to evaluate and improve movement and function of the body, with particular emphasis on physical mobility, balance, posture, fatigue, and pain. Many factors affect the abilities of people with MS to be as physically active as they would like to be. Physical therapy (PT) has as its goal to help people meet the mobility challenges and physical demands in their family, work, and social lives while accommodating the physical changes brought about by the disease.

In PT, the therapist and person with MS work as a team to minimize limitations imposed by MS, maximize functional ability and overall quality of life, and prevent debilitating injuries and complications. The therapist recommends various treatment strategies following a thorough physical and functional evaluation. The individual provides the determination and commitment to follow through with the treatment regimen as well as valuable feedback to the therapist. It is only with this feedback that the therapist can accurately determine if the treatment is working effectively and make any necessary revisions in the treatment plan. There are three important components to a successful PT program:

◇ education for people with MS and their family members about the physical symptoms caused by the disease, and the steps that can be taken to alleviate current problems and prevent unnecessary complications;

◇ an individualized exercise program designed to deal with these problems; and

◇ mobility enhancement and energy conservation through the use of a variety of mobility aids, adaptive equipment for the home, office, and automobile, and education about community resources.

Evaluation

How will I know if I need to be seen by a physical therapist?

Your first contact with a physical therapist is likely to be initiated by your physician. Typically, the physician refers a person with MS to physical therapy for an exercise regimen designed to help one or more symptoms. If your physician has not yet mentioned PT to you, you can ask whether it would be beneficial for you and if it is available in your area. It is never too early in the course of MS to have a consultation with a physical therapist, since PT can help you maintain your comfort and flexibility, reduce the impact of MS-related fatigue, and prevent unnecessary injury and complications. Many people maintain intermittent contact with the physical therapist over the course of their MS, consulting the therapist for treatment recommendations as specific physical problems become bothersome and affect their ability to engage in normal activity. Periodic evaluation by a physical therapist is helpful not only in managing current problems but also in identifying and preventing potential ones.

How do I get in touch with a physical therapist?

When referring you for physical therapy, your physician will probably select a therapist in your area and tell you how to make contact. Many physical therapists work in health care facilities such as hospitals, community health centers, and rehabilitation centers. Others have a private practice, seeing patients in their office or in the patients' homes. Depending on where the therapist works, most PT services are covered, at least in part, by

Medicare, Medicaid, or a private insurance plan. In Canada, PT is covered by the provincial health care plan or private insurance plans. Some private practitioners who work in an outpatient center or in the home are available only on a fee-for-service basis.

How will the physical therapist evaluate my problems?

The physical therapist will perform a thorough physical and functional assessment of your:

◇ posture and body movements
◇ fatigue level
◇ muscle strength
◇ muscle, tendon and joint flexibility
◇ ability to discriminate sensations such as heat and cold, pain, pressure, touch, and movement
◇ safety and mobility at work, at home, and in the community.

Mobility is an area of specialty for most physical therapists—improving your ability to get around is the therapist's primary objective. The therapist performs a gait analysis to assess your capabilities in walking and mobility; this involves observing how you walk and identifying causes of change in your normal walking pattern. In gait analysis, as in posture assessment, actions and interactions of various body parts are studied. The actions of each leg individually and both legs in sequence, are observed, together with such factors as speed, rhythm, stride length, step length, and distance. The therapist will also note what type of walking device (if any) you are using, and under what circumstances.

The assessment also includes taking a comprehensive history focusing on the impact of your illness on role performance and satisfaction at home and at work, as well as overall quality of life. Family members, friends, and caregivers can provide useful background information and share their perspectives on the impact of MS on your daily life. However, each individual with MS is unique in being able to describe his or her own frustrations and limitations and in setting personal goals for physical therapy.

Both the therapist's assessment and your personal history are essential when determining the factors that contribute to any existing or potential problems. Together they form the basis of the physical therapist's plan of action, the strategies that the therapist will work with you to implement in order to maximize your mobility and enhance your physical and functional capabilities.

The Role of Exercise

Are there different types of exercise?

There is wide variation in the types of exercise that a physical therapist may recommend.

◇ *Strengthening exercises* are designed to make the body stronger. Weights, exercise elastic, or machines may be used to provide resistance so that your muscles have to work harder. Regular workouts build up muscle size and increase your ability to perform exercise. The physical therapist will design an exercise program to strengthen specific muscles that may have become weakened by disuse. Depending on the strength of these muscles, weights or other forms of resistance may be recommended.

◇ *Range of motion exercises* are performed to ensure that each joint is moved throughout the full range of available movement, with the objective being to maintain joint flexibility. Joint mobility is dependent on many factors; tightness of the joint capsule, ligaments, and tendons may individually or in combination restrict joint movements. Joint stiffness may occur when swelling is present or after an injury. If movement of the joint does not occur on a regular basis, the joint will become stiff and interfere with normal movement.

◇ *Stretching exercises* are recommended for muscles and tendons that have lost their elasticity. When muscles and tendons around a joint lose this elasticity, the person feels stiff and finds it difficult to move. These exercises help to maintain the elasticity or stretchability of tissues and to prevent **contractures.**

◇ *Resisted exercises* are performed against some form of resistance, e.g., weights or exercise elastic, and help promote and maintain strength.

◇ *Fitness exercises* are designed to maintain general health and well-being rather than for a specific problem or symptom.

◇ *Aerobic exercises for cardiovascular fitness* are designed to increase heart rate and thereby improve blood circulation and aerobic function, and reduce fatigue.

The exercises prescribed by the physical therapist can also be divided according to the degree of assistance required by the person performing them: *active exercises* are performed completely independently; *active assisted exercises* require some assistance by another person; *passive exercises* are performed by a helper (therapist or caregiver) if a person is unable to perform them independently. Thus, a person performing *active range of motion* exercises might do leg extensions at a variety of angles; the person engaged in *passive range of motion exercises* would need the therapist or caregiver to move the leg into the appropriate positions.

In what ways will exercise help my MS?

Exercises can help your MS by developing and strengthening those muscles that continue to have adequate nerve conduction and by helping to maintain the tone of those with inadequate nerve conduction. Exercise will train your muscles to work better individually and together and may thereby improve coordination in your arms and legs. Thus, an exercise program can help you learn ways of walking and moving that compensate somewhat for the neurologic changes caused by MS. Exercises are also used to improve range of motion and to help relieve mild **spasticity**, balance problems, and some types of pain. Regular aerobic exercise, tailored to your individual abilities and limitations, has been shown to reduce fatigue and depression, promote strength and fitness, and help control weight. Weight-bearing exercise can reduce the risk of **osteoporosis** in those who have become less mobile. It is important to remember, however, that exercise cannot reverse the disease process or undo damage that has been done to the nervous system.

I was recently diagnosed with MS. Should I continue to participate in the aerobic exercise class that I always attended?

Research in MS has shown that a regular aerobic exercise program can reduce fatigue and depression and increase cardiovascular fitness. Therefore, you should try to maintain your current activity level unless you find it too tiring or uncomfortable. Your physician or physical therapist will be able to guide you in determining the amount of exercise that is appropriate. Since MS symptoms can be temporarily worsened by external heat and/or elevated body temperature, it is important to exercise in a cool environment, drink plenty of fluids before, during, and after exercise, and work at a pace that does not allow you to become extremely overheated.

How can I find out what type of exercise is best for me?

Exercises designed to address your particular needs are best prescribed by your neurologist or physical therapist. Trainers in a fitness or health club can develop a general fitness program for you, but keep in mind that they probably do not understand MS and the ways in which neurologic changes affect your body. Be sure to check with your physician before beginning any type of exercise program.

Are there any types of exercise that are harmful to me now that I have MS?

No specific exercises are harmful to individuals with MS, however you should check with your physician before beginning any new exercise program. Common sense will be your best ally here. In general, your body will tell you how it is responding to exercise and will certainly let you know if it cannot tolerate the exercise program you have chosen. Be careful not to exert yourself to the point of exhaustion or raise your body temperature so much that you activate your MS symptoms. Although these momentary symptoms are indicative of being overheated rather than of any kind of disease activity or progression, they can be uncomfortable and unnerving. Regular, moderate exercise in a cool environment, with periodic rest breaks, will enable you to get maximum benefit from your exercise program and avoid unnecessary discomfort.

Is weight training helpful for the weakness that I feel in my arms and legs?

The weakness you are experiencing in your arms and legs is primarily the result of impaired nerve conduction to the muscles involved, rather than any weakness of the muscles themselves. Weight training cannot improve nerve conduction and thus will not improve this type of neurologically-based weakness. Weight training is good for developing and strengthening muscles that *do* have adequate nerve conduction, and for toning muscles that have been weakened by disuse. Your neurologist can evaluate the weakness in various parts of your body and advise you as to its causes. A physical therapist can then design a fitness program that specifically addresses the types of weakness you are experiencing.

How can I exercise effectively now that I have lost so much strength in my arms and legs?

If you are unable to perform active exercise because of problems with weakness, spasticity, or imbalance, the physical therapist can work with you on assisted and passive exercises that are more appropriate for your needs. It is important to remember that not all exercise programs are designed for strength or endurance; exercise is equally important for maintaining flexibility, range of motion, posture, and muscle tone.

I feel so fatigued most of the time that my regular daily activities use up all the energy I have. How can I possibly exercise when I feel so tired?

Reduced energy level and endurance are common problems for people with MS. The fatigue that is so common in MS can have a variety of causes. The physical therapist can help you understand the various causes of your fatigue and explore with you ways of optimizing your energy and reducing fatigue. You may be able to conserve energy and minimize tiredness by doing various activities in a slightly different way, making more effective use of tools or strategies to save time and reduce unnecessary effort, or creating small rest periods in your day. Walking or mobility aids are sometimes prescribed to increase a person's ability to cover greater distances with less fatigue. Additionally, the physical therapist can teach you types of exercises that are less physically strenuous and demanding than ones you might have done in the past. Regular aerobic exercise has been shown to reduce fatigue in MS. Keep in mind that exercise does not have to be fast or vigorous in order to provide you with substantial benefit. In fact, an important benefit of some exercises is increased relaxation.

Should I join a health club or an exercise class to get my exercise?

Some general fitness exercises can be performed in a health club or an exercise class setting. Specific benefits of exercising outside the home include socialization, encouragement and feedback from the instructor and fellow participants, and the guidance of a structured program. Getting yourself out to participate can also enhance continuity and commitment. Keep in mind, however, that the staff members in a health club are generally not trained to understand or treat neurologic symptoms. Consult with your physician before beginning any exercise program. If you require an exercise program that is more appropriate to your physical symptoms, your physician will refer you to a physical therapist.

Is swimming a good exercise for me?

Water is an excellent medium for exercise. It allows weakened muscles to move more easily while providing sufficient resistance to help strengthen other muscles. Water also helps to stabilize a person who has balance problems. Because swimming is a highly coordinated physical activity involving the whole body, it helps to regulate breathing and build endurance. In addition, your physical therapist can develop a personalized exercise program for you to do in the water, even if you do not like or know how to swim. Water-walking, as well as other types of exercises for the arms and legs, can be very beneficial.

It is advisable to gather some information before you go to a swimming pool. How far is it from the changing room and the toilet to the pool? Is someone available to provide assistance in and out of the pool if necessary? What is the temperature of the water? Although people react differently to water temperature, many with MS cannot tolerate heat. A water temperature of 81–85° F seems to be the most comfortable for individuals with MS. The temperature of a "therapeutic pool" is frequently too hot.

If you are experiencing any MS-related bladder symptoms that might interfere with your comfort in the swimming pool, talk them over with your neurologist or nurse before beginning a swimming program.

Is there any reason for me to stop playing the recreational sports that I enjoy?

The answer to this question depends on the symptoms of MS that you are experiencing and their impact on your enjoyment of any particular sport. If you can physically play the sport, even if not as well as before, then you should probably continue to do so. Too many people stop playing sports as soon as they are diagnosed or because they can't play as well as they did in the past. There is no reason to stop playing your sport unless you feel that you are putting yourself (or someone else) at risk of injury. Stopping prematurely will deny you recreation and enjoyment, as well as the benefits of exercise and the continued challenge to your body. The point is to adapt to change, not to stop living because of it.

There are many types of exercise equipment advertised and sold in sport stores. How can I figure out which equipment is right for me?

It is important to check with your doctor and/or physical therapist before starting any type of exercise program or purchasing any exercise equipment. They can work with you to identify your particular needs and goals and find the programs and equipment most suited to your physical condition. The pieces of exercise equipment differ not only in their uses, but in the demands they make on your stamina, coordination, and balance. For example, you can increase endurance and heart fitness by using either a treadmill or a recumbent bicycle, but one type of equipment may be more appropriate for you than another, depending on your particular symptoms and degree of mobility.

Keep in mind that when you exercise certain parts of your body (e.g., your legs to pedal a bicycle), those body parts do not work in isolation. Muscles from other parts of your body (e.g. heart and trunk) work in tandem to provide support for your efforts. Because greater exertion also increases the demand for oxygen to all those muscles, you will breathe more deeply and rapidly. This will expand your lungs and increase oxygen in your blood. Due to the increased pumping of the heart, there is an increase in blood circulation throughout the body. Thus, most types of physical exercise will help to improve heart health, blood circulation, and general fitness. Expensive equipment is not necessary for exercising or fitness training. Walking at a fast pace or aerobic exercise in the standing position can achieve similar results.

I recently saw an advertisement for a motorized bicycle. Will this type of bicycle keep my muscles from getting smaller?

In the motorized bicycle, the motor is driving the bicycle movement, which in turn moves your legs. Therefore, your own muscles are not required to work. Since your own muscles are not providing the power for movement, you will not derive the same benefits as you would from active muscle work on a regular or recumbent bicycle. In order to increase or maintain muscle mass, which contributes to the size of the muscle, you will need to utilize equipment that requires your own muscles to do the work.

Some people use the motorized bicycle to move their legs passively. The machine will cause bending and extending movements at your hips, knees, and some movements at your ankles. The movements generated by the bicycle are by no means the full range of possible movements at these joints. Some individuals find the movements from the machine relaxing but this side result does not occur to everyone who uses the machine. You have to balance the possible benefits gained from the machine to the cost of purchasing the machine, of needing assistance to get on and off the machine and to secure your feet to the foot pedals. Also because the machine does not move your joints to the fullness of range, you still need to do other exercises to achieve that goal.

Because of MS, I'm not getting as much exercise as I used to and I'm putting on weight. What should I do?

Weight control is an issue of concern for almost everyone, and becomes more challenging when symptoms of MS make a person less mobile and more fatigued. Three sessions of aerobic exercise per week have been shown to promote strength and fitness, help control weight, and reduce fatigue and depression in MS. Numerous exercise programs are offered by community Parks and Recreation Programs, the local YMCA, or health clubs. With the help of your physician or physical therapist, choose the type of exercise that meets your needs and interests. If your endurance and ability are limited, you might consider a senior's fitness program, water-walking, yoga, or Tai-Chi as other options. Keep in mind as well that certain types of hobbies, such as gardening, can also provide very beneficial exercise. It may also be necessary to reduce your food intake somewhat in order to compensate for your decreased activity level. Ask your physician to recommend a balanced, low-fat diet that can help you control the weight gain.

My posture seems to have changed since I've had MS. Are there exercises that will improve my posture?

Posture is a key area in the PT assessment. The therapist will observe the position of your head, neck, shoulders, torso, pelvis, hips, knees, ankles, and feet. Standing posture and seating posture, as well as posture during movement, are noted. The physical therapist is able to identify areas of muscle weakness and/or stiffness and develop corrective movements targeting these areas. Maintaining good posture is important not only for the sake of your appearance, but also to prevent uncomfortable muscle and joint strain and secondary back problems that can arise from standing, sitting, and moving improperly.

Why are correct positioning and correct posture so important?

Injury is not limited to the damage caused by something or someone doing harm to you. Injury to the body can also result from incorrect positioning of the body parts, incorrect posture, or repetitive strain. For example, "repetitive strain injury" refers to chronic pain caused by doing certain types of muscle work on a repetitive and prolonged basis, without any single incident of injury. Wrist pain due to prolonged computer work is a common example of a repetitive strain injury. People who spend a lot of time at a computer must be alert to the way they are sitting in relation to the desk and keypad, and to the positioning of their backs, legs, wrists, and forearms.

Similarly, people who use various types of mobility aids for walking need to be sure that the devices are measured and designed accurately, and that they are being used appropriately. For example, pain or injury can result from using a cane that is too short or too long because a cane of improper length can distort a person's posture and gait. These types of distortions eventually lead to back, hip, and leg pain. A person who sits in a wheelchair that does not provide proper back, leg, and foot support will also begin to experience neck, back and leg pain. The physical therapist assesses a person's needs, prescribes the mobility devices that are most suited to those needs, and provides instruction in how to use them safely and effectively.

Is yoga helpful to a person who has MS?

Yoga is an excellent form of exercise for people with MS because it involves a lot of stretching exercises for the whole body. The controlled breathing exercises promote relaxation of the mind and the body and help people to be more in tune with their bodies. As with any other form of exercise, it is important that the yoga exercises be tailored to your particular physical needs and limitations.

Is Tai-Chi a good form of exercise for someone with MS?

Tai-Chi is another excellent form of exercise for individuals with MS. In a recent study, people with MS who participated in a Tai-Chi program demonstrated improved walking ability and enhanced quality of life. Tai-Chi movements are slow and controlled with periodic changes in position. Many of the movements in Tai-Chi require good balance; try to perform your exercise routine close to a grab bar or railing in case you need to steady yourself. Once learned, performing Tai-Chi can also be relaxing. This form of exercise requires mental discipline and controlled breathing.

I have been experiencing a lot of pain with my MS. Can physical therapy help me to manage this pain? How can exercises help without causing me more pain than I'm already having?

There are several types of pain that can be associated with MS (see Chapter 2). In addition to primary (**neurogenic**) pain resulting directly from demyelinating lesions in the central nervous system, a person can experience pain that is secondary to other symptoms such as spasticity and weakness. The initial step in pain management, therefore, is to consult with your physician and/or physical therapist to identify the source(s) of the pain you are experiencing.

Physical therapists use a variety of strategies to help reduce pain, including the application of heat or ice, exercise, and teaching proper positioning or support for the body. Problems with balance and ambulation often cause changes in posture, and these postural changes can gradually result in secondary pain in the lower back, hips, and knees. The use of *ambulation aids* such as crutches or walkers can also contribute to secondary pain in the shoulders and upper back. If the pain is a result of changes in your posture, balance, or gait (i.e., if you have begun to sit or walk differently because of weakness or spasticity), the therapist may design a treatment regimen that involves education about the mechanism of your problem as well as exercises designed to improve the impaired functions that are contributing to the pain. Rather than giving you additional pain, the exercises involved will actually reduce pain by alleviating its causes. Additionally, the therapist may recommend the use of a new or different mechanical aid, such as a cane, walker, or wheelchair, if any of these would contribute to a reduction in the pain you are experiencing. If the pain is a result of spasticity and the inactivity resulting from it, the physical therapist will prescribe a daily regimen of range of motion exercises designed to reduce stiffness and enhance flexibility.

Can exercise help me with my balance problems?

Balance and safety are areas of primary concern for the physical therapist and common problems for many with MS. Impaired balance in MS results primarily from **plaques** in the **cerebellum** and **brainstem**, but can also be caused by impaired sensation in the soles of the feet and weakness and/or stiffness of any part of the leg. Even vision impairment may contribute to poor equilibrium. The physical therapist will assess your balance in the standing, sitting, and kneeling positions, as well as while you are walking. Balance problems that are caused by damage in the cerebellum and brainstem cannot be corrected by exercise. However, the therapist can recommend particular exercises designed to maximize your ability to maintain your balance or help you to compensate for changes in your ability to balance. The therapist may also prescribe a walking aid such as a cane or a walker. Safety is a primary concern since impaired balance can lead to falls resulting in bruising, swelling, pain, and even fractures.

Since my last exacerbation I have been unable to walk. Will exercising my legs help me to walk again?

Walking is a complex motor activity that is dependent on many functions working in a coordinated fashion. Exercising your legs will maintain flexibility of the joints and muscles, encourage the muscles to work to their best potential, and prevent further muscle deterioration. Therefore, depending on the degree and location of **demyelination** that occurred during your last exacerbation and the amount of spontaneous recovery you experience, leg exercises might facilitate your efforts to walk again. However, there is no guarantee since exercise cannot correct neurologic damage done by the disease. Even if walking is not possible, exercising your legs will help you to sit properly and thereby prevent the pain and stiffness that can result from prolonged sitting.

Can exercise help a person who is unable to walk and spends most of the time in a wheelchair?

Exercise is extremely important for the person who is no longer able to walk. In its various forms, exercise enhances flexibility, posture, strength, and endurance, each of which contributes to comfort and physical well-being. Stiffness in the legs affects a person's ability to sit upright with proper foot positioning. Passive range of motion and stretching exercises can help to relieve this type of stiffness. Exercises for the arms, upper body, and trunk are very important for maintaining good posture, which, in turn, reduces the risk of back and hip strain. Weight training to maintain upper body strength also facilitates transfers in and out of the wheelchair or bed and promotes cardiac health. Additionally, upper body exercises can strengthen the neck or torso and thereby increase a person's ability to sit comfortably for longer periods of time. Any exercise regimen that enhances the mobility of the person in a wheelchair also reduces the risk of skin breakdown (see Chapter 4). People who spend long periods of time in a wheelchair are taught specific exercises designed to shift their weight and thus relieve pressure on areas of the body that are particularly prone to skin breakdown. They are also taught to stand (if possible) for brief periods of time each day in order to allow the force of gravity to slow the reduction in bone density (osteoporosis) that can result from reduced mobility and inadequate amounts of weight-bearing exercise. This is critically important since a reduction in bone density contributes to the risk of bone fractures.

Since I have begun to spend much more time sitting down, I have swelling in my feet and ankles, especially by late afternoon. What can I do about it?

Since leg swelling can result from a variety of causes, it is important to consult with your physician to make sure that there are no other medical conditions that need to be addressed. Once other causes have been ruled out, you can utilize various strategies to reduce any swelling that results from reduced mobility. During walking and standing, the activity of the muscles in the legs helps to pump the blood in the legs back up to the heart. In the sitting position, the force of gravity draws the blood down toward the feet. With prolonged sitting, there is insufficient muscle activity in the legs to counteract the force of gravity and pump the blood back up to the heart. Try, if possible, to stand up for at least five minutes of every hour. This will relieve the prolonged pressure on your buttocks and allow the leg muscles to pump some of the blood back to your heart. If standing is very difficult, raise your legs after every two hours of sitting, and rest them on a chair or a stool that is at least as high as your hips. While your feet are elevated, try to do some foot and ankle exercises to help pump the blood back to your heart. Keep your feet elevated above the level of your hips for at least thirty minutes. For severe swelling, it may be necessary to lie down for some portion of each day with your feet elevated above the level of your heart. An additional strategy to control lower leg swelling involves wearing pressure stockings that need to be prescribed and specially fitted for you.

My foot is turning in. Are there exercises that can make this better?

When a foot "turns in," the muscles and tendons on the inside of the foot become shortened and the muscles turning the foot out are weakened due to disuse. Without exercise, the ankle joint can become stiff. Passive and active exercises for the muscles controlling ankle movements are vitally important in this situation. The physician or physical therapist may also suggest a special type of leg brace to help with this problem. The key is to begin the treatment regimen before changes to the muscles and joints become permanent.

What exercises can I do to relieve the stiffness I feel in my body?

Stiffness in MS is most often related to the common symptom of spasticity, which is caused by a dysregulation of nerve impulses in the spinal cord (see Chapter 2). Very mild spasticity in MS can often be managed effectively with a regimen of stretching and range of motion exercises. These exercises are very important for maintaining flexibility of the muscles and tendons and thereby reducing further stiffness and other complications. The physical therapist will design a specific stretching program for you. Keep in mind, however, that exercises alone may not be sufficient to treat your spasticity. If the stiffness continues or worsens, or if the exercises become too difficult or uncomfortable for you to do, your physician will probably recommend that you use medication in combination with exercise to manage the spasticity.

Walking and Mobility Aids

I've begun to stagger so much when I walk that people think I'm drunk. What can I do about this problem?

Staggering is a symptom of poor balance that is usually caused by disease activity in the cerebellum or brainstem. At this time,

no medication or other treatment is very effective for this problem. There are two major consequences of impaired balance: the
first is the risk of potentially dangerous falls; the second, unfortunately, is that others often perceive the person who staggers to
have a drinking problem. Depending on the cause and extent of
your balance problems, your physician or physical therapist will
probably recommend a mobility aid such as a cane, forearm
(**Lofstrand**) crutch, or walker (see Fig. 5-1). The use of a mobility aid will provide you with extra stability and will also send a
clear signal to any observer that there is a medical cause for your
staggering.

The physical therapist will determine which type of aid is
most beneficial for you by evaluating how much additional stability you need. A single cane, for example, adds a point of stability only on one side of your body. A **quad cane**, which has
four short legs attached to a small platform at its end, provides
greater stability by giving you a broader base on which to lean.

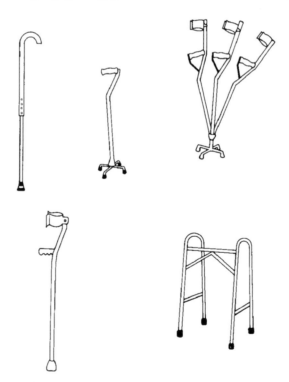

Figure 5-1. Walking aids. Left to right: straight cane, quad cane, quad
cane with swivel-action base, forearm crutch, and walker.

The therapist may recommend that you use two canes or crutches if you would benefit from a stabilizing point on each side of your body. If these do not provide sufficient stability, the therapist may recommend a walker. Because a walker moves directly in front of you, it provides greater stability and also reduces fatigue. Bear in mind that as your needs change, the type of aid that is recommended for you will change as well. Be sure to consult the therapist if you are experiencing more difficulty even with using your walking aid.

I seem to trip a lot and I've even had a few falls. Why is this happening?

Weakness of your foot, ankle, or hip muscles, stiffness in your legs, fatigue, and poor balance could, individually or in combination, contribute to tripping and falling. Since falls can have major consequences, the first step in the management of this problem is to identify its source. Having diagnosed the problem, your physician will provide the necessary treatment and/or make the appropriate referral. If, for example, your falls are primarily the result of *foot drop*, you will probably be referred to an *orthotist* or physical therapist for an *ankle-foot orthosis (AFO)* (see Fig. 5-2).

The AFO is a plastic brace that supports a weakened ankle so that you can walk with a heel-to-toe motion and avoid catching your toe on the ground. If tripping is primarily the result of leg weakness, you will probably be referred to a physical therapist for a treatment regimen of exercises and evaluation for a mobility aid such as a cane or walker. If the tripping and falling occur primarily when you are already tired from overexertion, the physical therapist may recommend that you use a mobility aid such as a motorized scooter when you need to cover longer distances.

How will I know if I need to use a walker?

Most people seem to feel that a walker makes them look more disabled, and would therefore prefer to try various types of unilateral supports, e.g., a cane, forearm crutch, or quad cane, before having to switch to a walker. The physician or physical therapist will recommend that you use a walker if you need more stability in order to maintain balance and avoid hazardous falls. A walker also requires less energy. Some walkers have (two or four) wheels, hand brakes, a seat, and a basket for carrying

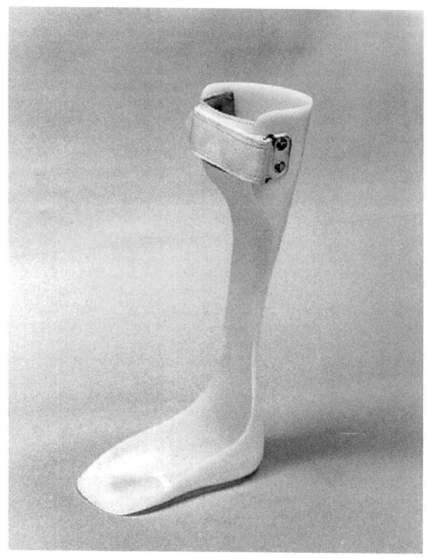

Figure 5-2.   A plastic ankle-foot orthosis.

things. The specific walker should be selected with special attention to your individual needs. You may find that a particular type of equipment works best for you in one situation while another type of aid is more useful in a different situation; the major objectives are to maintain stability and safety, conserve energy, and get the job done.

If I use a leg splint or brace, will my leg muscles become weak or useless?

A foot or leg splint is generally prescribed because of muscle weakness. In other words, the splint does not cause weakness; rather it substitutes for muscles that are already weakened due to lack of adequate nerve **innervation**. Since it is true that certain muscles in the foot are not required to work as hard when a splint is used, the physical therapist always prescribes stretching and active exercises to be done during the hours the splint is off. This will ensure the preservation of normal movement, which will, in turn, promote normal muscle action in both legs as well as the rest of the body.

Although I can walk around the house, I can't walk more than a block without getting weak. What should I do? I don't want to be stuck at home all the time.

Weakness and fatigue are limiting your ability to walk distances. Depending on your physical needs, the type of neighborhood in which you live, and your regular mode of transportation, a mobility aid such as a wheelchair or motorized scooter could greatly enhance your mobility and ability to enjoy life outside your home. People often believe that as long as they can walk at all, they have no use for this type of equipment. As a result, they use all of their available energy just getting from point A to point B and then have no energy left to enjoy themselves or get back again! A scooter is actually designed for use by a person who is independent, ambulatory, and on the go. By using a scooter to get from place to place, you conserve your energy and also get more things accomplished once you arrive at your destination.

You will probably find that your family and friends are very supportive of your decision to use a mobility aid. You will once again be able to participate with them in a variety of activities that previously felt too difficult, too tiring, and too slow, including trips to restaurants, the shopping mall, the zoo, a museum—and even Disney World.

Do not buy any piece of equipment without first consulting with a health care professional. Your physician can help you identify the exact nature of your walking problem and energy shortage. If your needs can be met with a mobility aid, a physical therapist can help you choose the type that would be most useful. Too much money is involved to make any decisions based solely on the advice of a salesperson, no matter how well-intentioned he or she may be. Equipment should meet your current needs as well as your future needs. A salesperson does not understand your medical condition and the potential changes you may experience in the future, and therefore cannot and should not advise you on what is the best equipment for you.

What is the difference between a manual wheelchair, a motorized scooter, and an electric wheelchair? How do I know which is best for me? Does insurance pay for any of them?

A manual wheelchair is a nonmotorized mobility device (see Fig. 5-3). A person who wants to use this type of wheelchair without assistance from another person needs to have sufficient upper body strength to propel the chair. If you have significant upper body weakness or fatigue, another person will need to assist you. The advantage of this type of mobility aid is that it is collapsible and hence easy to transport. Some people who are quite ambulatory most of the time keep a lightweight, portable wheelchair in the trunk of the car for use in places like shopping malls that have great distances to cover.

A motorized scooter is a vehicle that resembles a golf cart. It typically has three or four wheels, runs on rechargeable batteries, and is driven by a thumb push mechanism. To use a scooter effectively, you need to be able to stand and transfer into the seat. This requires standing ability, a fairly high degree of mobility, and adequate balance. Electric scooters can be disassembled and put into your car. Depending on the size and style of your car, it is possible to install an electric lift that will raise the heaviest parts of the scooter into the trunk. Scooters now come in a bewildering variety of styles, sizes, and weights. Some are designed primarily for indoor use while others can travel very well over outdoor terrain. All can be taken on an airplane as checked baggage.

A motorized wheelchair has a battery and is driven with a stick control by the person sitting in the wheelchair. This type of chair is useful for the person who cannot stand and transfer independently, and needs more seating support than is provided by the seat of an electric scooter. Its major limitation is that

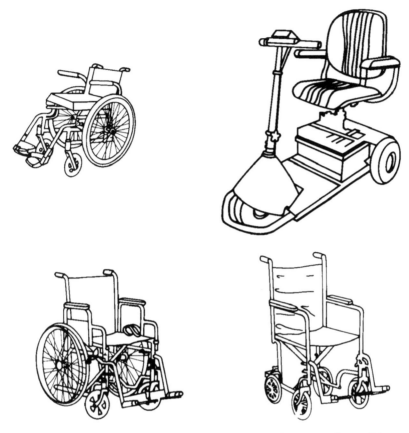

Figure 5-3.   Different types of wheelchairs. (**A**) sports chair, (**B**) scooter, (**C**) standard wheelchair, and (**D**) chair with small wheels, which must be pushed.

it is not collapsible or easily transportable. The person who wants to use an electric wheelchair independently within the community will probably need a wheelchair-equipped van for transportation. Both the scooter and the motorized wheelchair are good alternatives for someone who does not like the feeling of being pushed from behind. It is quite easy to "wheel" alongside a companion, carrying on a conversation and feeling completely independent.

Many factors must be considered before deciding what equipment is best for you. Your physician and physical therapist can evaluate your physical requirements and tell you which option(s) would be best for you. Once you know which types of equipment would meet your needs safely, the physical therapist will assist you to think through the following questions:

◇ Where do I want to be able to use this equipment?
◇ Where will I store the equipment when I am not using it?
◇ How will I transport it from one place to another?
◇ Will I be able to get the equipment in and out of my home?
◇ Will I be able to use this equipment independently or will I need someone else's help?

Answering these questions will help you to select the particular equipment that meets your needs most effectively.

Some government agencies and insurance plans pay the entire cost or a portion of the cost of mobility equipment. Since physical therapists are aware of the different funding sources and their requirements, they may be able to help you to apply for funding.

If I start to use a wheelchair to go long distances, will I lose the ability to walk?

No. Inability to walk is caused by demyelination and/or damage to the axons, not by using a wheelchair. Due to increased fatigue or diminishing endurance, you may wish to use a wheelchair or scooter to increase your mobility at work or in the community. Or you may begin to use a mobility aid for high-energy outings such as trips to malls, museums, or the zoo. Using the mobility equipment to enhance your life and broaden your scope of activities will not cause your symptoms to worsen. A mobility aid is not the cause of weakness or fatigue—it is the solution to these two common problems.

Should I purchase a secondhand wheelchair?

Like eyeglasses, mobility equipment is prescribed specifically to fit you. Each person has a different physical build as well as different MS symptoms that must be accommodated. A tall, heavy person with balance problems and a weak right side would need a very different size and style of equipment than a small person whose primary symptom is severe fatigue. Since your prescription for mobility equipment is based on a thorough seating evaluation that takes into account all of your specific physical characteristics and symptoms, your mobility aid is not interchangeable with that of another person.

It is difficult for me to get around town to do my errands and take care of household business without having someone to help me. Can a physical therapist be of help with this problem?

In addition to recommending the appropriate mobility equipment, the physical therapist is one of several possible sources of information (including MS Care Centers, your local chapter of the National Multiple Sclerosis Society, and other members of your health care team) about transportation in your community. The therapist may help you to obtain a disabled license plate from the local motor vehicle department, which will enable you to make use of handicapped parking spaces. The therapist can also show you how to apply for access to any available public transit programs for the disabled, or for a designated disabled parking spot near your home, school, or work place.

This is only a sample of the questions commonly asked of physical therapists. Questions more specific to your own situation should be directed to your own therapist. Although two individuals with MS may seem to have the same symptoms, the underlying causes of these symptoms may be quite different. It is best to get an individual assessment of your particular situation.

Recommended Readings

Blonsky R. *The Exercise Program (2nd edition)*. New York: Demos, 1988.

Kraft GH, Catanzaro M. *Living with Multiple Sclerosis: A Wellness Approach (2nd edition)*. New York: Demos Medical Publishing, 2000.

Schapiro R. *Symptom Management in Multiple Sclerosis (3rd edition)*. New York: Demos Medical Publishing, 1998.

Selected materials available from your local chapter of the National Multiple Sclerosis Society (800-FIGHT-MS):

◇ *Managing MS Through Rehabilitation* (ECS 6022)
◇ *Exercise as Part of Everyday Life* (ES 6008)

◇ *At Home with MS: Adapting Your Environment* (ECS 6035)

◇ *Controlling Spasticity* (ECS 6037)

◇ *Facts and Issues* (reprints of articles from the National Multiple Sclerosis Society magazine, *Inside MS*, covering such topics as fatigue, energy management, and gait problems).

◇ *MS and Wellness*—Jane Brunette, R.N., M.S.N. & Diane Reaves, B.S. Workbook in a series entitled *Living Well with MS* that was written for, and by, people who have been living with MS for some time.

◇ *Considering Assistive Devices*—Mary Elizabeth McNary, M.A., CRC. Workbook in a series entitled "Living Well with MS" that was written for, and by, people who have been living with MS for some time.

Reprints available from the Canadian Multiple Sclerosis Society (416-922-6065):

◇ *Coping with Fatigue in MS Takes Understanding and Planning*—Alexander Burnfield, M.B., M.R.C. Psych.

Recommended Resources

(See Recommended Resources at the end of Chapter 6.)

6

Occupational Therapy

Jean Hietpas, O.T.R., L.C.S.W.

Due to the nature of the disease process, the symptoms of multiple sclerosis can vary greatly from one individual to another. For some, the symptoms may be slight, such as tingling in the hands or mild weakness. For others, the symptoms may be more severe, possibly including problems such as paresis (weakness), balance problems, alterations in sensation, fatigue, difficulty with coordination, vision loss, speech disturbances, and cognitive impairment.

In addition to the variety of symptoms, a person with MS can also experience variation in the progression of symptoms. Some people experience fluctuations between periods of **remission** (recovery) and episodes of **exacerbation** (worsening). Others experience increasingly severe symptoms over the course of time with little or no remission (see Chapter 2).

Occupational therapy assists individuals to manage both the variety of symptoms and the variations in symptom progression. The therapy focuses on energy conservation and the maintenance of everyday skills that are essential for productive, independent living, such as dressing, bathing, grooming, meal preparation, writing, and driving. The **occupational therapist** (OT) tailors treatment to specific individual needs and deficits. From the time of diagnosis, the goal of treatment is to develop and support individual **abilities** and **adaptations** that promote functional independence in everyday living and enhance quality of life.

The OT addresses four major areas that are essential to maintaining independence:

◇ upper body strength, movement, and coordination;

◇ aids to independent living (including practice with *activities of daily living (ADL)* skills and equipment, mobility devices, assistive technology for the home and office, and environmental modifications for greater accessibility);

◇ compensatory strategies for cognitive impairments, sensation problems, or vision loss;

◇ fatigue management through education about energy conservation, work simplification, environmental adaptations at home and in the workplace, and stress management.

The OT uses both assessment and treatment tools to manage MS-related problems. Assessment, which is often an ongoing process, involves both the expertise of the OT and the active participation of the person with MS. As part of the assessment process, you will be asked about your home and work environment, including your ability to maneuver around your kitchen, bathroom, living area, and work space, as well as access in and out of your home or place of employment. The OT will also evaluate your sitting and standing abilities, as well as the strength and ease of upper body movement. Once problem areas have been identified, the OT will work with you to develop a treatment plan to correct or manage these problems.

I'm experiencing increasing weakness in my hands and fingers. Will exercise make my hands strong again? What exercises are best for this problem?

Our hands are the "doing" centers for many of our everyday tasks. Many of the jobs we need to do become frustrating and difficult when hand strength and coordination decrease. The hand weakness you experience as a result of MS is due to reduced nerve conduction rather than weakened muscles.

Therefore, the primary goal is not necessarily to increase hand strength (although for some people the hands do become stronger), but to maintain existing dexterity and muscle strength and, to the extent possible, prevent further deterioration. Your OT will prescribe active range of motion exercises such as opening and closing the hands, and mild resistance exercises such as a thera-putty exercise program. The exercise program needs to be individualized so that the appropriate muscles are involved, especially if you are experiencing stiffness or *spasticity.*

It seems to take so much effort just to get up in the morning and deal with bathing, dressing, and breakfast. Is there something I can do to make those tasks easier and less tiring?

The principles to keep in mind with all of your activities of daily living (ADLs) are to simplify your life and conserve energy. When MS fatigue interferes with your ability to perform the basic physical tasks, take time to think about your routine. Experiment with ways to simplify and reorganize your routine to conserve your energy. Examples of energy conservation might include such simple changes as taking a shower in the evening so that you have less to do in the morning, and building two-to three-minute rests into your schedule so that you do not get overly exhausted. If you are heat-sensitive, consider taking a cool or lukewarm shower rather than a possibly fatigue-producing hot shower. Consider selecting your clothes for the next day and putting them on a bedside chair before you go to bed in the evening. As you purchase clothes now and in the future, try to select items that are easy to take on and off and require a minimum of energy to maintain. Similarly, plan your breakfast the night before, and leave the nonperishable items and dishes on the counter or table so that they are ready to use in the morning.

I enjoy my work, but am finding it increasingly difficult to maneuver around my office and manage my fatigue over the course of the working day. I'm afraid I won't be able to stay at this job if it gets any worse.

Work simplification is the key to enhancing comfort and productivity on the job. Work simplification involves:

◇ making sure that your work space, furniture, and office equipment are designed and situated in such a way as to promote your physical comfort and reduce fatigue;

◇ organizing your workspace to eliminate unnecessary reaching, lifting, and walking;

◇ re-examining your approach to tasks to ensure that you are doing them in the simplest, most energy-efficient, and least time-consuming way;

◇ becoming familiar with the tools and/or adaptive devices that are available to simplify your tasks and enhance your comfort;

◇ arranging your schedule to make the best use of high-energy times and build in short rest periods.

You can schedule an appointment with an occupational therapist to visit your workplace and recommend ways to simplify your tasks and help you be more comfortable and productive on the job. Many of the adaptations he or she might suggest are considered "reasonable accommodations" under the Americans with Disabilities Act (see Chapter 14). The OT can help you formulate your requests for accommodations from your employer.

My hands feel weak and clumsy most of the time. Is there anything to help tie my shoes and button my shirt?

A variety of products are now available (see ADL equipment in the Recommended Resources) to help with frustrating tasks such as tying shoes and buttoning shirts. There are several options available if you are able to bend over and reach your shoes, including "no-bows," a spring-loaded lace tightener; velcro shoe closures; and even one-handed shoe-tying techniques. If you are not able to reach your feet, you can replace your cotton shoelaces with elastic ones that will turn your tie shoes into slip-ons. Once the elastic laces are tied in place, have a shoemaker stitch the shoe tongue to the top of the shoe so it won't move around, and use a long-handled shoehorn to put on your shoes. A shoemaker can also sew a loop on the back of the shoe so you can pull it on with a long-handled hook. Another simple solution is a well-fitting pair of slip-on shoes. If you are also finding it tiring and difficult to pull on socks, there is a gadget called a sock-aide that helps to pull the sock over the toes and up the calf of your leg.

Buttoning is made simpler with a buttonhook, which is used to pull the button through the buttonhole with a minimum of strength and dexterity. Some people prefer to wear shirts with large, easy to grasp buttons, pullovers, or polo-type shirts that have very few buttons. Mail-order catalogues and Internet Web sites containing these and other products are available for consumers. See "Shop-At-Home Catalogs" in the Recommended Resources. You will discover numerous ways to streamline many aspects of your daily routines as you begin to look for ways to conserve time and energy.

Dressing is becoming a tiring and time-consuming task. What kinds of clothing are simple to put on, simple to take care of, and still look good enough for me to wear to work?

Energy conservation is important to consider in the dressing process. Generally, oversized clothes or shirts and blouses with large buttons down the front are easier to get on and off. Likewise, loose-fitting slacks with an elastic waist are comfortable and easy to pull on and off (see Clothing in the Recommended Resources). Adaptive aids such as dressing sticks, sock aids, and long-handled shoehorns can be helpful when you are trained by an OT to be proficient in their use (see ADL equipment in the Recommended Resources).

Women can add a scarf or jewelry to almost any kind of pullover shirt or sweater to enhance it. Men may find it useful to wear clip-on ties or to leave their neckties tied so that they need only be slipped over the head and tightened. Dress shirts can remain permanently buttoned except for the top buttons. This allows the shirt to be simply slipped over your head. Another strategy is to remove the buttons, close the buttonholes, and reattach the buttons on top of the buttonholes. Velcro pieces can then be sewn behind the buttonholes and on the original button sites for easy closure.

What underwear can a man get on and off without standing up that is also convenient for bathroom functions?

Several companies specialize in adaptive clothing for health care needs. A man's velcro-closure underpants can be taken on and off from a seated position. The President's Committee on Employment of People with Disabilities created a resource list of clothing for people with disabilities (see Clothing in the Recommended

Resources). Many companies have free or minimal-charge catalogs for mail order shopping.

Getting on and (especially) off the toilet has become difficult. Are there any modifications I can make that will ease this problem?

Several modifications can be made to facilitate toileting, some having to do with your body mechanics, others with adaptive equipment. It is important to pay attention to the placement of both your arms and feet when changing from the seated to standing position. With your feet placed firmly in front of you, use your hands and arms to push off from the toilet seat. To go from a standing to a sitting position, place yourself squarely in front of the toilet seat, bend your knees until you can touch each side of the toilet seat with your hands, and then lower yourself slowly to the seat.

The simplest mechanical aid to help you get on and off the toilet is a secure grab bar on the wall next to the toilet. Obviously, this is only effective if the toilet is adjacent to a wall. An over-the-toilet commode frame allows for adjustability in the height of the seat and provides bilateral armrests to assist you in lowering and raising your body (see Figure 6-1). A number of other medical equipment items such as an elevated toilet seat and side rails can be helpful. These items are available through a local medical supplier or through the ADL equipment companies referenced at the end of this chapter. An OT can be helpful in determining which piece of equipment best suits your needs.

I'm concerned that I'm not adequately cleaning myself after toileting. Are there ways to do this more effectively?

Independence in toileting is a very personal matter, yet one that can be problematic because of poor sitting balance or limited use of the hands. Try using a wet washcloth or disposable baby wipe to clean yourself or have a squeeze bottle with lukewarm water to rinse yourself after toileting. Several toileting aids, such as a toilet paper holder, are available through ADL equipment suppliers (see Recommended Resources). Also available are portable or permanently installed bidets that rinse and, in some models, dry the genital area of the body.

Getting in and out of the shower-tub combination has become difficult for me. Do you have any suggestions for making this task easier and safer?

It is important to make sure that the transition or transfer in and out of the shower stall or tub-shower is safe. Adequate balance and a certain amount of strength are both necessary for safe transfers. If your balance is in question, the easiest solution is to install a grab bar to hold onto during the transfer. Grab bars should be permanently mounted to a stud in the wall (your local hardware store can recommend a handyman to install them). Your physician or an OT can assess your upper body strength to determine if you are able to use a grab bar to assist with the transfer safely and independently. If your upper body strength is not sufficient, or if your lower body is too weak, an OT may recommend a tub transfer bench for a seated transfer in and out of the tub-shower (see Figure 6-1).

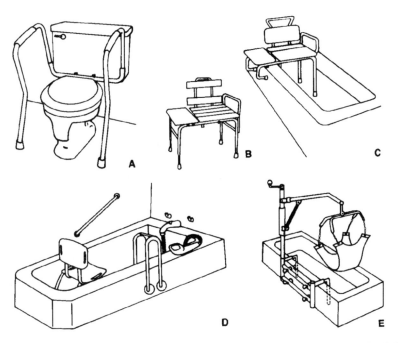

Figure 6-1. Bathroom aids. (**A**) toilet frame, (**B**) transfer bench, (**C**) bathing bench, (**D**) shower chair, lifeguard rail, diagonal grab bar, and hand-held shower hose, and (**E**) patient lifter and bath attachment.

A shower chair or bench is the answer if your standing balance and endurance are not sufficient to allow you to stand confidently during your shower. This type of equipment is available through your local medical supply company, and can usually be found in the Yellow Pages under medical equipment. A shower chair should be adjustable in height so you can set it to your comfort. A hand-held shower hose, mounted on a height-adjustable, wall-mounted rod, will make a seated shower more enjoyable. A non-slip mat in the tub or shower stall will help prevent a fall.

Getting up and out of a chair is becoming harder for me. What is the best type of chair for me to sit in, and are there any recommended techniques or gadgets that will make it easier for me to get up again?

The best type of chair is one that is relatively high off the ground and has solid arms. The height of the chair is critical because it is always more difficult to get out of low, soft chairs than higher ones that are firmer. Chairs generally measure 17 or 18 inches from the floor to the top of the seat. You can add a two-to-three-inch foam cushion to raise the height of your chair, or add leg extenders (rubber cups that fit on the legs of the chair) to raise the seat height. It will be easier to get up from the seat if you scoot forward first and then use your hands to push up from the arms of the chair. If these adaptations are not sufficient, there are portable lifter cushions that you can place on your own chair, or chairs with built-in lifter seats, that will gently propel you out of a seated position. Many of the companies that offer these products are referenced at the end of the chapter under chair lifts or ADL equipment suppliers.

My bed is so low that I have a hard time getting out of it. Are there ways to modify my bed that will solve this problem?

Getting up from low surfaces can be difficult. First, pay attention to your body mechanics: try rolling onto your side, facing the edge of the bed, and pushing yourself up with your bottom arm while swinging your legs over the side of the bed. If you have trouble rolling over onto your side, you can purchase sheets with fabric pull-strips sewn onto them, or grab bars that can be attached to the sides of your mattress. Once in a sitting position on the edge of the bed, try to push yourself up with your hands. If the bed is too low or too soft for you to be able to push yourself upright, you can raise the height of the bed by placing it on wood blocks. A strategically-placed grab bar on the wall next to your bed, bed handles, or a floor-to-ceiling pole next to the bed, can allow you to pull yourself from a sitting position to a standing position. Bed handles and floor-to-ceiling poles are available through your local medical equipment suppliers listed in the Yellow Pages of your telephone directory.

I'm looking for a new car. Is there anything in particular I should take into consideration when selecting one?

Take your time when selecting a new car. Try to anticipate what your needs might be in the future as well as thinking carefully about your present needs. For example, a stick shift or standard transmission car might seem more appealing to you now, but can cause future difficulties if you develop weakness or incoordination in your left foot. Compare the ease with which you can get in and out of different models. Operate the door handles, gear shift, turn signal, windshield wipers, horn, cruise control, radio, air conditioning, parking brake, and seat adjustments to see how easy to manipulate and accessible they are. Always purchase air conditioning in the automobile to prevent fatigue on a hot day. Consider a tilt steering wheel and power seats to give you maximum adjustability and comfort.

Try lifting packages in and out of the back seat and the trunk of the car. Large parcels, grocery bags, a small child, and possibly a wheelchair or other piece of adaptive equipment are examples of the "cargo" that people often need to be able to maneuver in their cars. Vehicles with a lower trunk opening allow you to take items in and out without having to lift them as high off the ground. You may find that a four-door sedan allows easier access to back-seat storage space for crutches or a wheelchair, or that a station wagon or hatch-back vehicle better fits your needs. A minivan or van is also an option to consider if you currently use a power mobility device such as an electric scooter, or anticipate using one in the future. Refer to the list of recommended resources at the end of the chapter for further information about vehicles and vehicle modifications.

Being able to drive my car is very important to me, but my right leg doesn't move as quickly and reliably between pedals as it used to. I've heard about hand controls and I'm wondering whether they could work for me.

Thousands of people operate vehicles with the use of hand controls. They work well for someone who has good upper body control but limited lower body function. Since safe driving depends on a variety of functions, including eye-hand coordination, head and neck flexibility, adequate vision, and reasonable reaction time, it would be well worth your while to seek a driving evaluation before investing in equipment for your car. Ask your physician, OT, or the local chapter of the National MS Society for the name of the nearest driver evaluation program. The major car companies also offer listings of driver evaluation programs as well as the names of companies that will perform adaptive modifications on your car (see Vehicle Modifications under Recommended Resources).

Hand controls come in a variety of styles and configurations. They most often are attached to the steering column and look like additional sticks protruding from it. Acceleration and braking are accomplished by pulling the control toward you or pushing it away from you. If turning the steering wheel has become more difficult because of hand or arm weakness, a round knob can be attached to the steering wheel. Be sure to check with your state Department of Motor Vehicles to find out the local procedures for obtaining these adaptive devices.

When I do the laundry, I have to carry it up and down fourteen stairs. Is there anything I can do to make this process easier and safer?

Carrying items can be dangerous if your standing balance is unstable. Break the task into small, light loads rather than carrying one large load. Or put the laundry in a bag with a drawstring and pull it up and down the stairs behind you. Depending on your staircase, you may be able to create a simple pulley system that allows you to pull the laundry bag up and down the stairs with a minimum amount of strength and exertion. Another solution might be for a family member or neighbor to carry the laundry up and down the stairs. Do not hesitate to recruit assistance for tasks that become too difficult or too dangerous for you to do

alone. You may want to consider relocating your laundry equipment to the main living area such as the kitchen or closet on the
main floor.

Some people find that the sorting and folding of laundry is
time-consuming and tiring. Ask family members to presort their
own clothes into dark and light piles before bringing them to the
washing machine, and to make sure that each item is turned right
side out. You can also tell them that anything that is given to you
turned inside out will be given back to them clean but still inside
out. Depending on the ages of your family members, you might
even ask each person to take care of his or her own laundry!

**We are planning to redo the bathroom and kitchen in our home.
What kinds of modifications would you recommend?**

Accessibility and ease of use are the main factors to consider in
making home modifications. Several good references to home
modifications are available (see Environmental Adaptations in
Appendix E).

When designing for accessibility in the bathroom, important
features to consider include:

◇ door width
◇ adequacy of space in which to maneuver
◇ height, shape, and mounting of the sink and toilet
◇ accessibility of the medicine cabinet and other storage areas
◇ access to the shower stall
◇ shape and style of faucets and shower heads.

Likewise, a well-designed kitchen can make meal preparation
more pleasurable and less exhausting. Carefully placed appliances, counters, sinks, cabinets, and work areas should be considered and discussed when remodeling your kitchen. You will
want to be able to reach the items you need without having to do
a great deal of walking back and forth or reaching. *As with any
other long-term, expensive decisions and purchases, try to think
not only about your present needs but your potential needs in
the future as well.* You might plan for your countertops to be
lower than usual in case you want or need to do more of your
cooking from a seated position. Similarly, you might want to
consider overhanging countertops that would allow space for

your legs if you were working from a seated position. You are well-advised to consult with an OT as well as a general contractor or architect who is knowledgeable about accessibility before proceeding.

I want to remain in my current home but have to admit that is has become difficult getting up and down the entrance steps.

There are several options available to provide safe access in and out of your home. Solidly mounted hand rails on both sides of the stairs can help with getting up and down the stairs. A physical therapist (PT) can assess your ability to use stairs safely using the hand rails for support. If you are not able to maneuver the steps safely, you will want to consider a ramp or mechanical lift. Ramps require 12 feet of ramp for every 12 inches of rise plus 5′ x 5′ at the top and bottom of the ramp for landings. A lift or small elevator requires less space, saves energy, and is often less expensive than the cost of a ramp.

I enjoy cooking but find that I get worn-out from the effort and weakened by the heat. Do you have any suggestions for solving these problems?

There are now available many nutritious and easy-to-prepare foods that require less preparation time. For example, instant oatmeal provides a nutritious and tasty breakfast, and items such as instant rice, instant potatoes, instant soups, frozen vegetables, and frozen meals are easy to prepare.

A microwave, convection oven, or toaster oven create little or no heat and reduce meal preparation time. If you are now using a standard oven or doing a lot of stove-top cooking that makes the kitchen overly warm, you might want to consider the use of a "cool vest." This handy garment looks like an outdoor vest designed to hold frozen gel packs. Wearing this vest during cooking or any other uncomfortably warm activity can keep you cool and reduce heat-induced fatigue that is so common in MS.

Make sure that the kitchen is organized, clean, and neat so you have an open work area. Having a stool in the kitchen to sit on during meal preparation and clean-up assists in conserving your energy. Use a dishwasher for clean-up or recruit family assistance for tasks that are difficult for you.

We eat a lot of fresh vegetables and make salads for our meals, but peeling, chopping, and cutting have become difficult. Are there any techniques or gadgets that will make this task less difficult?

Many types of blenders and food processors are available at your local hardware or department store. These devices save on the effort and time needed to prepare vegetables. Select kitchen knives that have a good solid grip and are easy to maneuver. The Good Grips® knife, for example, has a built-up handle with a non-slip surface and a serrated edge on the blade. Dycem® is a non-slip material designed to anchor bowls and cutting boards while you work. Some cutting boards are designed to hold or stabilize the item you are cutting (see ADL equipment under Recommended Resources). You might also ask a family member to help you wash and cut a two- or three-day supply of vegetables at one time and store them in plastic containers or bags in the refrigerator. Another solution might be to take advantage of the convenience packs of ready-to-eat salad vegetables now carried by many grocery stores.

In addition to using proper utensils and convenience foods, try to conserve your energy by gathering all the items you need for the job in one place before starting to do your food preparation.

I enjoy talking on the telephone, especially since it has become more difficult for me to get out and see family and friends. Holding the phone is starting to become tiring and awkward. Is there anything I can do to make my time on the phone more comfortable?

Several good telecommunication products and services are available that will make talking on the phone easy and enjoyable. Speaker phones permit hands-free operation so that you can speak and listen without having to hold the receiver. If you wish to have a private conversation, try a hands-free telephone headset (available at Radio Shack). The telephone company also offers an operator-assisted service for disabled individuals who are unable to dial a telephone number.

If you are experiencing problems with your hearing or vision that interfere with independent phone use, your phone company has various no-charge services. Contact your local phone service to find out if you would benefit from any of these programs, or see the reference list under Communications at the end of this chapter.

Going to the grocery store is a major ordeal. The aisles are crowded, I can't reach many of the items I need, and getting the grocery bags into my house is exhausting. There must be an easier way!

Grocery shopping can be a major ordeal for many people, and it is compounded for those with physical problems. Plan what you need and make a list prior to going to the store. Photocopy a master grocery list and simply check the items you need for that shopping trip. Try to shop during off-peak times when the store is less crowded. Know your grocery store (some stores have printed maps indicating which products are stocked in each aisle) and bypass the aisles you do not need. Request shopping assistance at customer service for items that are out of your reach. Often an employee will accompany you while you shop, or the requested items will be waiting for you at customer service. Although you may initially feel reluctant to ask for this kind of help, most people find that store employees and other shoppers are more than happy to provide assistance.

A few grocery stores have electric scooters available for public use and some stores provide a delivery service. In most supermarkets, a store employee is available to carry the groceries to your car. When you return home, ask a family member to carry the groceries from the car, or carry the perishable items in a separate bag or backpack and leave the other items for later, when you have more energy.

If getting to the grocery store becomes impossible, call your local stores and ask if they will take a telephone order for delivery. While it can be very frustrating to have to rely on someone at the store to pick out your items (particularly fresh fruits and vegetables), you will probably find that the process works fairly well once you and the store's employees have gone through it a few times. Or grocery shop on the internet through *www.peapod.com* or similar on-line grocery sites.

I've belonged to a bridge group for years. Lately I haven't gone to the group because I'm afraid of dropping the cards. Do I have to give up card playing?

It is important not to give up the things that you love to do. Card holders come in a variety of shapes and sizes for different kinds of card games. The card holder called Four Suiter® is popular and attractive. Playing cards with large numbers and symbols are readily available and a card shuffler may be helpful as well (see ADL equipment under Recommended Resources).

Numbness and tingling in one of my hands causes me to drop things. Is there anything I can do about this problem?

Sensory symptoms that include numbness and tingling have a tendency to come and go intermittently in MS (see Chapter 2). At the present time, no available treatment is likely to have any lasting impact on the numbness and tingling that you are experiencing. The best approach is to learn how to accommodate these symptoms in order to protect yourself from burns or other injuries, and your possessions from unnecessary breakage.

The decreased sensation and dexterity that often accompany numbness and tingling are the likely cause of your tendency to drop things. You drop something because you are less able to feel it in your hand. Visual contact with the object in or near your hands is very important to compensate for this decreased sensation and dexterity, so try to keep an eye on what you are doing. Use cups with large handles that accommodate your whole hand rather than one or two fingers. Also, using a coffee mug with a lid, such as the kind used for travel, will help avoid painful burns. Try using a pen that has a thicker body and perhaps a rougher surface. Slow down enough to make sure that you have a good grip on dishes and other breakable items, and consider purchasing a set of unbreakable dinnerware. You may find that you need to carry each item with two hands in order to ensure its safety and yours. Isotoner® gloves or rubber gloves are useful for some tasks to improve your grip and compensate for sensation loss.

I feel tightness in my neck and arm muscles. Are there stretches or other exercises that might help me with this?

Maintaining flexibility and range of motion in the neck and arms is very important to ease discomfort and prevent tightness. Stretching and range of motion exercises are the best strategy for enhancing arm mobility and comfort. An OT or PT can assist you in creating the right program for your particular needs.

Exercise can be fun and may include activities such as swimming, yoga, Tai-Chi, and exercise groups. It is very important to create a program that you enjoy and can commit to do on a regular basis (see Chapter 5).

**Shortly after my baby was born I began experiencing a great
deal of fatigue and weakness in my arms and legs. I don't have
much help available and need to learn how to handle my
daughter safely, particularly as she becomes more active. Do
you have any suggestions?**

Principles of energy conservation and good body mechanics will
be important as you analyze the various tasks you must perform
to take care of your daughter safely. Instead of carrying the baby
in your arms, experiment with a sling or infant carrier that you
can strap to your torso. If carrying your baby in this manner is
too tiring, explore what options you have for child equipment
with wheels, such as a bassinet, stroller, or portable crib. Wash,
change, and dress your baby at counter height, and use a safety
belt on the changing table. Kneel while washing her in the bathtub and use an infant-size, lightweight tub with a non-slip surface inside the big tub when the child is young. Consider using
disposable diapers as well as easy-on and easy-off clothing with
few fasteners.

Learn to rest when your child rests. Prioritize tasks and spread
the more difficult jobs throughout the week. Remember to relax
and take care of yourself as well as your new baby.

**I've heard that a home computer can be very useful for some-
one who is disabled. How could a computer help me and where
should I go to find out which computer would best meet my
needs?**

The most important question to ask yourself is, "how could a
computer be useful for me?" You might, for example, come up
with a list of tasks that includes the following: letter writing; fil-
ing information and creating mailing lists; bookkeeping and
finances; electronic mail and online communication; drawing
graphics; sending and receiving information via fax; playing
computer games. The next step is to try using a computer. Take
a computer literacy course, and talk to friends about ways in
which they use their computers. In other words, try to find out
whether you are likely to be able to enjoy and make effective
use of a computer before you go to the expense of purchasing
one.

Now you are ready to go to a computer store and spend time
with a salesperson that can explain the jargon and describe the
various types of equipment and accessories that are available. It

is very helpful to have a friend along, preferably someone who knows more about computers than you do. When talking with the salesperson, it is important that you be quite specific about your disability. A computer system can be adapted for many kinds of visual, sensory, and motor problems. If you find that the salesperson is simply trying to sell you a computer without taking time to understand your needs, try a different salesperson or a different store. References and resources listed at the end of the chapter can also direct you to materials describing various adaptations such as screen magnification to help with decreased vision, keyboard adaptations, and voice recognition to compensate for upper extremity incoordination.

I have a significant tremor in both of my hands, which makes it difficult for me to write legibly or eat without making a mess. It's very important to me to be able to continue doing these things independently. Are there any gadgets that would help with this problem?

Tremor is one of the most difficult and frustrating of MS symptoms (see Chapter 2). Fortunately, a number of well-designed writing and eating aids can alleviate some of the problems it can cause in your daily life. The first step is to try dampening the tremor with weights. A weighted pen with a good grip might help improve your handwriting. A weighted mug and weighted spoon or fork can help you get food to your mouth more smoothly and with less spillage. Wearing a one- or two-pound velcro closure wrist weight during such activities as writing and eating might also be helpful. However, weighted utensils and wrist weights will not be particularly useful if you tire easily or if your arms are extremely weak. A signature stamp can be made for signing letters, checks and legal documents. Some people find that a pen holder compensates for the tremor and improves legibility. One such holder resembles a rounded paperweight with a hole for your pen and grooves for your fingers. You write by grasping the molded holder with your entire hand and moving it along the page. Plastic writing "guides" are also available to help you write in straighter, more legible lines. Similarly, dinner plates with a curved edge will contain the food and prevent it from scattering onto the table. Drinking glasses are available with lids to prevent spillage.

Recommended Readings

Bell L, Seyfer E. *Gentle Yoga: A Guide to Gentle Exercise.* Berkeley, CA: Celestial Arts, 1987.

Garee B (ed.). *Parenting: Tips from Parents (Who Happen to Have a Disability) on Raising Children.* Bloomington, IL: Accent Press, 1989.

Holland N, Halper J (eds.). *Multiple Sclerosis: A Self-Care Guide to Wellness.* Washington, D.C.: Paralyzed Veterans of America, 1998.

Peterman Schwarz S. *300 Tips for Making Life with Multiple Sclerosis Easier.* New York: Demos Medical Publishing, 1999.

Rogers J, Matsumura M. *Mother to Be: A Guide to Pregnancy and Birth for Women with Disabilities.* New York: Demos, 1990.

Schapiro R. *Symptom Management in Multiple Sclerosis (3rd edition).* New York: Demos Medical Publishing, 1998.

Webster B. *All of a Piece: A Life with Multiple Sclerosis.* Baltimore: Johns Hopkins, 1989.

Wolf J. *Fall Down Seven, Get Up Eight.* Rutland, VT: Academy Books, 1991.

Wolf J. *Mastering Multiple Sclerosis: A Guide to Management (2nd edition).* Rutland, VT: Academy Books, 1987.

Publications available from the National Multiple Sclerosis Society:

◇ *At Home with MS: Adapting Your Environment* (ECS 6035)

◇ *Considering Adaptive Devices*—Mary Elizabeth McNary, M.A., CRC. Workbook in a series entitled *Living Well with MS,* written for, and by, people who have been living with MS for some time.

◇ *Coping with Change*—Mary Elizabeth McNary, M.A., CRC. Workbook in a series entitled *Living Well with MS,* written for, and by, people who have been living with MS for some time.

Recommended Resources

ASSISTIVE EQUIPMENT & DEVICES
(With permission of the National Multiple Sclerosis Society)

Please Note: The National Multiple Sclerosis Society does not endorse or recommend any products, services or manufacturers. The National MS Society assumes no liability whatsoever for the use, contents, or performance of any products listed below.

UNIQUE & NEWSWORTHY

The *CRUISER DELUXE* by Nova
A new lightweight 4-wheeled rolling Walker with light-touch hand brake, basket and a seat.

The *TRAVELER* by Nova
A new lightweight, stable 3-wheeled rolling Walker. Very maneuverable, it features large wheels, a basket and pouch and folds to 9″.

Both Nova Products available through:
Ortho-Med, Inc.
Tel: 800 557-6682
Website: www.novaortho-med.com

The *3000 IBOT TRANSPORTER*
Innovative, motorized, standing wheelchair able to climb stairs.
Available in the year 2000–2001
Independence Technology
Div. of Johnson & Johnson
Tel: 888 463-3000
Website: www.indetech.com

The *TravelMate*™
The first folding motorized scooter.
Amigo Mobility International, Inc.
Tel: 517 777 0910
Website: www.myamigo.com

COMMUNICATION

• Telephone Devices

Access Solutions for the Hearing
  Disabled
Tel: 800 445-9968
Website: www.harcmercantile.com

ATT Telephone &
  Telecommunications
Lucent Technologies
Tel: 800 233-1222 (maintenance)
800 222-3111
888 708-0874 (sales)
Website: www.telephones.att.com

Crestwood Co.
6625 N. Sidney Place
Milwaukee, WI 53209-3259
Tel: 414 352-5678
Fax: 414 352-5679
Email: Crestcomm@aol.com
Website:
  www.communicationsaid.com

Extensions for Independence
555 Saturn Blvd., # B-368
San Diego, CA 92154
Tel: 619 423-7709
Fax: 619 423-7709
Website: mouthsticks.net

Maxi-Aids
Tel: 800 522-6294
Website: www.hearmore.com

Prentke Romich Co.
Tel: 800 262-1984
 800 262-1933 (sales)
Website: www.prentrom.com

The Radio Shack
Tel: 800 843-7422
Website: www.radioshack.com

Making TDD (Telephone Device for
  the Deaf) Calls:
Call the Relay Operator to place calls
Tel: 800 421-1220

HOME

• Bathroom Equipment

Automatic Bidet

Lubidet USA
1980 S. Quebec St #4
Denver, Co 80231-3234
Tel: 800 582-4338
Fax: 303 368-0812
Email: info@lubidet.com
Website: www.lubidet.com

Portable Bidet

Andermac, Inc.
2626 Live Oak Blvd.
Yuba City, CA 95991
Tel: 800 824-0214
530 674-8450
Fax: 530 674-1806
Website: www.hygenique.com

Bath and Shower Chairs

ActiveAid
PO Box 359
Redwood Falls MN 56283
Tel: 800 533-5330
Fax: 507 644-2468
Website:www.activeaid.com

Diversified Fiberglass Fabricators
Tel: 704 435-9586
Fax: 704 435-9596
Website: www.dffinc.com

Innovative Products, Unlimited
2120 Industrial Drive
Niles, MI 49120
Tel: 800 833-2826
414 738-9090
Website: www.ipuproducts.com

Ortho-Kinetics, Inc.
PO Box 1647
Waukesha, WI 53187
Tel: 800 824-1068
Fax: 414 542-3990
Website: www.orthokinetics.com

R.D.Equipment,Inc.
230 Percival Drive
W. Barnstable, MA 02668
Tel/Fax: 508-362-7498
Email: rdequip@capecod.net
Website: www.rdequipment.com

Wheelchairs of Kansas
PO Box 320
Ellis, KS 67037
Tel: 800 537-6454
Website:
    wwww.wheelchairsofkansas.com

Bath Lifts

Clark Medical Products
Tel: 800 889-5295
905 238-6163
Fax: 905 624-3161
Website: www.clarkmedical.com

R.D.Equipment,Inc.
See listing under Bath and Shower
    Chairs

Grab Bars/Railings

Invacare Corp.
899 Cleveland St.
Elyria OH 44036
Tel: 800 333-6900
440 329-6000
Fax: 800 272-2822
Website: www.invacare.com

Lumex, Inc
Division of Graham Field, Inc.
Tel: 800 645-5272
Fax: 800 545-8639
Website: www.grahamfield.com

Shampoos

Bumble & Bumble Dry Shampoo
146 East 56th Street
New York, NY 10022
Tel: 800 728-6253

N/R Laboratories
Tel: 800 223-9348
Fax: 937 433-0779

Jergens Body Washes
Tel: 800 222-3553
Website: www.drugemporium.com

Shampoo Sinks

Durable Medical Equipment & Supply
3600 Fifth Ave South
Birmingham, AL 35222
Tel: 800 545-0641
Fax: 205 591-3734
Website: www.dmequip.bellsouth.net

Homecare Products
Tel: 800 451-1903
Fax: 253 630-8196
Website: www.homecareproducts.com

Toilet Risers

HMT Enterprises
547 Haymore Avenue
So. Worthington, OH 43085
Tel: 614 885-9172
Website:
    www.citywideguide.com/hmtent

Medway Corp.
Tel: 800 817-3118
Fax: 614 846-2056
Website: www.medwaycorp.com

Mobile Aid
Tel: 800 727-8483
Fax: 248 366-8969
Website: www.mobilaid.com

Toilet Seats

Gendron, Inc.
400 E. Lughill Rd.
Archbold OH 43502
Tel: 800 537-2521
Fax: 419 446-2631
Website: www.gendroninc.com

Invacare Corp.
See listing under Grab Bars and
    Railings

Lumex
See listing under Grab Bars and
    Railings

Maddak, Inc.
6 Industrial Blvd.
Pequannock, NJ 07440-1993
Tel: 800 443-4926
973 628-7600
Fax: 973 305-0841
Email: custservice@maddak.com
Website: www.maddak.com

Rubbermaid
3124 Valley Ave.
Winchester, VA 22601
Tel: 800 526-8051
Fax: 800 331-3291
Website: www.rubbermaid.com

Sani-Med
Div. of Sanderson Plumbing Prod.
PO Box 1367
Columbus, MS 39705
Tel: 800 647-1042
662 328-4000
Website: www.sppi.com

Tubular Fabricators Industry Inc.
600 W. Wythe St.
Petersburg, VA 23803
Tel: 800 526-0178
804 733-4000
Website: wwwtfihealthcare.com

Tubs and Showers

Assistive Technology Inc.
530 Whittaker St. #240
New Buffalo, MI 49117
Tel: 800 478-2363
219 522-7201
Fax: 219 293-0202
Email: info@pvcdme.com
Website: www.pvcdme.com

Diversified Fiberglass Fabricators
See listing under Bath and Shower
   Chairs

Electric Mobility Corp.
591 Mantua Blvd.
Sewell NJ 08080
Tel: 800 662-4548
Website: www.electricmobility.com

The Kohler Co.
Tel: 800 456-4537
Website: www.kohlerco.com

Porta shower of America, Inc.
134D, Route 111
Hampstead, NH 03841
Tel: 800 422-0098
617 886-9247
Fax: 617 270-9543

Silcraft Corp.
739 Goddard Avenue
Chesterfield, MO 63005
Tel: 800 347-5440
Fax: 800 797-8402
Website: www.invacare-ccq.com

The Tub-master Corp.
Fax: 800 327-1911

• **Eating Utensils**

Sammons Preston, Inc.
PO Box 5071
Boling Brook, IL 60440-5071
Tel: 800 323-5547
Fax: 800 547-4333
Website: www.sammonspreston.com

• **Plug-in Remote Controls**

Radio Shack
Tel: 800 843-7422
Website: www.radioshck.com

• **Elevators and Ramps**

Alumiramp
90 Taylor Street
Quincy, MI 49082
Tel: 800 800 3864
517 639-8778
Fax: 800 753-7267
Website: www.alumiramp.com

American Ramp Systems
202 W. First Street
S. Boston, MA 02127-1110
Tel: 800 649-5215
617 269-5679
Fax: 617 268-3701
Website: www.americanramp.com

The Braun Corporation
1014 S. Monticello
P.O. Box 310
Winamac, IN 46996
Tel: 800 843 5438
219 946 6153
Fax: 219 946 4670
Website: www.braunlift.com

Bruno Independent Living Aids
1780 Executive Drive
PO Box 84
Oconomowoc, WI 53066
Tel: 800 882-8183
Website: www.bruno.com

Homecare Products
See listing under Shampoo Sinks

Inclinator Co. of America
PO Box 1557
Harrisburg, PA 17105-1557
Tel: 800 343-9007
Fax: 717 234-0941
Website: www.inclinator.com

Mac's Lift Gate, Inc.
2801 South Street
Long Beach, CA 90805
Tel: 310 634-5962

Porta-Ramp
1616 Marlborough Ave
Riverside, CA 92507
Tel: 800 654-7267
Fax: 909 788-0609
Website: wwwportaramp.com

Automatic Door Openers

Power Access Corp.
PO Box 235
Collinsville, CT 06022
Tel: 800 344-0088
Fax: 860 693-0641
Website: www.power-access.com

Bed Handles

Bed Handles, Inc.
4825 S. Tierney Drive
Independence, MO 64055
Tel: 800 725-6903
Fax: 816 478-4324
Website: www.bedhandles.com

Standing Devices

Altimate Medical Inc.
262 W. First St.
Morton MN 56270
Tel: 800 342-8968
507 697-6393
Fax: 507 697-6900
Email: info@easystand.com
Website: www.easystand.com

Stair Climbers

Inclinator Co.
See listing under Elevators and Ramps

Trays and Tables

G E Miller Inc.
540 Nepperhan Ave.
Yonkers, NY 10701
Tel: 800 431-2924
914 969-4036
Fax: 914-969-3511

MOBILITY/TRANSPORTATION

• **Automotive and Van Adaptations**

Abilities Unlimited
49 E. Industry Court
Deer Park, NY11729
Tel: 800 664-8434
Fax: 516 254-4059
Website: www.abilitiesunltd.com

Access Wheels
Tel: 800 631-5791
Fax: 623 435-1518
Website: www.accesswheels.com

Action Vehicles
Servicing NJ, NY and CT
Tel: 888 323-9200
Fax: 914 381-4319

Arcola Mobility
51 Kero Road
Carlstadt, NJ 07072
Tel: 800 272-6521
Fax: 201 507-5372

Associated Handicapable Vans
6591 W. Highway 13
Savage, MN 55378
Tel: 612 890 7851
800 956 6668
Fax: 612 890 1903
Website: www.rollxvans.com

The Braun Corporation
See listing under Elevators and Ramps

Brunswick Automotive Professionals
1490 Route 1
N. Brunswick, NJ 08902
Tel: 732 545-6300
Website:
    www.brunswickautomotive.com

J. Busani, Inc.
500 Central Avenue
Bethpage, NY 11714
Tel: 516 938-5207
Fax: 516 938-5263
Website: www.jbusani@aol.com

Causeway Ford Mobility
375 Route 72
Manahawkin, NJ 08050
Tel: 877 Causeway
609 597-8083
Fax: 609 597-6089
Email: causeway4u@aol.com
Website: www.causewayford.com

Central Jersey Mobility Services, Inc.
436 W. Commodore Blvd., Rte. 526
Jackson, NJ 08527
Tel: 732 833-9700
Fax: 732 833-9705
Email: INFO@adaptiveservices.com
Website: www.adaptiveservices.com

Daimler Chrysler Corp./Auto Program
PO Box 3124
Bloomfield Hills, MI 48302-3124
Tel: 800 255-9877
Website:
    www.automobility.chrysler.com

Ford Mobility Motoring Program
PO Box 529
Bloomfield Hills, MI 48303
Tel: 800 952-2248
Website: www.ford.com

4 Wheel Driveline Systems
1168 Castleton Avenue
Staten Island, NY 10310
Tel: 800 794-8220
718 447-3038
Fax: 718 447-1565

Freedom Motors USA, Inc.
923 E Michigan Ave
Battle Creek, MO 49014
Tel: 888 625-6335
616 660-1002
Fax: 616 660-1296
Website: www.freedommotors.com

Fun Truck'n
82 Midland Avenue
Saddlebrook, NJ 07663
Tel: 888 467-4376
973 546-1900
Website: www.funtruckn.com

GM Mobility Assistance Ctr.
PO Box 100
Detroit, MI 48202
Tel: 800 323-9935
Website: www.gm.com

Independent Mobility Systems, Inc
Tel: 800 467-8267
Fax: 505 326-4846
Website: www.ims-vans.com

Monmouth Vans Acess & Mobility
5105 Rts. 33/34
Farmingdale, (Wall) NJ 07727
Tel: 800 221-0034
Fax: 732 919-0256
Website: www.monmouthvans.com

National Mobility Equipment Dealers Assn
For referrals to Dealers.
909 East Skagway Avenue
Tampa, FL 33604-1747
Tel: 800 823-0427
Fax: 813 931-4683
Website: www.nmeda.org

Personal Mobility Inc.
191 Tilghman St.
Allentown, PA 18102
Tel: 877 435-7600
Fax: 610 437-4611
Website: www.personalmobility.com

Tempe Dodge
7975 S. Autoplex Loop
Tempe, AZ 85284
Tel: 800 525-7142
480 598-2341
Fax: 480 496-6478
Email: Wcampell5@prodigy.net

Vantage Mobility International
5202 South 28th Place
Phoenix, AZ 85040
Tel: 800 348-82
Fax: 602 304-3290
Website: www.vantagemobility.com

Hand Controls

Central Jersey Mobility Services, Inc.
See listing under Automotive and Van Adaptation

4 Wheel Driveline Systems
See listing under Automotive and Van Adaptation

Leasing/Renting of Handicapable Vans

Associated Leasing
Div. of: Associated Handicapable Vans
See listing under Automotive and Van Adaptation

Caraleasing. Inc.
PO Box 265
White Plains, NY 10603
Tel: 914 288-9123
Fax: 914 761-1664

Wheelchair Getaways
NYC/ **New Jerse**y - Tel: 800 344-5005
YC/ Long Island -Tel: 800 379-3750

• **Golf Carts**
Ortho-Kinetics, Inc.
Website: www.fairwaygolfcars.com
See listing under Bath and Shower Chairs

• **Scooters**
Advanced Care, Inc
334 Main St., corner Rtes 79 / 516
Matawan, NJ 07747
Tel: 888 654-2273
Website: wwwadvancedcare.com

Amigo Mobility Intl Inc.
6693 Dixie Highway
Bridgeport, MI 48722-0402
Tel: 800 692-6446
Fax: 517 777-8184
Website: www.myamigo.com

The Braun Corporation
See listing under Elevators and Ramps

Bruno Independent Living Aids
See listing under Elevators and Ramps

Durable Medical Equipment & Supply
See listing under Shampoo Sinks

Electric Cart & Wheelchair Co.
415 N. Mulberry St.
Elizabethtown, KY 42701
Tel/Fax: 800 227-1919
Email: heartland99@hotmail.com

Electric Mobility
See listing under Tubs and Showers

Everest & Jennings, Inc.
Div. of Graham-Field, Inc.
3601 Rider Trail South
Earth City, MO 63045
Tel: 800 245-4661
Fax: 800 542-3567
Website:
   www.coast-
   resources.com/everestandjennings/

Lark Of America
Div.of Ortho-Kinetics, Inc.
See listing under Bath and Shower
   Chairs

Leisure Lift
Tel: 800 255-0285
Fax: 913 722-2614
Website: www.pacesaver.com

Mobilectrics
4014 Bardstown Road
Louisville, KY 40218
Tel: 800 876-6846
Website: www.mobilectrics.com

Palmer Industries, Inc
PO Box 5707JF
Endicott, NY 13763
Tel: 800 847-1304
Website: www.palmrind.com

Ranger Corp.
Tel: 800 225-3811
Website: www.rangerallseasons.com

The Scooter Store
1551 N. Walnut Ave., No.16
New Braunfels, TX 78130
Tel: 800 723-4535
Fax: 830 620-7291
Website: www.thescooterstore.com

Wheelcare
800 Avenida Acaso, Ste.E
Camarillo, CA 93012-8758
Tel: 888 910-2273
Website: www.wheelcare-inc.com

Accessories for Scooters

Diestco Manuf. Co.
P.O. Box 6504
Chico, CA 95927
Tel: 800 795-2392
Website: www.diestco.com

Homecare Products
See listing under Shampoo Sinks

Travel Scooters

Amigo Mobility Int'l
See listing under Scooters

• **Transfer Devices**

A.D.A. Solutions
601 Upland Avenue
Upland, PA 19015
Tel: 800 716-4662
610 876-5975
Fax: 610 876-5977
Website: www.adasolutions.com

Advanced Care, Inc
See listing under Scooters

Bailey Manufacturing Co.
118 Lee Street
Lodi, OH 44254
Tel: 330 948-1080
800 321-8372
Website: www.baileymfg.com

Bruno Independent Living Aids
See listing under Automotive and
   Van Adaptation

The Braun Corporation
See listing under Elevators and
   Ramps

J. Busani, Inc.
See listing under Automotive and
   Van Adaptation

Causeway Mobility
See listing under Automotive and
   Van Adaptation

4 Wheel Driveline Systems
See listing under Automotive and
   Van Adaptation

Invacare, Inc.
See listing under Grab Bars and
   Railings

Moving Solution
Tel: 800 228-7980
Email: movngsolns@aol.com

Personal Mobility Inc.
See listing under Automotive and
   Van Adaptation

Rand-Scot Inc.
Ft. Collins, CO 80524
Tel: 800 467-7967
970 484-7967
Fax: 970 484-3800
Email: easypivot@aol.com
Website: www.easypivot.com

Rubbermaid Health Care Products
See listing under Toilet seats

Sears Healthcare Catalog
Sears Tower, Dept. 608
Chicago, IL 60684
Tel: 800 326-1750
Fax: 800 278-8808
Website: www.sears.com

Spri Medical & Rehab Corp.
642 Anthony Trail
Northbook, IL 60062
Tel: 800 345-3456
847 272-7211
Fax: 847 272-0420

Sunrise Medical Co.
7477 B East Dry Creek Pkwy.
Longmont, CO 80503
Tel: 888 333-2572
Website: www.sunrisemedical.com

SureHands International
Tel: 800 724-5305
Email: surehand@warwick.net
Website: www.surehands.com

Therafin Corp.
19747 Wolf Road
Mokena, IL 60448
Tel: 708 479-7300
800 843-7234
Fax: 888 479-1515
Website: www.therafin.com

• **Walkers and Canes**

Walkers

Artistic Medical Supply
1872 Star Batt Drive
Rochester Hills, MI 48309
Tel: 800 667-5660
Fax: 248 852-1730
Email sales@HeatherMedical.com

Durable Medical Equipment & Supply
See listing under Shampoo Sinks

Gendron, Inc.
See listing under Toilet seats

Innovative Products, Unlimited
See listing under Bath and Shower
   Chairs

Invacare Inc.
See listing under Grab Bars/Railings

Noble Motion Inc.
6741 Reynolds Street
Pittsburgh, PA 15206
Tel: 800 234-9255
412 363-3550
Fax: 412 363-7189
Website: www.noblemotion.com

Rubbermaid
See listing under Toilet seats

Sunrise Medical Co.
See listing under Transfer Devices

Tubular Fabricators Industry, Inc.
See listing under Toilet Seats

Wenzelite
Tel: 800 706-9255
Fax: 718 768-8020
Email: wenzelite@aol.com

Walker Accessories

Homecare Products
See listing under Shampoo Sinks

Sammons Preston, Inc.
See listing under Eating Utensils

Canes

Artistic Medical Supply
See listing under Walkers

The Braun Corporation
See listing under Elevators and
    Ramps

Canes and Such
Tel: 888 383-2263
Fax: 352 495-3270
Website: www.canesandsuch.com

Durable Medical Equipment &
    Supply
See listing under Shampoo Sinks

Raising Cane
Tel: 888 854-3452
Website: www.raisingcane.qpg.com

Rubbermaid
See listing under Toilet Seats

Sammons Preston Inc.
See listing under Eating Utensils

Tubular Fabricators Industry, Inc.
See listing under Toilet Seats

Cane Accessories

Ableware Homecare Catalog
Div of Maddak, Inc.
6 Industrial Road
Pequannock, NJ 07440-1993
Tel: 973 628-7600
Website: www.ableware.com

• **Wheelchairs**

*Durable Medical
Equipment & Supply*

See listing under Shampoo Sinks

Electric Cart & Wheelchair Co.
See listing under Scooters

Everest & Jennings, Inc.
Div. of Graham-Field, Inc
Graham Field, Inc
81 Spence St.
Bay Shore, NY
Tel: 800 645-5272
516 273-2200
Website: www.grahamfield.com

Gendron, Inc.
See listing under Toilet seats

Gunnell, Inc.
8440 State St., PO Box 308
Millington MI 48746
Tel: 800 551-0055

Invacare Corp.
See listing under Grab Bars/Railings

Redman Powerchairs
3840 S. Palo Verde
Tucson, AZ 85714
Tel: 800 727-6684
Fax: 602 294-8836

Sammons Preston, Inc.
See listing under Eating Utensils

Sears Healthcare
See listing under Transfer Devices

Sunrise Medical Inc.
See listing under Transfer Devices

Theradyne Health Corp.
395 Ervine Industrial Dr.
Jordan MN 55352
Tel: 612 502-6190
Fax: 612 492-3442
Website: www.kurt.com

Wheelchairs of Kansas
See listing under Bath and Shower
    Chairs

Wheelchair Warehouse
100 E. Sierra, Ste. #3309
Fresno, CA 93710
Tel: 800 829-0202
209 436-6147
Accessories for Wheelchairs

Diestco Manuf. Co.
See listing under Scooters

Homecare Products
See listing under Shampoo Sinks

Invacare
See listing under Grab Bars and
  Railings

Sammons Preston, Inc.
See listing under Eating Utensils

All-Terrain Wheelchairs

Natural Access
PO Box 2222
Princeton, NJ 08543
Tel: 800 411-7789
Fax: 609-588-9836
Website: www.natural-
  access.com/home

Lifts for Wheelchairs

Inclinator Co
See listing under Elevators and Ramps

The Braun Corporation
See listing under Elevators and Ramps

Ranger Corp.
See listing under Scooters

Standing Wheelchairs

Stand-N-Go, Inc.
RT. 5, Box 22A
Fergus Falls, MN 56537
Tel: 218 739-5252
Fax: 218 739-5262

Travel Wheelchair

Travel Light, Inc.
PO Box 27740
Las Vegas, NV 89126
Tel: 800 995-5541

PERSONAL

• Clothing

Birmingham Limb & Brace
Tel: 800 762-9850
205 595-9850

Shelley Peterman Schwartz
Author of *Book on Dressing Tips*
933 Chapel Hill Road
Madison, WI 53711
Tel: 608 824-0402
Website: www.makinglifeeasier.com

Undergarments

Duraline Medical Products, Inc
324 Werner St.
PO Box 67
Leipsic, OH 45856
Tel: 800 654-3376

Home Delivery Incontinent Supplies
9385 Dielman Industrial Drive
Olivette, MO 63132
Tel: 800 269-4663
314 997-8771
Fax: 888 874-4347
Website: www.hdisnet.com

Woodbury Products
3580 Oceanside Road
Oceanside, NY 11572
Tel: 800 777-1111
516 594-8100
Website: www.woodburycares.com

Cooling Devices

Body Cooler
Tel: 800 209-2665
Website: www.bodycooler.com

MicroClimate Systems, Inc.
965 E. Saginaw Road
Sanford, MI 48657
Tel: 800 642-9077
Website: www.microclimate.com

The Sharper Image
Tel: 800 344-4444 (code 11053)
Website: www.sharperimage.com

Steele Inc.
26112 Iowa Avenue NE
PO Box 7304
Kingston, WA 98346
Tel: 888 783-3538
360 297-4555
Fax: 360 297-2816
Website: www.steelevest.com

Exercise and Therapy Equipment

Endless Pools, Inc.
200 E Dutton Mill Rd., Dept.387
Aston, PA 19014
Tel: 800 233-0741

Ex N' Flex International
Tel: 888 298-9922
Fax: 250 658-2350
Email: info@exnflex.com
Website: www.exnflex.com

Flaghouse Inc.
601 Flaghouse Drive
Hasbrouck Heights, NJ 07604
Tel: 800 793-7900
201 288-7600
Website: www.flaghouse.com

North Coast Medical
18305 Sutter Blvd.
Morgan Hill. CA 95037-2845
Tel: 800 821-9319
Fax: 877 213-9300
Website: www.ncmedical.com

NuStep by LifePlus, Inc.
3770 Plaza Drive
Ann Arbor, MI
Tel: 800 322-2209
Fax: 734 769-8180
Website: www.nustep.com

Oakworks Inc.
PO Box 99
34 Main Street
Glen Rock, PA 17327-0099
Tel: 800 558-8850
717 235-6807
Fax: 717 235-6798
Website: www.oakworksinc.com

Sammons Preston, Inc.
See listing under Eating Utensils

Sears Healthcare Catalog
See listing under Transfer Devices

Sinties Scientific, Inc
5616A 122 E Avenue
Tulsa, OK 74146-6913
Tel: 800 852-6869
Fax: 918 254-4189

Sundance Spas
Tel: 800 899-7727
Website: www.sundancespas.com

Therafin Corp.
See listing under Transfer Devices

The Therapy Machine
389 Pointes Drive East
Shelton, WA 98584
Tel: 800 314-4851
360 427-5511
Fax: 360 427-4564
Website: www.therapymachine.com

Service Dogs

Canine Partners for Life
Box 170
Cocranville, PA 19330
Tel: 610 869-4902
Fax: 610 869-9785
Website: www.chesco.com/k94life

Delta Society's Nat'l. Serv. Dog Ctr.
Tel: 800 869-6898
Fax: 425 235-1076
Website: www.deltasociety.org

Independence Dogs, Inc.
Provides referrals only
146 State Line Road
Chadds Ford, PA 19317
Tel: 610 358-2723
Website: www.independencedogs.org

Internat'l Assoc.of Assistance Dog
  Partners (IAADP)
For referrals
PO Box 1326
Sterling Heights, MI 48311
Tel: 810 826-3938
Fax: 810 977-0079
Website: www.iaadp.org

Nat'l Education for Assistance Dog
  Services, Inc. (NEADS)
PO Box 213
West Boylston, MA 01583
Tel: 978 422-9064 (voice/tty)
Website: www.neadsdogs@aol.com

Shop-At-Home Catalogs

Can-Do Products
Independent Living Aids Inc.
Tel: 800 537-2118
Fax: 516 752-3135
Website:
  www.independentliving.com

CAT/UB Publications & Media
  Catalog
See listing under Technology
  Information

Crestwood Co.
See listing under Telephone Devices

Durable Medical Equipment, Inc.
See listing under Shampoo Sinks

Enrichments for Better Living
  Catalog
PO Box 5050
Bolingbrook IL 60440
Tel: 800 323-5547
Website: www.sammonspreston.com

Health Plus
24310 Multon Pkwy., Suite G
Laguna Woods, CA 92653
Tel: 949 859-4440
Fax: 949 580-1723

The Lighthouse International
Low Vision Customer Catalog
Tel: 800 453-4923

Maddak, Inc.

See listing under Toilet Seats

MaxiAids Catalog
Tel: 800 522-6294
Website: www.maxiaids.com

Sears Healthcare Catalog
Tel: 800 326-1750

Smith & Nephew
Rehabilitation Division
1 Quality Drive
PO Box 1005
Germantown, WI 53022-8205
Tel: 800 558-8633
Fax: 800 545-7758
Website: www.americasdoctors.com

TECHNOLOGY INFORMATION

Abledata
8455 Colesville Road, Ste. 935
Silver Spring, MD 20910
Tel: 800 227-0216
301 588-9284
Fax: 301 587-1967
Email: abledata@maccromt.com

Adaptive Environments Center
374 Congress Street, Ste.301
Boston, MA 02210
Tel: 617 695-1225
Website: adaptenv.org

American Academy of Orthopedic
  Surgeons
Assorted Free Booklets
Tel: 800 824-2663

American Assoc. of Retired Persons
  (AARP)
Consumer Affairs Section
601 E Street, NW
Washington, DC 20049
Tel: 800 424-3410
Website: www.aarp.org

American Occupational Therapy
  Association
4720 Montgomery Lane
Bethesda, MD 20824
Tel: 301 652-2682
Website: www.aota.org

The Arthritis Foundation
PO Box 1900
Atlanta, GA 30326
Tel: 800 283-7800

Center for Assistive Technology
  (CAT)
Jennifer Weir- Information
  Coordinator
515 Kimball Tower
Buffalo, NY 14214-3079
Tel: 800 628-2281 (TDD/TTY)
716 829-3141
Fax: 716 829-3217
Website:
  http://wings.buffalo.edu/ot/cat

The Center for Universal Design
North Carolina State Univ.
Box 8613, Raleigh, NC 27695-8613
Tel: 800 647-6777
Website: www.design.ncsu.deu/cud

The Complete Directory for People
  with Disabilities
Exceptional Parent Library
PO Box 1807
Englewood Cliffs, NJ 07632
Tel: 800 535-1910
Fax: 201 947-9376
Website: www.eplibrary.com

IDEA: Center for Inclusive Design &
  Environmental Access
School of Architecture & Planning
SUNY at Buffalo – Room 378
Buffalo, NY 14214-3087
Tel: 716 829-3485 ext 329
Fax: 716 829-3861
Website: www.ap.buffalo.edu/ ~idea

Metropolitan Center for Independent
  Living
1600 University Ave West, Suite 16
St. Paul MN 55104-3825
Tel: 651 646-8342
Fax: 651 603-2006
Website: www.macil.org/mcil

National Council on Independent
  Living
1916 Wilson Blvd., Suite 209
Arlington, VA 22201
Tel: 703 525-3406
Fax: 703 525-3409

National Rehabilitative Information
  Center (NARIC)
1010 Wayne Ave. Suite 800
Silver Spring, MD 20910
Tel: 800 346-2742
301 562-2400
Fax: 301 562-2401
Website: www.naric.com

Project LINK
Karen Inman – Information Coordinator
Same info as CAT—listed above
Website: http://wings.buffalo.edu/
  ot/cat/rerca-link.htm

The Simon Foundation for
  Incontinence
Tel: 800 252-3337
Fax: 847 864-9758
Website: www.simonfoundation.org

Technology Related Assistance for
  Individuals w/ Disabilities
For TRIAD Centers and info on this
  program, contact:
NY State Office of Advocate for
  Persons w/ Disabilities
1 Empire State Plaza, Suite 1001
Albany, NY 12223-1150
Tel: 800 522-4369 (voice and TTY)
518 473-4129
Fax: 518 473-6005
BBS: 800 943-2323
Email: info@oapwd.state.ny.us
Website:
  www.state.ny.us/disabledadvocate

Trace Research & Development
  Center
5901 Research Park Blvd.
Madison, WI 53719-1252
Tel: 608 262-6966
Fax: 608 262-8848
Website: trace.wisc.edu

NOTE: Check the BLUE PAGES OF
  GOVERNMENT listings in your
  local telephone book for
  "Disability Services" and your
  local Independent Living Center
  for more information.

WORK ENVIRONMENT

• **Adaptive Desks**

Extensions for Independence
See listing under Telephone Devices

Fellowes Worcester

PO Box 60

Belcamp, MD 21017
Tel: 410 273-0330
Fax: 410 273-0338
Website: www.fellowes.com

Accessories

Fellowes Worcester
See listing under Adaptive Desks

AliMed Products
Tel: 800 225-2610
Fax: 800 437-2966
Website: www.alimed.com

Lap Boards

Posture Mate, Inc.
139 Burke Lane
Kneeland, CA 95549
Tel: 707 445-4841

Rifton Equipment
Route 213, PO Box 901
Rifton, NY 12471-0901
Tel: 800 777-4244
914 658-8799
Fax: 800 336-5948

Salmons Preston Inc.
See listing under Eating Utensils

Work Stations Inc.
11 Silver Street
So. Hadley, MA 01075
Tel: 800 759-6948
413 535-3340
Fax: 413 535-3345

Page Turners

Touch Turner Co.
13621 103rd Ave NE
Arlington, WA 98223
Tel: 888 811-1963
360 651-1962
Fax: 360 658-9380
Website: www.coast-
  resources.com/touchturner/

Computer Devices

Extensions for Indepence
See listing under Telephone Devices

Infogrip, Inc.
1141 East Main St.
Ventura, CA 93001
Tel: 800 397-0921
Fax: 805 652-0880
Website: www.infogroup.com

In Touch Systems
11 Westview Rd.
Spring Valley, NY 10977
Tel: 800 332-6244
914 354-7431
Website:
  www.magicwandkeyboard.com

7

Speech and Voice Disorders

Pam Sorensen, M.A., C.C.C.-SLP

MS lesions in the brain can interfere with muscle control in the lips, tongue, soft palate (the soft muscle tissue extending back from the roof of the mouth), vocal cords, and diaphragm (the dome-like muscle under the lungs that plays an important role in breathing). These muscles control speech production and voice quality as well as the process of swallowing. A person who develops problems with speech or swallowing is usually referred by his or her physician to a *speech/language pathologist*, who specializes in the diagnosis and treatment of speech and swallowing disorders. The evaluation and treatment of problems with speech production and voice quality are discussed in this chapter while MS-related swallowing difficulties are the subject of Chapter 8.

The speech/language pathologist can also evaluate and treat cognitive-communication symptoms, including problems with attention, memory, finding the words to express ideas while speaking or writing, and processing or remembering what is heard or read. Cognitive-communication disorders are discussed in Chapter 9.

Normal speech and voice production is complex, requiring the following five systems to work smoothly together:

◇ *Respiration*—using the diaphragm to fill the lungs fully, followed by slow, controlled exhalation for speech.

◇ *Phonation*—using the vocal cords and airflow to produce voice of different pitch (highness or lowness of tone), loudness, and quality.

◇ *Resonance*—raising and lowering the soft palate to direct the voice to vibrate in either the mouth or nose and further affect quality.

◇ *Articulation*—making quick, precise movements of the lips, tongue, and soft palate for clarity of speech.

◇ *Prosody*—combining all of the above elements for a natural flow of speech, with adequate speaking rate, appropriate pauses, and variations in loudness and emphasis to enhance meaning.

Approximately 25 percent to 40 percent of people with MS experience speech and voice disorders during the course of the disease. The disorders are caused by spasticity, weakness, slowness, and incoordination of the muscles in the tongue, lips, soft palate, vocal cords, and diaphragm.

Dysarthria is the term used to describe motor speech disorders that result in the slurred or unclear articulation of words. Impairments in volume control, articulation, and emphasis have been reported as the three most common features of dysarthria.

◇ Impaired volume control refers to a voice that is too quiet, too loud, or tends to fluctuate because of poor breath support and control.

◇ Poor articulation results in speech that is slurred and sometimes difficult to understand in conversation.

◇ Problems with emphasis result in speech that is slowed or unnatural because of inappropriate pauses, placement of excess and equal stress on each word, or difficulty varying pitch and loudness to emphasize important words.

The term **dysphonia** refers to disorders of voice quality. Dysphonia commonly involves the following features:

◇ Harsh voice quality resulting from spasticity or too much muscle tone in the vocal cords that gives the voice a strained, brassy sound.

◇ Impaired pitch control due to tremor or spasticity in the vocal cords, which results either in pitch breaks (similar to the "cracking" that is heard in an adolescent whose voice is changing), or in a monotone or flat voice (lacking the pitch variation that produces a natural line of melody while speaking).

◇ Hypernasality is a nasal speech quality caused by weakness, slowness, or incoordination of the soft palate that allows too much air to resonate in the nasal cavity.

◇ A pitch level that is higher or lower than usual (caused by changes in muscle tone) or an uneven, gravelly voice quality (caused by trying to speak when there is very little air left in the lungs).

◇ Breathiness (caused by vocal cords that allow too much air to escape).

◇ Hoarseness (resulting from vocal cords that fluctuate between coming together too tightly and too loosely) that sounds similar to laryngitis.

Problems with speech and voice can come and go. They sometimes worsen temporarily with MS exacerbations or during bouts of severe fatigue, and then gradually improve. Depending on the course that the disease is following, these symptoms may also progressively worsen. Anyone who experiences problems with speech or voice that interfere with everyday communication should request a physician's referral to a speech/language pathologist, who is trained to evaluate symptoms and design an individualized treatment program. Therapy can alleviate many types of speech and voice problems; the sooner that therapy is begun, the greater the improvement is likely to be.

What will the speech/language pathologist do to evaluate my voice and speech?

The speech/language pathologist will first complete an *oral peripheral examination*. This examination includes:

◇ An assessment of the oral muscles necessary for speech (lips, tongue, and soft palate) in terms of strength, speed, range, accuracy, timing, and coordination. In order to evaluate the strength and control of your tongue muscles, for example, you may be asked to stick out your tongue, wag your tongue from side to side as quickly as you can, and lick your lips around in a circle and then change directions. To evaluate the functioning of your lips and soft palate, you may be asked to puff up your cheeks with your lips tightly closed, and resist pressure on your cheeks so that no air is allowed to be released. You may also be asked to show your teeth, pucker your lips, and alternate between a pucker and a smile. In order to determine how quickly you can coordinate the lip and tongue movements necessary for speech, you may be asked to say "pataka" as quickly and evenly as you can.

◇ An examination of your teeth and hard palate.

The speech/language pathologist will also do a *voice evaluation* to assess the function of the vocal cords, respiratory muscles, and soft palate as they relate to pitch, loudness, and voice quality.

◇ To assess respiratory function for speech, you may be asked to fill your lungs deeply, say "ahhh" for as long as you can; repeat "ah" many times quickly; and count as high as you can in one breath.

◇ To determine how well you can control pitch and loudness, you may be asked to sing up the scale ("do, re, mi . . .") or count from one to ten while gradually increasing your volume from a whisper to a shout.

◇ Referrals to an otolaryngologist (also known as an ear, nose, and throat (ENT) specialist) for examination of the vocal cords, or to a pulmonologist for a baseline pulmonary (lung) function test may also be indicated.

A *motor speech evaluation* will be done to assess how well all systems work together: breath support and control, voice production, resonance, articulation, and flow of speech.

◇ The precision of your pronunciation (articulation) and the ease with which you are understood by others (intelligibility) are measured at the sound, word, sentence, and conversational levels.

◇ A baseline sample of your speech may be tape-recorded.

◇ Conversational speech may be analyzed for its natural flow (prosody): Are there appropriate pauses or do they occur too often or at illogical places? Are important words emphasized with more loudness and higher pitch to enhance meaning, or are all words spoken with the same or no emphasis?

◇ The rate at which you speak may also be measured in order to determine if your speech is too fast or too slow when compared with the norm.

The speech/language pathologist will also complete a *communication profile* to assess your everyday communication needs, and the adequacy of your speech and voice at home, at work, and in the community. For example, the communication requirements of a public speaker, teacher, and retired, single parent may be very different. The profile evaluates the complexity of your typical speaking situations (the familiarity and size of the audience, and the demand for speed and intelligibility). It also assesses the perceptions and responses of your primary communication partners. What is their attitude? How well do they understand you? What do they do to help the communication? The ultimate goal of speech and voice therapy is to improve the intelligibility, rate, and naturalness of your speech in order to enhance your communication with others, in whatever setting you find yourself. Information from the communication profile provides the overall framework within which treatment planning on specific speech and voice problems occurs.

A *brief assessment of cognitive function* may also be included in the speech/language evaluation. Information about any problems you may be having with attention, memory, verbal fluency, and problem solving will be useful to the speech/language pathologist in designing a treatment plan and determining appropriate treatment goals, since problems in any of these areas could impact your progress. The results of the brief cognitive assessment can guide the choice of learning and memory strategies to be used in the therapy, and may also help to predict how much improvement to expect.

An *audiological assessment* may be necessary to determine if there is a hearing loss or problem with auditory discrimination. It is important to rule out hearing problems since they may influence clarity of speech as well as the ability to self-monitor and self-correct errors. Your hearing may be screened by the speech/language pathologist, using pure tone audiometry, or you may be referred to an audiologist for a complete evaluation.

Determining the status of *fatigue and visual-motor skills* also has important implications for treatment planning.

◇ Fatigue is a common MS symptom that can temporarily interfere with speech and voice production. You may be asked to describe the frequency and severity of your fatigue, the conditions or activities that seem to precipitate it, its impact on your speech, and the strategies you use to manage your fatigue.

◇ Motor problems, such as spasticity and tremor, and visual problems such as optic neuritis, nystagmus (jiggly eye movements), double vision, and visual scanning difficulties, can also occur with MS. Information about visual-motor abilities is helpful when planning the visual and written material to use in therapy, and when selecting the appropriate type of alternative communication device.

What is involved in the treatment of speech and voice problems?

Therapy is recommended with a speech/language pathologist if speech or voice problems interfere with everyday communication needs. The type and amount of treatment will vary with each individual. A treatment plan can be devised based on the person's specific problem areas and communication needs. Therapy usually begins with learning about normal speech and voice production. Daily home exercises for the lips, tongue, soft palate, vocal cords, and diaphragm are taught to strengthen and improve coordination in these muscles. Active self-monitoring is essential and can be enhanced with the use of a tape recorder, Voice Lite® (an instrument that becomes brighter as loudness increases), spirometer (an instrument that measures how completely the lungs are filled), and speech analysis computer software.

The person may be taught new strategies and compensatory techniques for improving the clarity of speech, including slowing down, overarticulation (exaggerated enunciation), phrasing, strategic pauses, and syllable tapping (tapping as you say each syllable). Practicing these techniques in increasingly more difficult and less structured speaking situations, during individual and then group therapy sessions, can help a person stabilize these new skills. Training family members in ways to provide useful cues can help promote treatment carryover outside the therapy sessions.

Home programs to enhance progress can be developed that incorporate, for example, the use of a mirror during oral exercises, and the use of a tape recorder while practicing and self-evaluating the new speaking strategies and compensatory techniques.

Training in the use of an augmentative or alternative communication (AAC) device can be provided for any person who is unable to speak loudly or clearly enough to be understood by others. For example, a simple voice amplifier (with headset microphone, loudness control, and speaker) can enhance one-to-one or even room-to-room communication for those who cannot speak loudly enough to be heard, or who become easily fatigued by the effort to do so. For those who are unable to articulate clearly enough to be understood, there are AAC devices ranging from a simple alphabet board to computer-assisted, electronic communication systems.

Referrals may also be made to other members of the medical team, based on individual needs, including a neurologist, otolaryngologist (or ENT specialist), pulmonologist, respiratory therapist, or occupational therapist.

My thoughts still flow as well as they used to, but I can't speak as quickly and clearly now. It sounds as though I have a mouthful of marbles. What is causing my speech to sound so slurred?

Feeling "out of sync," as if your mouth is unable to keep up with your thoughts, is a common complaint. Clear speech requires precise, rapid, coordinated movements of your lips, tongue, and soft palate. MS can cause the mouth and throat muscles to become weaker and less coordinated, resulting in the neuromuscular speech disorder called **dysarthria.** Slurred speech or imprecise articulation is a common feature of dysarthria. It can occasionally become severe enough to interfere with the ability of others to understand what you are saying.

A speech/language pathologist can help you improve the clarity of your speech. First, it is important to become consistent in identifying when your speech sounds slurred. This may require you to improve your self-monitoring skills by evaluating your own tape-recorded speech samples. Hearing the problem is the necessary first step to being able to make adjustments. The following techniques are helpful in improving speech clarity:

◇ *Slow down.* Do not try to speak as quickly as you did before. Your oral muscles and breathing probably cannot keep up with your thought process and the rate at which you want to say words. Concentrate on a slower speaking rate.

◇ *Overarticulate.* Open your mouth a little more while talking, and exaggerate the movements of your tongue, lips, and jaw.

◇ *Pause strategically.* Instead of trying to say too many words at once, it is better to utilize a strategy called "phrasing," by which you learn to pause at logical places in long sentences. This takes extra time and planning, but can promote clear speech.

Talking seems to take much more effort than it used to. I can get very tired and not have enough breath to say complete sentences loudly enough for others to understand me. Why is this happening? What can I do about it?

Talking is a complex activity that we take for granted until something like MS interferes. Clear, audible speech requires physical effort and precise timing by many muscle groups. Speaking for extended periods can thus be quite tiring, particularly for those individuals who also experience MS-related fatigue. A speech/language pathologist can help you become efficient at speaking loudly while simultaneously learning to pace yourself.

Adequate breath support and control are needed for loud speech. Air is the "gasoline" needed to drive the necessary muscles. You start by completely filling your lungs, using your diaphragm to inhale quickly and deeply. Then slowly extend your exhalation to produce words. It is important to identify how many words are loud enough before you run out of air and lose necessary volume. Then you can begin to modify your speech and breathing patterns to raise your volume and improve audibility. Plan pauses for breathing rather than saying too many words in one breath—a technique called "phrasing." For example, you may find that breaking sentences into five-word breath units helps you to maintain adequate loudness.

Besides teaching diaphragmatic breathing exercises and phrasing techniques, the speech/language pathologist can provide other options, as needed. For example, the "push technique" requires you to push down with your elbows on the armrests of your chair while talking. This can help your vocal cords come together more strongly and therefore help create a louder voice. Using a spirometer can assist you in observing and measuring how fully you are filling your lungs. A tape recorder, Voice Lite®, and computer programs that analyze speech volume can give feedback on how loud you sound and if you are reaching the goals set in therapy. Voice amplifiers with headset, collar, or neck loop microphones are sometimes recommended when loudness cannot be improved to a functionally adequate level. However, a speech/language pathologist should first evaluate the problem, recommend the most appropriate equipment, and then train you in its use.

Sometimes I avoid talking to others because it feels bad not to be understood. People seem to lose interest because it takes more time to listen to me. Sometimes they even nod when I know they do not understand what I'm saying. What should I do?

You are not alone in your frustration. People with MS who have moderate to severe dysarthria often experience similar feelings. Some also express resentment that their impaired speech causes others to "talk down" to them in the mistaken belief that they are not capable or intelligent. A useful strategy is to let people know about your speech difficulty and explain what assistance you need from them. It takes time and practice to feel comfortable asserting yourself in these ways. You might try out the following explanation: "The reason my speech is slow and hard to understand is because of my MS. My brain works fine, but my lips and tongue don't always cooperate." You can then give your listener guidance in how to respond to you by saying, "I am trying to speak clearly, but please tell me when you don't understand." These simple statements will help you and your listeners to feel more comfortable because they give your listeners permission to talk about any difficulty they might have in understanding what you are saying.

We live in a fast-paced world. Assess the situation and watch the body language of your listeners. This will enable you to judge which people and situations can allow the extra time that you need. Estimate the time needed and ask first: "Do you have . . . minutes to talk about . . .?" It is important that you do not avoid talking to others. It can be a challenge, but you have a right as a speaker to be understood and a responsibility to let listeners know what you need from them. A speech/language pathologist can help you become comfortable and proficient in this process. It is best to build your comfort level gradually with this new approach, first with a therapist and then family and close friends, before trying it with strangers.

If my speech gets any worse, even my family will not understand what I am saying. Are there other ways of communicating that I can learn?

The speech problems typical of MS can usually be improved with therapy. Although your speech may not be as loud, precise, fast, or flowing as it was, learning the appropriate techniques will usually allow you to be adequately understood by others. However, alternative modes of communication are necessary in certain situations. Many options are available, ranging from the simple to the "high tech." Selection depends on your specific needs, abilities, and financial resources. Some of the simpler communication aids include light and buzzer switches to get the attention of others; yes/no signals, eye blink systems, alphabet charts to spell out messages with finger or eye movements, and picture/word communication charts.

Many electronic and computer-assisted forms of communication are also available. They vary in size, portability, complexity, function, input, output, and cost. Some are laptop size for you to type in the message and have it printed out. Others can be programmed so that one keystroke produces a frequently used complete sentence. Some computers actually speak the messages you program in or type. Because of the variety and complexity of the available technology, you should be evaluated by a speech/language pathology and occupational therapy team that has expertise in this area. This specialty team can help you identify the type of equipment best suited to your needs by taking into account whatever physical limitations you may have, as well as your visual-motor, cognitive, and communication skills.

You can then purchase or construct the appropriate communication aid and be properly trained in its use.

Do speech and voice problems caused by MS ever remit like other MS symptoms?

If you experience slurred speech only during times of fatigue, you have probably noticed that the problem disappears once you are rested. If you experience the kind of MS-related fatigue that persists in spite of adequate sleep or rest, an occupational therapist can teach you energy conservation techniques to help manage your fatigue. A physician may also prescribe medication (e.g., amantadine, pemoline (Cylert®), or fluoxetine (Prozac®), to help control the fatigue (see Chapter 2 and Appendix B). Speech and voice problems that occur during an MS exacerbation may improve or resolve following treatment with high-dose steroids. Thus, managing fatigue and treating MS exacerbations can at times help speech and voice symptoms to remit. However, referral to a speech/language pathologist is recommended if symptoms persist even when you are rested, or one month after medical treatment is received for an MS exacerbation.

Why doesn't my voice sound the way it used to? Sometimes it seems hoarse, as if I have laryngitis. Other times it sounds strained or harsh.

Your voice quality is largely determined by how your vocal cords function. MS can cause spasticity, weakness, slowness, and incoordination of any muscle group. Your vocal cords are muscles, too, and can therefore undergo these changes. This can occur temporarily during MS exacerbations or more continuously as a result of disease progression. The types of voice problems or *dysphonia* that are characteristic of MS include harshness, hoarseness, breathiness, and hypernasality.

A harsh, strained voice quality occurs when there is too much muscle tone or tightness in the vocal cords due to MS-related spasticity. Baclofen (Lioresal®), a medication to relieve spasticity (see Chapter 2 and Appendix B), may be helpful. A speech/language pathologist can help you and the prescribing physician monitor the effectiveness of the antispasticity medication on your voice and speech quality. Voice therapy can help to reduce harshness by emphasizing relaxation techniques for your throat and vocal cords, improving breath support, promoting "easy onset" of your voicing, and a breathier speech quality. The "yawn-sigh" approach, in which the vocal cords are automatically relaxed during a yawn to promote a softer voice quality during the exhaled sigh, may also help with this problem.

A hoarse voice quality results when something interferes with the way your vocal cords come together during speaking. Hoarseness is a combination of harsh and breathy voice qualities. Your vocal cords may fluctuate between coming together too tightly (harsh) and too loosely (breathy), resulting in hoarseness. When hoarseness lasts more than 7 to 10 days, it is important to have an otolaryngologist or ENT specialist evaluate medical causes that can be treated, such as colds, allergies, abnormal growths, and paralysis. After these are ruled out, voice therapy that emphasizes increasing breath support and loudness, lowering your usual pitch, and self-monitoring for a "clear" target voice quality may reduce the problem.

What causes my voice to fluctuate so much? It doesn't seem to be within my control. Sometimes I have bursts of loudness. Other times my pitch changes or my voice turns off mid-sentence.

Such wide variations in pitch, loudness, and voice control are probably due to MS lesions in the cerebellum, the part of the brain responsible for regulating and coordinating complex voluntary movements. Either fine tremor or wide, jerking, shaking movements, also called *cerebellar tremor* or ataxia, may be seen in MS. Tremor can be one of the most disabling symptoms of MS. It may affect a variety of muscle groups (including the arms, legs, trunk, head, vocal cords, jaw, lips, and tongue) and interfere significantly with the daily activities of walking, self care, sitting balance, head control, writing, swallowing, speech and voice.

Cerebellar lesions can interfere with the vocal cord action required to produce vocalizations. You may experience sudden changes in pitch because of uncontrolled fluctuations between vocal cord elongation (high pitch) and contraction (low pitch). Bursts of loudness may result from abrupt vocal cord tension and diaphragm contraction. Intermittent aphonia (the loss of voice in mid-sentence) may occur because of unexpected parting of the vocal folds, when they should be vibrating together to produce voice. Continuous vocal cord tremors may interrupt the smoothness of your voice quality.

Problems with cerebellar tremor or ataxia are very difficult to treat (see Chapter 2). No medication has been developed specifically for tremor control. However, some medications designed to treat other conditions have been found to have secondary anti-tremor properties. Muscle relaxants, antiseizure medications, and certain beta blockers have been tried on individuals with MS. A speech/language pathologist can help evaluate the effectiveness of a medication on your speech and voice. Other treatment approaches for reducing the impact of cerebellar tremor on speech and voice include: improving sitting posture, trunk stabilization and head control; learning relaxation techniques and EMG/ biofeedback to enhance muscle control for smoother respiration and voicing; and using a tape recorder, Voice Lite®, or speech lab computer software to monitor pitch, loudness, and voice quality. Therapy that emphasizes active self-monitoring, practicing the new vocal skills while reading aloud and conversing, and reducing physical effort during speech, may also be beneficial.

How often and for how long will I need to see the therapist?

The frequency and duration of your therapy depends on the type and severity of your problems and your communication needs. Individualized treatment planning may also be impacted by insurance coverage. However, there is typically much that can be accomplished in twice-weekly outpatient therapy, with a re-evaluation and update of goals after two or three months. Involving the primary communication partner in treatment sessions, and diligently following the home program are essential for successful carryover of techniques.

Recommended Readings

Beukelman D, Kraft G, Freal J. Expressive communication disorders in persons with multiple sclerosis: A survey. *Arch Phys Med Rehabil* 1985;10:675–77.

Colton R, Casper J. *Understanding Voice Problems—A Physiological Perspective for Diagnosis and Treatment.* Baltimore: Williams & Wilkins, 1990.

Darley F, Brown J, Goldstein N. Dysarthria in multiple sclerosis. *J Speech Hearing Research* 1972;15:229–45.

Farmakides M, Boone D. Speech problems of patients with multiple sclerosis. *J Speech Hearing Disorders* 1960;25:385–89.

Glennen S, DeCoste D. *Handbook of Augmentative and Alternative Communication.* San Diego: Singular Publishing, 1997.

Hartelius L, Svensson P. Speech and swallowing symptoms associated with parkinson's disease and multiple sclerosis: A survey. *Folia Phoniat Logop* 1994;46:9–17.

Interactive Therapeutics. *A Guide for the Patient and Family* (Interactive Therapeutics, Inc., P.O. Box 1805, Stow, OH 44224-0805 tel: 800-253-5111).

Robertson SJ, Tanner B, & Young F. *Dysarthria Sourcebook: Exercises to Photocopy.* Bicester, Oxon: Winslow Press, 1986.

Silverman, FH. *Communication for the Speechless.* Boston: Allyn & Bacon Publishing, 1995.

Sorensen P, Brown S, Logemann J, Wilson K, Herndon R. Communication disorders and dysphagia. *J Neuro Rehab* 1994;8:137–43.

Yorkston K, Beukelman D, Bell K. *Clinical Management of Dysarthric Speakers.* Boston: College-Hill Publications, 1988.

Yorkston K, Bombardier C. *The Communication Profile for Speakers with Motor Speech Disorders and the Communication Profile for Spouses of Speakers with Motor Speech Disorders.* Unpublished questionnaires, University of Washington, Seattle, 1992.

8

Swallowing

Jeri A. Logemann, Ph.D.

In addition to the problems with speech and language discussed in the previous chapter, the *speech-language pathologist* is also trained to diagnose and treat symptoms related to the swallowing mechanism. Normal swallowing is a rapid, safe, and efficient process that occurs in four stages:

◆ *Stage One—Oral Preparation*

When food is placed in the mouth, chewing reduces it to a consistency appropriate for swallowing. Chewing requires the coordinated action of lip, tongue, and jaw muscles to move the food onto the teeth, pick up the food as it falls from the teeth, mix it with saliva, and replace it onto the teeth. The saliva that is mixed into the food during chewing helps with the digestion process and acts as a natural acid neutralizer. Chewing takes a variable amount of time depending on the amount and thickness of food put in the mouth. When chewing has reduced the food to a consistency appropriate for swallowing, the tongue subdivides it and forms a ball or bolus of the right size to be swallowed. The thicker or more viscous the food, the less a person can swallow at one time. Trying to swallow too much food at one time is uncomfortable and may result in gagging.

◆ Stage Two—Oral Stage

The tongue pushes the bolus of food up and backward through the mouth, applying pressure to the tail end of the bolus. As the tongue pressure pushes the food backward, the movements of the tongue and bolus stimulate sensory nerve endings; these, in turn, signal the brain to trigger a series of muscle contractions in the pharynx (throat), called the "pharyngeal swallow." Figure 8-1 illustrates the oral stage of swallow.

◆ Stage Three—Pharyngeal Stage

The triggering of the pharyngeal swallow sets in motion a series of neuromuscular actions. The soft palate (the soft portion at the back of the roof of the mouth) lifts and closes the back entrance to the nose, preventing food or liquid from entering the nasal passages. The larynx (voice box) lifts up and closes to help prevent food or liquid from entering the trachea (windpipe). The base of the tongue and the walls of the throat move toward each other until they touch. This movement generates the pressure needed to push the food through the throat. The airway (to the lungs) automatically closes to prevent accidental **aspiration** of food or liquid into the lungs. The valve at the bottom of the throat relaxes and opens to allow the bolus to pass easily into the esophagus (food canal leading down to the stomach). Figure 8-2 shows the onset of the pharyngeal stage of swallow. Figure 8-3 illustrates the middle of the pharyngeal stage of swallow.

◆ Stage Four—Esophageal Stage

Muscle contractions in the walls of the esophagus propel the bolus through the esophagus, and the valve at the bottom of the esophagus opens to let the food enter the stomach.

In normal swallowing, it takes approximately two seconds for the food to move through the mouth and throat before entering the esophagus. Once in the esophagus, it takes anywhere from eight to twenty seconds for the food to travel to the stomach. When the swallowing mechanism is working normally and effi-

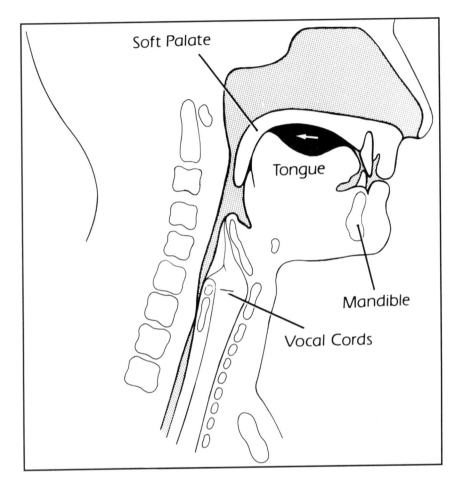

Figure 8-1. This side view of the mouth and throat shows the mouth containing the bolus with the tongue applying pressure to the food.

ciently, food particles and liquids seldom make their way into the airway or windpipe. This usually happens only when someone is doing two things at once, such as talking or laughing while trying to swallow. A person who tries to talk while eating may begin to cough or choke because a small or large particle of food has slipped into the airway. Once a normal swallow is completed, very little food is left in the mouth, throat, or esophagus.

What is dysphagia?

Dysphagia means difficulty swallowing. Approximately thirty muscles in the mouth and throat and eight *cranial nerves* are

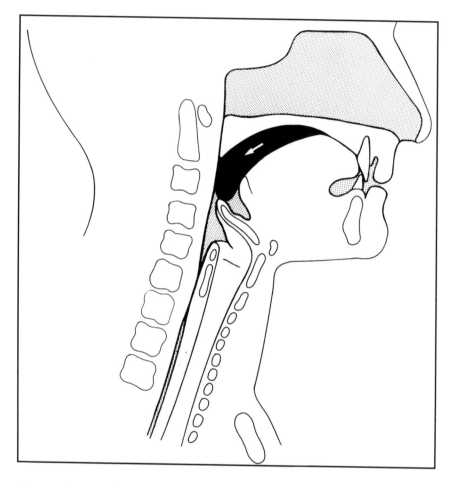

Figure 8-2. This side view of the mouth and pharynx shows the tongue pushing the food (bolus) out of the mouth. The entrance to the nose is closed and the airway is closing.

involved in the swallowing process. **Lesions** in various parts of the brain including the **brainstem** and/or the cranial nerves can cause problems at any point in the swallowing process, from the time the food enters the mouth until it reaches the stomach. A slowing of the nerve impulses that control the mechanisms of swallowing can interfere with the voluntary movements involved in chewing, with the initiation of the pharyngeal swallow, or with the strength or range of movements that are required to push the food through the mouth, throat, or esophagus. Reduced muscle strength or coordination can allow food parti-

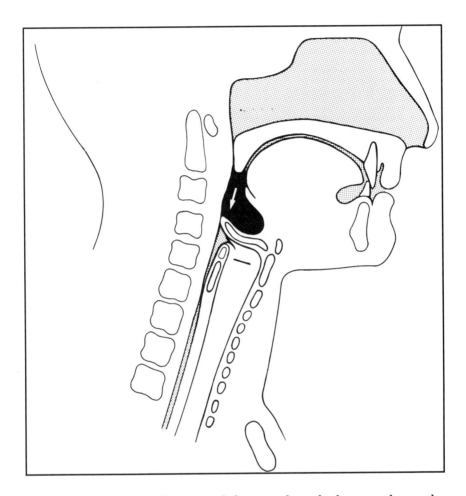

Figure 8-3.   This side view of the mouth and pharynx shows the food at the base of the tongue. The entrance to the nose is still closed. The airway is closed. The junction into the esophagus is almost open.

cles to remain in the mouth, throat, or esophagus after the swallow is completed. Food particles remaining in the mouth and throat may be accidentally aspirated into the lungs after the swallow when breathing resumes. If there is a delay in triggering the pharyngeal swallow, the airway to the lungs remains open and the food can fall into the airway before the pharyngeal swallow triggers. Food or liquid can also escape into the nose or windpipe during the pharyngeal swallow if there is a malfunction in the valves in the throat. The type of dysphagia a person develops will depend on the particular neuromuscular actions that are impaired. The problems most commonly seen in MS are a delay in the initiation of the pharyngeal swallow and a slowing of the passage of food through the pharynx.

What are the chances that I will develop a swallowing problem?

Most people with MS never experience this type of symptom over the course of the illness. Whether or not you develop a swallowing problem will depend entirely on the location of demyelinating lesions. Dysphagia can result if muscles of the mouth, throat, or esophagus are affected by the neurologic disease process. We do not know the exact percentage of people with MS who develop a swallowing problem, nor do we know if there are any specific characteristics that will predict whether someone will develop a swallowing problem. You should talk with your doctor about seeing a speech-language pathologist for a swallowing evaluation if you are finding it more difficult to chew or swallow your food, or seem to be coughing or choking during or after meals.

I have been referred for a swallowing evaluation. How is the evaluation done and what will the test be able to tell me about my swallowing problem?

A speech-language pathologist usually conducts the swallowing evaluation. The speech-language pathologist will take a complete clinical history and evaluate your ability to control the muscles of your mouth and throat. During this examination, you will be asked to move your lips, tongue, and soft palate in various ways and to produce speech samples that require different types of muscle control. You will also be asked questions about your diet, the kinds of foods that are difficult for you to eat, and the problems you have noticed in eating or swallowing. You may be asked, for example, about:

◇ episodes of coughing or choking during or after a meal
◇ how long it usually takes you to eat a meal
◇ whether your voice becomes hoarse or gurgly during or after eating
◇ the frequency with which you get respiratory infections
◇ whether you experience frequent heartburn or indigestion

Typically, the swallowing assessment also involves a radiographic study called *videofluoroscopy* (modified barium swallow). The barium you are given to swallow makes the structures of your mouth, throat, and esophagus visible on X-ray. The movements of these structures as you swallow different types of foods are recorded on videotape. During this examination, you will be asked to swallow varying amounts of liquids and solid foods with different consistencies. You may also be asked to chew and swallow a cookie with a small amount of barium on top.

The modified barium swallow is designed to help you, the speech-language pathologist, and your physician understand the specific nature of your swallowing problem. Depending on the results of the test, the speech-language pathologist may ask you to do various swallowing exercises in an attempt to improve or strengthen your swallow. You also may be given instructions on the safest ways to eat (e.g., optimal positioning of your head and neck, the size and frequency of meals, the correct way to chew) as well as the safest kinds of foods to eat (e.g., blenderized food, thickened liquids). The goal of this intervention is to identify ways to make it easier for you to continue to eat safely and comfortably.

What other specialized tests are available besides the modified barium swallow and why might they be used?

The modified barium swallow is the best assessment of the overall function of the mouth and pharynx when swallowing difficulties are thought to be present. If there might also be esophageal problems, then the doctor may order a barium swallow, an x-ray test designed to examine the function of the esophagus. Larger amounts of liquid are swallowed during the barium swallow than during the modified barium swallow. Another possible test is the endoscopic examination of swallowing, which involves the placement of a small fiberoptic tube through the nose and over the soft palate into the pharynx. This study does not involve x-ray but looks only at the pharynx, or throat, before and after the swallow. Because MS can cause oral problems, pharyngeal problems, or the two in combination, and because the relationship between the movements in the mouth and in the pharynx is so important, the endoscopic examination is not usually the swallowing examination of choice. However, the equipment is portable and can be taken to the person's bedside more easily than the modified barium swallow test that requires x-ray equipment. So, if a person is in a hospital or nurs-

ing home and needs an assessment of swallow, a fiberoptic endoscopic examination may be used.

If you are having difficulty with food coming back up from
the stomach after it is swallowed, a gastroenterologist (a doctor
specializing in the esophagus, stomach and the rest of the GI
tract) may examine you with a test called reflux monitoring.
Reflux monitoring involves a tube placed through the nose
down into the throat and esophagus. The purpose of the test is
to identify how many events of reflux (food coming from the
stomach back into the esophagus or throat) occur during a day,
and whether or not the food comes all the way up into the
throat. There are many medications that can be helpful for this
problem.

When should I ask the doctor for a swallowing evaluation?

If you are experiencing slowness of eating, difficulty in swallowing particular foods, or coughing associated with swallowing
either during a meal or after a meal, you should discuss these
symptoms with your doctor and ask about a swallowing assessment. Similarly, if you find that food sticks in your throat or in
your chest, you should ask your doctor for a swallowing assessment. Slow eating, the feeling of food catching, or coughing or
throat clearing frequently during a meal, can all be indications
of a swallowing problem.

I have heard that some medical facilities have a dysphagia team. Who makes up the dysphagia team and what does each member of the team offer?

The dysphagia team will differ somewhat from one facility to
another, but usually includes the person's physician, a speech-
language pathologist as the team coordinator, an occupational
therapist, a physical therapist, a dietitian, and sometimes a
dentist. Each professional offers different information and
types of care. Generally, the physician oversees the information
coming from all of the team members and makes the final decisions about what types of management should be used. The
speech-language pathologist typically does the swallowing
assessments and treatments, and coordinates the team interventions. The occupational therapist usually recommends any
adaptive eating utensils that may be needed for the person to
be able to eat comfortably and independently. The physical
therapist typically assists the person in optimal positioning

and postural readiness for eating. The dietitian is very important in assessing the person's nutritional requirements, and
determining the type of diet which best meets the person's
nutritional needs and eating abilities.

If the speech-language pathologist recommends swallowing therapy, what does this treatment involve and for how long am I likely to need it?

Swallowing therapy usually involves exercises to strengthen the
muscles used in swallowing and to improve the coordination of
muscles during swallowing. Therapy often involves practicing
muscle movements and learning safe swallowing strategies. Each
person is different, so the exercises and techniques you are given
may differ from those prescribed for someone else. The length of
time swallowing therapy needs to be continued will also vary
from one individual to another. Generally, however, a month or
so of twice-weekly therapy sessions will provide you with
enough training to proceed independently with your swallowing
practice. Some people need to continue to exercise daily to keep
their muscles operating at maximum strength and efficiency.

What are some of the exercises and swallowing strategies that a speech-language pathologist may teach me?

A speech-language pathologist may teach you how to coordinate
your breathing and swallowing and/or protect your windpipe
during swallowing so no food or liquid goes into your lungs. You
may also be given specific exercises to strengthen your tongue
and lip function and/or make the swallow come faster.

Why can't this book tell me how I should swallow?

Multiple sclerosis can affect swallowing in many different ways.
What works to improve swallowing in one individual may actually make swallowing worse for another. Therefore, the safest,
most effective strategy is to see a speech-language pathologist for
a thorough swallowing assessment and development of a personalized treatment plan.

If I start having trouble with my swallowing, how often will the doctor want a swallowing evaluation?

There is no set schedule for swallowing evaluations. Generally,
the evaluation should be repeated if you have had a change in
your symptoms. For example, you will need a reevaluation if

you begin to cough more frequently or have a gurgly voice during or after eating. Sometimes your doctor will want regular reevaluations of swallowing to see if a particular medication has a positive effect on your swallowing ability. You may also ask for a reevaluation if you notice changes in your swallowing ability. Even though you may not cough or have a gurgly voice, you may notice, for example, that swallowing is more difficult, or that it requires more energy and effort to swallow, or more time to eat a meal. If you feel your swallowing has changed, it is a good idea to ask your physician for a swallowing reevaluation.

Why do I sometimes have trouble swallowing liquids but have no trouble at all with solid foods?

Some people have more difficulty swallowing liquids, particularly if there is a delay between the end of the oral stage of swallowing (the movement of food through the mouth) and the beginning of the pharyngeal stage of swallowing (the movement of the food through the throat or pharynx). Since the airway remains open until the pharyngeal stage of swallowing has actually begun, the longer the delay, the greater the chance that liquid can slip into the airway and lungs. Because liquids have a thinner consistency than solids, they generally move faster and with less muscle effort than solids. Liquids are therefore likely to find their way into the open airway before solid foods do. People with multiple sclerosis sometimes develop a problem in triggering the pharyngeal stage of swallowing. When this occurs, they may have a tendency to cough or choke when trying to swallow liquids. Adding a thickening agent to the liquids you drink can often help to alleviate this problem.

Why are some solid foods more difficult than others for me to swallow?

Because solid foods are thicker in texture than liquids, they require a great deal more pressure to push backward through the mouth and throat. Some solid foods are naturally thicker than others (peanut butter is the worst, of course). Generating more pressure requires greater muscle strength. If neurologic changes are impeding the muscle action in your mouth, the resulting weakness may affect your ability to swallow solid foods. You will probably have more trouble swallowing the thickest foods and less trouble with thinner ones.

Weakness in the muscles used for chewing can also affect your ability to swallow. If chewing is difficult or tiring, you may be trying to swallow foods that are only half chewed. These half-chewed foods are much more difficult to swallow than foods that have been broken down to a softer consistency. If you are having trouble chewing, you may benefit from chewing exercises or from chopping or blenderizing the food before putting it on your plate. If you notice that your chewing gets weaker throughout a meal, you may want to eat five smaller meals rather than three larger ones.

I seem to have a mouthful of saliva much more often than I used to, and I sometimes start to choke on it. Is there anything I can do about this problem?

A mouthful of saliva that is not easily swallowed may result from a delay in triggering the pharyngeal swallow. You may benefit from swallowing therapy designed to improve the triggering mechanism and reduce the delay. You should talk with your speech-language pathologist about exercises for this problem. Excess saliva may also occur when you are not paying attention to the need to swallow or are unable to feel it. In that event, it may be helpful to train yourself to swallow more often and to receive cues from others. You may also want to keep a lozenge in your mouth to stimulate more saliva, which will, in turn, stimulate more swallows. A sour candy may naturally stimulate more swallows than a milder or less tasty lozenge.

I used to swallow automatically, without even having to think about it. Now I'm having a problem starting and finishing the swallow. Sometimes I even feel as though I haven't swallowed everything that needs to go down. Why is this happening and can I do anything about it?

This problem probably indicates both a delay in the pharyngeal stage of swallowing and muscle weakness that allows food particles to remain in your mouth or throat following each swallow. These problems can sometimes be alleviated with swallowing therapy: Certain icing techniques can help trigger the pharyngeal stage of swallowing. Exercises may strengthen muscles used during swallowing. Sucking on a sour candy or taking a very small sip of sour lemonade between every few bites of food may help you to trigger these swallows more efficiently. A safe swallow strategy such as "hold your breath, swallow, clear your throat, and swallow again for each bite or sip" can help to clear out leftover food or liquid from the throat.

What advice can you give my caregiver to use during mealtime?

Caregivers should observe their friend or family member during mealtime to determine whether swallowing and eating are slowing down or becoming more difficult. If so, the caregiver should remind the person about those strategies that have been recommended by the speech-language pathologist. Sometimes in the course of a meal, a person may forget the strategies he or she is supposed to be using. Head position, amount of food or liquid taken per swallow, time between swallows, and other variables can make a difference between a successful and unsuccessful swallow. Once the speech-language pathologist has recommended specific eating strategies, the caregiver can provide gentle reminders for the person to use these strategies.

What special equipment do you recommend to help a person eat independently?

Modified eating utensils may be needed to facilitate independent eating (see Chapter 6). An occupational therapist can recommend the devices that are most suited to your needs, and tell you where to get them.

Sometimes my husband chokes so badly, I get scared he might choke to death. What is the Heimlich maneuver and when should I give it?

The Heimlich maneuver is the best-known method of removing an object from the airway of a person who is choking. You can use it on yourself or someone else. If someone is choking and cannot breathe because food is blocking his or her airway, the Heimlich maneuver can be used to dislodge the food. Caregivers and the person with MS should be familiar with this intervention. The Heimlich maneuver should *not* be performed if the person is coughing, speaking, or breathing. If the person cannot cough, speak, or breathe, proceed as follows:

1. Stand behind the choking person and wrap your arms around his or her waist. Bend the person slightly forward.

2. Make a fist with one hand and place it slightly above the person's navel.
3. Grasp your fist with the other hand and press hard into the abdomen with a quick, upward thrust. Repeat this procedure until the object is expelled from the airway.

If you must perform this maneuver on yourself, position your own fist slightly above your navel. Grasp your fist with your other hand and thrust upward into your abdomen until the object is expelled.

If a person with MS requires the Heimlich maneuver, he or she is in need of a swallowing evaluation.

Can you give me some simple ways to make my swallowing better?

Because multiple sclerosis varies so much from one person to another, swallowing problems caused by multiple sclerosis also vary greatly. There is no single way to improve the swallow for everyone. In fact, any universal suggestions could be dangerous for some individuals. Therefore, the best way to manage your swallowing problem is to have a detailed evaluation of your swallowing and let a speech-language pathologist devise a therapy program for your particular swallowing problems.

I have been told to cut my food into very small pieces (or put it through a blender) and thicken all the liquids I drink because I am coughing or choking more often. The problem still seems to be getting worse. What will happen if I can't solve the choking problem?

If you cannot solve the choking problem with therapy, modified swallowing techniques, or changes in the consistency of your food, your doctor may recommend that you begin nonoral (not by mouth) feedings. Frequent coughing or choking is an indication that you may be aspirating food or liquids into your lungs, which can, in turn, increase your risk of getting pneumonia. In addition to the increased risk of aspiration and pneumonia, severe swallowing problems may deprive you of adequate nutrition and fluids. People who find it too tiring to eat properly, or whose eating is frequently interrupted by bouts of coughing or choking, may not be able to eat or drink sufficient amounts to maintain their weight. Your doctor may recommend nonoral feedings in order to ensure that you get adequate nutrition and liquids.

There are two basic types of nonoral feeding that allow food and liquids to be taken into the body without being swallowed. A *nasogastric tube* (that goes through the nose and throat and into the esophagus and stomach) is typically used on a very temporary basis (following surgery, for example) when the person is expected to be able to resume eating by mouth within a few days or weeks. The nasogastric tube can be irritating to the nose and throat if left in for a prolonged period. A *percutaneous endoscopic gastrostomy (PEG)* is used if nonoral feedings are likely to be needed for a longer time. The PEG involves the insertion of a feeding tube through the abdominal wall directly into the stomach. In this relatively simple bedside procedure, an endoscope (a special instrument designed to illuminate the inside of an internal organ) guides the placement of the tube through a tiny incision in the stomach wall. The tube remains in place as long as nonoral feeding is necessary, and a special dietary formula is pumped into the tube on a scheduled basis.

Both types of nonoral feeding tubes can be removed when and if your swallowing improves. Therefore, if your doctor recommends that you begin nonoral feedings, you do not have to feel that you are making a permanent decision. You can choose to have the feeding tube removed at any time. Keep in mind that being well-nourished and getting adequate liquids are important for maintaining your strength. Losing weight and getting weaker can, by themselves, cause swallowing problems, and your chances of regaining your swallowing abilities are better when you are strong and well-nourished. So, while it can be a big decision to take some or all nutrition and fluids by tube, that decision may help you to recover improved swallowing later. Do not put off taking good nutrition and liquids by nonoral means if your physician recommends them.

If I do start nonoral feeding, does that mean that I can never eat any food by mouth?

No. Even with nonoral feeding, you may be able to take certain kinds of foods by mouth. This will generally depend on the nature of your swallowing problem and the thickness of the foods you want to eat. Many individuals take nonoral tube feeding for part of their nutritional needs and eat certain foods orally. Sometimes people can safely and efficiently swallow some types of food but not others. If you are safely able to chew and swallow foods of a certain thickness or consistency, you will be given a list of foods that are safe for you to eat by mouth and the kinds of foods you should be sure to avoid. Generally, if you are able to manage one or two consistencies of food, your speech-language pathologist or physician will try to keep you eating those types of food by mouth. However, you may need total nonoral feeding if you are having difficulty swallowing all types of foods and liquids.

If I need to have a PEG now, does that mean I will always have to have one?

No. You may only need a PEG for a few months. If your swallowing improves due to swallowing therapy or a remission in the disease, your physician will probably recommend that you resume eating by mouth at least some of the time. If you have no further difficulties with swallowing, the PEG can be removed. It is important that you pay attention to your swallowing ability and report changes or improvements to your physician and speech-language pathologist. A reevaluation of your swallowing, probably including a repeat videofluoroscopy, will indicate whether or not it is safe for the PEG to be removed.

Is there any cure for my swallowing problems or will they just keep getting worse?

Some people with MS experience swallowing problems that gradually worsen over time. Others have a temporary problem with swallowing that gradually improves to the point that they can eat efficiently and safely by mouth. Once improved, the swallowing problems may or may not return. Your best strategy is to see your physician and speech-language pathologist any time you feel that your swallowing has changed so that they can provide you with the best kinds of exercises and management.

Recommended Readings

Groher ME. *Dysphagia: Diagnosis and Management.* Boston: Butterworth Publishers, 1984.

Jone, GW, Feldmann MC, Ireland JV, Reinhart R, Yozwiak A. *Dysphagia: A Manual for Use by Families.* Austin, TX: Pro-Ed, 1994.

Logemann JA. *Evaluation and Treatment of Swallowing Disorders (2nd edition).* Austin, TX: Pro-Ed, 1998.

Logemann JA. *Swallowing Problems: How Can They be Identified, Evaluated, and Treated: A Caregiver's Manual.* Menu Magic/ASHA, 1991.

Logemann JA. *A Professional's Guide to Swallowing Disorders.* Menu Magic/ASHA, 1992.

Schapiro, RT. *Symptom Management in Multiple Sclerosis (3rd edition).* New York: Demos Medical Publishing, 1998.

Recommended Websites

Mayo Foundation for Health Education and Research. First Aid: The Heimlich Maneuver. Mayo Website, 1999 (*http://209.67.220.19/mayo/firstaid/httm/fa5d.htm*).

NYLCare. Mastering the Heimlich Maneuver. NYLCare Website, 1999. (*http://www.nylcare.com/mchtak.html*)

9

Cognition

Nicholas G. LaRocca, Ph.D.
Pam Sorensen, M.A., C.C.C.-SLP
Jill Fischer, Ph.D.

Cognition refers to a variety of high-level functions carried out by the human brain. These include our ability to:

◇ understand and use language;
◇ accurately recognize objects (*visual perception*) and use these perceptions to draw, assemble things, and find our way around (*visual construction*);
◇ perform calculations;
◇ focus, maintain, and shift our attention as needed even when information is coming at us very rapidly (*information processing*);
◇ learn and remember information (*memory*); and
◇ perform complex tasks such as planning and carrying out activities in the proper order, solving problems, and monitoring our own behavior (*executive functions*).

It was believed for many years, even by MS specialists, that the disease rarely caused changes in cognitive function. Such changes were thought to occur only in the late stages of MS, if at all. Based on a number of research studies published since the early 1980s, however, it is clear that **cognitive impairment** is quite common in MS. The results of several large-scale, controlled studies suggest that approximately half of all people with MS experience changes in their cognitive function. Not surprisingly, cognitive impairment can have a profound effect on a person's ability to perform important daily activities related to work, social interactions, driving, preparing a simple meal, or even taking care of personal hygiene.

Just as MS can vary in terms of how it affects a person physically, there is considerable variability in the cognitive symptoms of MS. Some people experience cognitive changes as one of their earliest MS symptoms, while others who have had MS for many years may have no cognitive deficits at all. Typically, MS affects only some cognitive functions, while others remain relatively intact. Both research and clinical experience suggest that memory impairment is the most common cognitive symptom in MS. However, changes in information processing and executive functions occur nearly as often. Visuospatial deficits (i.e., impairment in visual perception and constructional abilities) are seen less frequently. Changes in calculation ability are relatively uncommon in MS, but a person may have difficulty doing activities involving calculation (such as balancing a checkbook) due to deficits in information processing, problem solving or organization.

Cognitive-based communication problems may also be seen in MS. Changes in the ability to comprehend or use high-level language skills, can result from problems with attention, speed and capacity of information processing, planning, reasoning, and self-monitoring. A person with MS may have difficulty comprehending information (either heard or read) that is too complex or presented too rapidly. Distractions in the environment can also interfere with comprehension of incoming information. A person may experience difficulty formulating thoughts and retrieving specific words to express ideas either verbally or in writing. While these problems are typically mild and tend to go unnoticed by most, they can at times interfere with communication at home, work, or in the community.

Cognitive dysfunction is only weakly related to disease course and duration of multiple sclerosis. In other words, a person can experience cognitive changes at any point over the course or the disease, regardless of the severity of his or her physical symptoms. At present, the best predictor of cognitive status appears to be brain MRI (*magnetic resonance imaging*). In general, the greater the number and the more extensive the *lesions* that can be seen on a person's brain MRI, the greater the likelihood that there will be changes in his or her cognitive function. However, this "rule of thumb" is imperfect. Cognitive impairment can be present even if few lesions are visible on MRI; conversely, some people whose MRIs show many MS lesions have few measurable cognitive deficits. Recent studies have shown that MS demyelinating lesions can be accompanied by *axonal loss* and *brain atrophy* even early in the course of the disease. These recent findings underscore the fact that deficits in cognitive abilities related to significant changes in the brain can occur at any time during the course of MS.

The location of MS lesions is also an important predictor of their effects on a person's function. Most MS lesions tend to cluster in the white matter around the fluid-filled ventricles in the brain (the *periventricular region*) and the bundle of fibers connecting the two cerebral hemispheres, the *corpus callosum*. This area of the brain is involved in those cognitive functions that are most susceptible to impairment in MS, including memory, information processing, and executive functions. However, isolated lesions can appear anywhere in the white matter or at the junction of the white and gray matter. Some of these may be in so-called "silent regions" of the brain and therefore have relatively little impact on cognitive function. Others may be located in very important brain regions, in which case a relatively small lesion may produce a striking cognitive deficit. Consequently, the only reliable way of determining whether a person has experienced cognitive changes due to MS is through the objective assessment of cognitive function. An objective assessment of the type and severity of cognitive involvement can then be used to guide treatment recommendations.

Cognitive function can be assessed using an extensive "battery" of tests. This type of assessment is typically carried out by a *neuropsychologist*, a *speech/language pathologist*, or an *occupational therapist*. While these specialists have somewhat different approaches to the assessment of cognitive impairment, and utilize different types of tests, their common goal is to identify changes in cognitive function that interfere with everyday

life. Most major medical centers and many **rehabilitation** facilities have qualified specialists in these areas. Evaluations of
cognitive function typically involve an interview and several
hours of testing because the functions being tested are quite
complex.

In order to determine whether a person's cognitive function
has changed as a result of MS, the examiner compares the individual's test performance with that of healthy adults who are
similar in terms of age, education, and other factors that can
affect test performance. If no changes have occurred, the individual's test performance should be comparable to that of this
reference, or normative, group. In general, the lower one's test
performance relative to these norms, the more severe the impairment in that particular cognitive function. Unless there are other
factors that could reasonably explain identified deficits, it is
assumed that they are attributable to MS.

Cognitive rehabilitation refers to techniques designed to
improve the functioning of people who have cognitive impairment due to MS and other central nervous system disorders.
Most of these techniques were developed for patients with acute
changes in their cognitive function due to traumatic brain injury
or stroke, but many are applicable to MS. Cognitive rehabilitation may be offered by different types of health care professionals, including neuropsychologists, speech/language pathologists, and occupational therapists.

There are two primary types of cognitive rehabilitation strategies, one aimed at restoring a function, the other focusing on
strategies to compensate for a deficit. Restorative strategies are
designed to improve the impaired function directly through
repetitive drills and practice. Examples of this would include
memory retraining strategies based on repetitive list-learning, or
attention retraining strategies based on practice and mastery of
progressively more challenging exercises. In contrast, compensatory strategies assume that the impaired function will not
improve. Consequently, the person is taught to compensate for
identified deficits through the use of such strategies as visual
imagery, techniques for minimizing distractions, or the use of a
personal organizer. The ultimate aim of any cognitive rehabilitation technique is to improve a person's ability to function as
independently and safely in his or daily activities as possible, in
spite of cognitive impairment.

Assessment

My wife and children keep telling me that I'm becoming forgetful. How can I tell if MS has affected my memory?

Unfortunately, people are often inaccurate in judging their own cognitive function. Those who are extremely distressed (depressed or anxious) are more likely to believe that their memory is worse than it actually is or to believe that they are having problems with many cognitive functions when they may only have deficits in one or two areas. Conversely, others may be unable to acknowledge their cognitive deficits because it is too emotionally painful for them to accept that MS can affect cognitive as well as physical function. Finally, individuals with extensive cognitive impairment may have only limited awareness of their deficits because they have lost the ability to monitor their behavior and performance.

The perceptions of family members and close friends can also be inaccurate. To be fair, subtle cognitive deficits are often hard to detect in the course of normal social interactions, even for experts. However, relatives and friends sometimes observe cognitive symptoms and misinterpret them as indications of "depression," "disinterest," or "laziness." Family members may be aware of cognitive deficits but feel reluctant to acknowledge them for fear that these deficits would require changes on their part (for example, in the distribution of household responsibilities). Conversely, some relatives and friends may become overly vigilant, interpreting even the most infrequent memory lapse as something abnormal, and therefore caused by MS.

An objective assessment can help determine whether cognitive impairment is present and, if so, its nature and extent. It often includes tests that measure specific areas typically affected by MS, such as attention, new learning, memory, information processing, word retrieval, verbal fluency, reasoning, and executive functions. Complex reading, writing, and other communication skills may also be examined. A psychological assessment of patient and family interactions can also yield helpful information. Such an in-depth assessment can lead to recommendations regarding treatments for underlying or related problems, be they cognitive, emotional, interpersonal, or some combination of these.

Can I be tested for cognitive problems while I'm taking medications? Can medications affect the way my memory works and therefore alter the test results?

The interpretation of test results is simpler if a person is not taking medications because there are no medication effects to confound or confuse those results. While you do not need to stop taking most medications in order to be evaluated, it is important to tell the examiner what drugs you are on and their dosages. This knowledge will enhance the examiner's ability to interpret the test results.

Many medications, such as antibiotics and medications used to treat spasticity and bladder problems in MS, have no known effects on the *central nervous system*, and therefore do not affect a person's cognitive function. Other medications, such as some that are used to treat hypertension and depression, have subtle effects on the performance of certain neuropsychological tests. However, the effects of these medications are small relative to the effects of MS, and the conditions for which they are prescribed can affect cognitive function as well.

Medications that pose the greatest problems for test interpretation are those which have known central nervous system effects. These include medications with sedative properties, such as tranquilizers and certain pain medications, and some treatments for MS exacerbations, such as methylprednisolone. If at all possible, a person should be tapered off these medications prior to cognitive assessment so that they do not confound the test interpretation.

Sometimes my memory and thinking seem much better than at other times. When I'm tired, my memory seems even worse than usual. Can fatigue affect cognitive function?

Many people with MS report that memory and other cognitive functions seem to fluctuate, getting worse in periods of increased sleepiness, fatigue, or stress. This is true of everyone, whether or not they have MS. However, this is a bigger issue for people with MS since they are at greater risk for disabling fatigue. The limited research available on fatigue and cognitive function suggests that fatigue affects cognitive test performance to a lesser extent than even MS experts would have predicted. However, if you find that fatigue adversely affects your memory, try to plan your activities in such a way that you use the times you are least fatigued to do your most demanding work. Place fewer demands on your memory at times when you are most likely to be fatigued. It is also important that you keep in mind that the adverse effects of fatigue are temporary and will reverse once you feel more rested—which for most people is within a few hours. You should also become familiar with the options available for managing your fatigue, such as regular aerobic exercise (see Chapter 5), energy conservation and work simplification techniques (see Chapter 6), and medications such as amantadine, pemoline (Cylert®), and fluoxetine (Prozac®) (see Chapter 2).

Does heat affect cognitive symptoms?

Many people with MS report that heat can adversely affect all of their symptoms, including cognitive function. This may be due in part to the fatigue that can result from prolonged exposure to high temperatures. Unfortunately, there have been no research studies on the effects of temperature changes on cognitive function in MS. Preliminary research suggests that cooling suits, vests, or cold baths may enhance certain physical abilities in persons with MS, at least for a few hours. These benefits have not as yet been clearly documented for cognitive abilities. Whatever the effects of heat and cooling on cognitive function, these effects are transient and will pass in a few hours. You may find that you feel better in general, and as a result think more clearly, if you stay out of the heat.

I know that there can be exacerbations and remissions of physical symptoms in MS. Are there exacerbations and remissions in cognitive symptoms?

Although there has been no formal research on cognitive **exacerbations** and **remissions**, it has been observed clinically that cognitive function may get worse during an exacerbation and improve during remission. In rare cases, cognitive function can become dramatically worse in a very short period of time and then may gradually improve. These dramatic changes are most likely the result of an **acute** inflammatory process. When MS is active, there is swelling in the central nervous system as the immune system attacks **myelin** and a person's symptoms are at their worst. As this acute stage nears its end, people often notice improvement in their symptoms. This process generally runs its course in a matter of weeks at most. If cognitive impairment has developed gradually and been present for months or years, it is unlikely to improve substantially on its own.

Recent tests by a neuropsychologist indicated some problems with my memory and concentration. Will my cognitive problems get worse?

Unfortunately, relatively little is known about the course of cognitive impairment in MS. Some recent longitudinal studies suggest that MS-related cognitive impairment may be more stable over time than physical disability, or at least may progress at a slower rate. Although cognitive problems are unlikely to remit, rapid deterioration is also rare. This is one of the reasons why there is increasing interest in the use of rehabilitative strategies for improving or compensating for cognitive deficits in people with MS. If, over the course of the next year or two, you notice that you are having more problems with your memory or concentration or new cognitive problems appear, you may find it worthwhile to be reassessed neuropsychologically to determine if there have been any objective changes in your cognitive function.

Do cognitive symptoms ever occur before physical symptoms in a person with MS?

Although physical symptoms are usually the first clue that a person has MS, there have been instances in which changes in cognitive function were the first observable MS symptom. Likewise, after a person has been diagnosed with MS, cognitive changes may signal disease activity before new physical symptoms develop. To the surprise of many MS experts, there is only a weak relationship between cognitive impairment and physical disability. A person with very little physical disability may have striking cognitive deficits, while one with severe physical disability may be intact cognitively. Although there is some evidence to suggest that cognitive impairment may be more common in those whose MS is following a progressive course, there are many exceptions to this rule. In short, knowing the extent of someone's physical disability tells you very little about that person's cognitive status.

Why am I able to remember things that I knew a long time ago better than things that just happened recently?

People use the term *memory* to refer to a number of cognitive processes that are actually quite different. MS is much more likely to interfere with a person's ability to lay down new memories than with the ability to summon up old ones from the distant past. This is because the processing of new information is often slowed in MS, making it more difficult to consolidate the new information in a meaningful way. Thus, you may be able to recall your high school years or your first job (drawing on your **remote memory**) much more readily than what occurred in a meeting you attended yesterday (**recent memory**) or at breakfast when you agreed to stop at the grocery store on the way home from work (**prospective memory**). This can be particularly puzzling to friends and family members, who may misinterpret this as a sign that you do not care enough to remember details of shared conversations or activities. However, once these memory problems are understood as a symptom of MS, a number of strategies can be used to help manage or compensate for them.

How are MS-related cognitive problems different from those in Alzheimer's disease?

MS-related cognitive problems differ from those in Alzheimer's disease in several important respects. Cognitive impairment is the *primary* symptom in Alzheimer's disease, whereas not everyone with MS experiences changes in cognitive function. This difference results from the fact that Alzheimer's is a disease of the brain characterized by dramatic changes in, and loss of, nerve cells (**neurons**) in the "gray matter" of the brain (**cortex**), while MS is a disease that primarily involves the white matter in the brain, optic nerve, and spinal cord (central nervous system). Although MS produces some loss of neurons and damage to the cortex, these effects are much less extensive than those observed in Alzheimer's disease. A diagnosis of Alzheimer's disease requires impairment of at least two cognitive functions, one of which must be memory, with progressive worsening of these functions over time. Even in its early stages, Alzheimer's disease typically involves severe impairment of memory (both recent and remote) and breakdown of language (primarily comprehension and word retrieval), as well as possible visuospatial deficits.

Ultimately, a person with Alzheimer's disease loses the ability to recognize family and friends and to perform even the most basic personal care. In contrast, MS exerts selective effects on cognitive function, typically involving recent memory, information processing, and/or executive functions. Furthermore, MS-related cognitive impairment appears to be relatively stable over time, so that a person may be able to function quite effectively for many years, given appropriate cognitive rehabilitation.

Can cognitive impairment affect my driving ability?

Driving is a very complex task, requiring integration of visual-motor and cognitive-perceptual skills. It involves understanding and following directions, planning and remembering a route, multitasking (i.e., doing more than one thing at a time), safe decision-making, and quick response time. There have been no formal studies of the effects of cognitive impairment on driving in MS. Based on clinical experience and the few studies that have been done in other patient populations, your driving ability may well be impaired if MS has affected your information processing, visuospatial abilities, and executive functions. Often, a person who is aware of having these deficits voluntarily restricts his or her driving or stops driving entirely. However, because driving is a major source of personal independence, this is often a difficult decision to make.

Unfortunately, the procedures used by state departments of motor vehicles are not designed to detect driving problems related to cognitive impairment, so a person's license may be renewed even if he or she is unsafe to drive. If you are concerned about your driving, the best approach would be to obtain an objective driver's evaluation (often done by an occupational therapist with specialized training) and a cognitive assessment so that you can find out the impact of both physical and cognitive symptoms of MS on your driving. Many major medical centers and rehabilitation facilities offer these services; your local chapter of the National Multiple Sclerosis Society can help you locate the one closest to you.

I know that I have begun experiencing some changes in my thinking and memory. What is the best way to explain these changes to my family and friends? People always seem to say "Oh, the same thing happens to me all the time—I can't remember a thing!"

Well-meaning family and friends often try to reassure a person by saying that they have a similar problem with memory or word-finding. This can be frustrating when you are trying to explain your MS symptoms and request their help. You can try explaining to them that, although you may have experienced some of these problems before you had MS, your cognitive problems are different now and much worse. Explain to them that these are a direct result of your MS, much like your physical symptoms. If you have had a cognitive assessment of some kind, you may want to share the results of that assessment with them so that they can begin to understand how MS-related memory problems are different from everyday forgetting. You may want to set up a family meeting with a psychologist, social worker, or speech/language pathologist who is knowledgeable about cognitive problems in MS, and can explain them to your family and friends. You might also want to include family members in the problem-solving portion of your cognitive rehabilitation sessions. Then you can work together to develop strategies to help you function better. Such strategies might include using a family calendar to keep track of appointments and social events, designating a specific place to store commonly used household objects, and speaking one at a time so that you can take in information more effectively.

How can I explain my cognitive problems to my children?

Children vary in their need to know about your illness, depending on their ages and the seriousness of your MS. They are usually able to take cognitive changes in stride as long as they understand that these are symptoms of MS, and the changes do not interfere too drastically with the flow of everyday life. Children will probably be more upset by your distress over these problems (especially if you are angry and irritable) than by the cognitive problems themselves. A matter-of-fact explanation is probably best, using words such as "MS has affected the way my brain works, just like it has affected my walking." Children may ask if this means that you are "stupid" or "crazy." The answer, of course, is that this is *not* the case.

Be open to questions, but avoid flooding your child with too much information. Younger children may need to be reassured that you are going to be okay and that what is happening is not their fault, while adolescents may need to be reminded that they should not take advantage of your memory problems (or any other symptom of your MS). If your cognitive problems are a major source of distress for your children, or if you find it too difficult to discuss these problems with them, you may want to seek professional help from a psychologist, social worker, or cognitive rehabilitation specialist. One or two family meetings is often enough to ease the way for better family communication about these problems.

Should I discuss my cognitive problems with my supervisor at work?

There is no easy answer to this question. Like the decision to disclose the diagnosis of MS, the decision to inform your supervisor that you have cognitive problems due to your MS is complex. One approach is to disclose the information on a "need to know" basis. There may be little reason to tell your supervisor if you have some mild memory problems for which you have effective compensatory strategies and which do not affect your job performance. On the other hand, if your work is beginning to suffer because of your cognitive changes, it may be to your advantage to set up a meeting to talk frankly with your supervisor. Otherwise, any problems with your performance could be misinterpreted as lack of motivation, sloppiness, or a host of other incorrect factors. People often fear that revealing the presence of cognitive symptoms may be a "kiss of death," stigmatizing them as impaired and incompetent. Such fears are generally unfounded; however, it is important to take into account your unique situation and the atmosphere of your workplace.

Many people find it helpful to work with a cognitive rehabilitation specialist or *vocational rehabilitation* counselor familiar with the cognitive symptoms of MS. A formal evaluation, including an assessment of the cognitive and communication requirements of your job tasks, can guide the rehabilitation process. Take the time to become familiar with the compliance guidelines of the Americans with Disabilities Act (ADA) concerning cognitive and communication disorders (see Chapter 14). Then, the rehabilitation or vocational specialist can meet with you and your supervisor to identify ways in which your job tasks or your work environment can be modified to enhance your effectiveness on the job. During the meeting with your supervisor to discuss the cognitive changes caused by your MS, be sure to emphasize your track record and strengths. Try to engage your supervisor in problem-solving about how you and your work environment could adapt to accommodate these changes.

My wife, who has MS, seems to be forgetting a lot lately. What is the best way to talk to her about this?

Family members are often reluctant to bring up concerns about memory or other cognitive problems with a person who has MS for fear that it will be upsetting. Often, however, it is a great relief to the person with MS when these concerns are raised because he or she can stop pretending that everything is okay. This can also open the door to a constructive discussion of ways that the person with MS and the family can adapt so that these problems do not "snowball" and cause major disruptions in family functioning.

You should plan to raise your concerns about your wife's memory at a time of day when you and she are well-rested, will not be interrupted, and will have plenty of time to talk things over. You may want to start out by asking her how MS has been affecting her recently to see whether she brings up concerns about her memory. If she does, you could offer your own observations and then talk about getting an objective memory assessment and recommendations about what can be done. If she does not mention memory problems on her own, you could offer some recent examples and then ask her whether she thinks MS could be affecting her memory. You might want to add your observations about how these memory lapses have affected her, as well as how they have affected you and other family members, and suggest that she undergo cognitive assessment to sort things out.

If your wife becomes irritated or defensive when you bring this up the first time, it is probably best to drop it and try again at another time. If you get a similar response the next time, it may be wise to call and inform her physician of your concerns so that he or she can raise the issue and recommend appropriate assessment. Memory problems can have several different causes, many of them treatable or amenable to rehabilitation once they have been properly assessed.

I have MS and memory problems. I am also experiencing symptoms of menopause. My friends who are also going through menopause tell me that they have lots of memory problems and that hormone replacement therapy can help. Can hormones help with my memory problems?

Approximately half the MS population is over 50, and two-thirds are women. The net result is that there are a lot of people with MS who are entering or in menopause. Because cognitive changes are known to accompany menopause, women with MS have a dual risk for memory problems. Hormone replacement therapy can have some benefits for menopause-related memory deficits. However, there are no studies documenting whether these benefits carry over into the MS population. Moreover, it may be very difficult to sort out whether certain deficits are related to MS, or to menopause, or to a combination of the two. Hormone replacement therapy is a complex and controversial intervention intended to address a number of the changes brought on by menopause. It would probably be a good idea to discusst the pros and cons of hormone replacement therapy with your primary care physician and your neurologist. In the meantime, you and your friends might find it useful to share strategies you have developed to deal with your day-to-day memory demands.

Treatment and Rehabilitation

Are there any medications to treat cognitive deficits?

At present, there are no medications that are generally accepted as improving cognitive function in MS. Physostigmine, a medication that was originally used experimentally in Alzheimer's disease, proved to be of some benefit in a pilot study with a small number of people with MS. However, the beneficial effects were seen on only a few memory measures and were not evident to family members who rated the person's everyday memory performance. A related medication, Aricept®, has been approved by the FDA for the treatment of memory disorders in Alzheimer's disease. There have been some positive anecdotal reports concerning Aricept® as a treatment for memory problems in MS. Preliminary studies of Aricept® in MS are underway, but no results have been reported thus far. There is a rationale in Alzheimer's disease for the use of medications such as physostigmine and Aricept® that increase the availability of a neurotransmitter called acetylcholine. Acetylcholine is thought to be important in memory processes and to be reduced in persons with Alzheimer's disease. However, there is no such rationale for their use in MS.

A different type of medication, pemoline (Cylert®), a psychostimulant that has been used to treat fatigue in MS (see Chapter 2 and Appendix B), is currently being studied to determine its effectiveness in treating MS-related information processing deficits. Results of this trial are not yet available. Another medication used to treat fatigue, amantadine, was shown to have some beneficial effects on information processing in persons with MS suffering from fatigue. A substance called 4-aminopyridine (4-AP), that is thought to improve nerve conduction, has also been shown to have modest effects on some neuropsychological measures. However, 4-AP is short-acting, has some problematic side-effects, and is not readily available (see Chapter 3). In the short run, rehabilitative strategies are the most promising method for improving the daily functioning of a person with MS-related cognitive problems.

Are the disease-modifying drugs effective against cognitive deficits?

The studies completed thus far of the various disease-modifying agents have not focused primarily on cognitive dysfunction. Cognitive function has only been examined by secondary outcome measures in such studies. Moreover, the people participating in these drug trials did not necessarily have any cognitive dysfunction; they were included based on the physical effects of their MS. As a result, the major clinical trials of disease-modifying agents have not been particularly sensitive tests of their effectiveness against cognitive dysfunction. Nevertheless, a few studies have indicated that some of the disease-modifying agents provide modest benefit compared to placebo in slowing the progression of cognitive dysfunction. There is some reason to believe that the disease-modifying drugs may be even more helpful for cognition than these limited results suggest. Avonex®, Betaseron®, and Copaxone® have all been shown to slow the development of new lesions on MRI. Since cognitive dysfunction is related to lesion number and volume, limiting new lesions should be beneficial for cognition over the long term. More recent clinical trials have been paying greater attention to cognitive changes and have used more sophisticated neuropsychological testing. As we learn more about the long-term effects of these medications with different populations, we will hope to obtain a clearer answer to your question.

On the World Wide Web I read that ginkgo biloba can improve memory. Can it help with my MS memory problems?

Ginkgo biloba is a dry extract made from the leaves of the ginkgo tree. The tree is a native of China, Japan, and Korea but is cultivated for ornamental purposes in many American cities because of its hardiness. It appears to have a variety of effects including reduction in cerebral edema (swelling), enhancement of the brain's ability to utilize certain neurotransmitters, and thinning of the blood. It has been shown to improve concentration and memory in patients suffering from peripheral arterial occlusive disease (a condition unrelated to MS in which certain parts of the brain experience a reduced blood supply because of partial blockage of arteries). There are no studies demonstrating any value of ginkgo biloba in MS and there is no evidence that arterial occlusion plays any role in MS.

Ginkgo biloba and other "natural" remedies are readily available in health-food and vitamin stores. It is often difficult to determine how standardized the dose of the active ingredients is in such products and many have been found to have impurities. In addition, many natural preparations may have unintended side-effects. Before taking any drug, dietary supplement, herbal treatment, or natural remedy, it is important to discuss your plan with you physician. Over-the-counter products can be dangerous and should be approached with care.

I would like to see if cognitive rehabilitation can help me with my memory problems. How can I find out where to get this type of treatment?

Cognitive rehabilitation by a neuropsychologist, speech/language pathologist, and/or occupational therapist may be offered at a comprehensive MS center, an outpatient rehabilitation facility, or by individual practitioners. It is preferable for the specialists to have experience in evaluation and treatment of mild cognitive impairment due to MS or other similar neurological conditions such as brain injury. Your physician or the local chapter of the MS Society can often refer you to such a facility or to individual practitioners in your area who have expertise in MS.

Depending on the cognitive rehabilitation specialist's assessment of your particular needs, one of three general approaches might be recommended:

1. a *general stimulation approach*, in which activities such as listening to stories and playing word games encourage cognitive processing at several levels;
2. a *process-specific approach*, in which a specific cognitive function is targeted for intervention through a hierarchical series of successively more difficult exercises; or
3. a *functional adaptation approach*, in which rehabilitation is performed in your own home or work environment.

Thus, some approaches to cognitive rehabilitation are very focused while others are part of a broader rehabilitative approach that may also include psychological counseling and other types of therapies. The cognitive rehabilitation specialist should give you the rationale for the approach that he or she recommends, as well as an estimate of what kind of results to expect and how many sessions this will take. Unfortunately, there are currently no published studies of cognitive rehabilitation in MS, so the clinical experience of the cognitive rehabilitation specialist is very important.

If cognitive rehabilitation is done by neuropsychologists, speech/language pathologists, and occupational therapists, how do I know which type of professional I should see?

Neuropsychologists became involved in cognitive assessment and retraining because of their interest in brain-behavior relationships. Speech/language pathologists offer cognitive rehabilitation because of their expertise in language- and communication-related problems. Occupational therapists direct their rehabilitation efforts at reducing the impact of cognitive impairment on a person's ability to carry out daily activities at home, work and in the community. For example, preparing a meal is a more cognitively complex activity than many realize. While each of these professionals brings to the rehabilitation process a somewhat different set of assessment tools and treatment strategies, they share a common goal of enabling people with MS to function comfortably and successfully in everyday life.

The type of professional you see for cognitive rehabilitation will probably be determined by the availability of these service providers in your area. Your physician will be able to refer you to the nearest agencies or individuals with expertise in cognitive rehabilitation in MS or other similar conditions such as brain injury. If you have the luxury of choice, you might want to discuss your situation with the available professionals and decide which individual(s) and which treatment approach(es) seem best suited to your particular needs and personality style. Ideally, an interdisciplinary team of professionals can work together toward your common goals, bringing different perspectives to the process.

How long will cognitive rehabilitation take?

There is no standard time frame for cognitive rehabilitation. Its duration will depend on the nature and severity of your cognitive problems. Cognitive rehabilitation techniques were originally developed in inpatient settings where sessions occurred daily or even more than once a day. Many of these techniques have been adapted for use in outpatient settings, with sessions occurring at least once a week (but preferably more often, to improve carryover) for several months.

You and your cognitive rehabilitation specialist should periodically review your progress together in order to revise or set new goals as needed. When you have achieved the goals you set, it is often a good idea to taper the frequency of cognitive rehabilitation sessions (i.e., gradually increase the length of time between sessions) rather than discontinuing them abruptly. Scheduling "booster sessions," much like dental checkups, can also help ensure that you continue to apply the techniques you have learned and identify any new problems before they become too disruptive. These periodic re-evaluations allow for updates of your therapy goals and revisions of your home-based practice program.

Can cognitive rehabilitation help me even if my memory and concentration are slowly getting worse?

Yes. Cognitive rehabilitation is designed to maximize your cognitive function and develop long-term strategies to compensate for functions that are not likely to respond to restorative treatments. In the course of cognitive rehabilitation, you will learn skills that you can use now and in the future, even if your problems get worse. In fact, there is probably some advantage to learning these skills early on, when it may be easier to assimilate them. For example, you may learn strategies for better regulating your attention and limiting environmental distractions—techniques that you can continue to apply if your concentration problems get worse. Or you may learn how to use an organizer notebook to record appointments, phone numbers, and things you need to remember to do. If your memory problems get worse, you can still use this notebook and perhaps add new sections, such as a diary in which to record the major events of the day so that you can review them at a later time. If your cognitive problems get worse or new problems arise, you may want to return to your cognitive rehabilitation specialist to review how you can get the most out of methods you learned in the past and identify new strategies that may be useful to you.

A friend told me that by changing the magnetic fields in my brain, my thinking and memory could be improved. Is that true and where would I go to get such treatment?

There has been increasing interest in recent years in "energy fields" and their effects on human health. Some people have hypothesized that physical and psychological symptoms can be caused by an imbalance in a person's energy fields. While it is true that in many neurologic disorders there are abnormalities in the electrical signals emanating from the brain (as measured on an *EEG)*, it is unclear how this relates to the concept of energy fields. At present, the concept of energy fields, and trying to put them into balance, is on the periphery of science. Solid research is lacking and there is no evidence to date that any technique related to the manipulation of magnetic fields or energy fields has any beneficial effects on cognition in MS.

My children keep accusing me of forgetting things that they have told me. Sometimes I remember these things once they remind me, but other times I don't recall them saying these things at all. I'm starting to wonder if they are telling the truth. How can we deal with this problem?

The first step in coming up with effective solutions is to obtain a thorough assessment of the problem. In a situation like this, it is important not only for you to have an objective cognitive assessment, but also for your family to meet with a social worker, psychologist, or other health care professional familiar with MS-related cognitive problems and their potential impact on family relationships.

If it turns out that you do have some identifiable cognitive problems, a cognitive rehabilitation specialist can work with you and your family to identify the circumstances under which these problems are most likely to occur and to modify them. For example, if your children are trying to talk with you while the television is on or while there is another conversation going on in the room, the cognitive rehabilitation specialist may suggest that the television be turned off during these discussions or that you and your child seek a quieter, less distracting place to talk. If you are having trouble remembering where your children have said they were going, the cognitive rehabilitation specialist may suggest a family "memo board" in a central location for everyone to record where they have gone and when they will be back. Often very simple changes can make a world of difference.

In some situations, however, cognitive changes are only a minor factor, and the real difficulty is an underlying family problem that has been present for some time. In such cases, working with a social worker or psychologist to address the underlying family problem is critical.

Recently I've noticed that I have a lot of trouble concentrating or following conversations, particularly when there is something else going on in the room. Is there anything that I can do about this problem?

It is not uncommon with MS to have difficulty ignoring background noise or distractions and, as a result, to have difficulty following social conversations. The ability to pay attention selectively to important information (i.e., what the person is saying to you) while ignoring unimportant information (such as other conversations in the room) is one aspect of information processing, often termed "selective attention." A cognitive rehabilitation specialist can work with you to improve this skill, teach you how to compensate for this problem, or both. For example, restorative strategies might include improving your selective attention through a series of gradually more difficult exercises in which you have to ignore competing background messages and attend only to what is important. Compensatory strategies might include learning ways to alter the environment so that it is easier for you to concentrate.

Communication is a cycle of "give and take" between speaker and listener. Some people are embarrassed when they cannot keep up with a conversation, so they nod and pretend they are following it. Others simply find excuses to avoid social situations in which they will be confronted with this problem. However, it is your responsibility and right as a listener to let others know what you need in order to participate successfully in a conversation. There are two ways to regulate input in this type of situation—quieting the background noise or moving away from it. For most people, it will take some practice to feel comfortable making requests such as "I'd appreciate it if you could lower the volume of the TV so that we can continue our conversation" (to quiet the background noise) or "Let's go to a quieter room so that we can talk without being interrupted" (to move away from the noise).

Other types of communication breakdowns may also occur. If you find that too much information is coming too quickly, or is "over your head," you might say one of the following: "Please repeat that—a little slower this time;" "Tell me a little at a time;" "Let's take a break and come back to this later;" "Please explain that in different words or give me an example." Often, when friends or family members understand the difficulties you may be experiencing, they automatically begin to modify their speech. In the long run, it is far better to learn strategies for regulating input than to allow a breakdown in communication.

I used to enjoy reading, but now I find that I have a lot of trouble remembering who the characters are and what the story line is. Are there strategies for dealing with this problem?

Problems with reading can have several different causes. First, reading requires you to see and use your eyes well. Visual problems typical of MS can interfere with the reading process, such as blurriness, double vision (**diplopia**), "jiggly eyes" (**nystagmus**), and difficulty with left-to-right scanning eye movements. Second, reading requires you to concentrate on the written material, understand what you are reading, and remember it later. People with MS report little or no difficulty understanding what they read. However, problems with concentration and memory result in frequent complaints such as "I cannot read for as long as I used to"; "I have to reread it many times"; "When I pick up a book to continue where I left off, I can't remember what I've already read."

A treatment plan can be developed following a thorough evaluation to determine the cause of your reading difficulties. If you have problems with eye movements and coordination, an occupational therapist or behavioral optometrist (an optometrist with additional expertise in eye training) can suggest eye movement exercises that may be helpful. The eye specialist will also make sure that you are fitted with the proper lenses.

If concentration and memory problems interfere with reading, a cognitive rehabilitation specialist may recommend exercises directed at the underlying attention/concentration problem, as well as specialized reading techniques such as the "four R's"— Read, Reread, Reorganize, and Review. The first phase of the "four R's" involves scanning the headings, pictures, and first and last paragraphs (of a newspaper article, for example) to get the "gist" or main idea. This builds a framework within which to organize new information as you then read each paragraph aloud. As you proceed to reread the entire article, it is helpful to highlight the key ideas, make notes, and continually relate the information in the new paragraph to the previous one. The next step is to reorganize the information by putting various elements into your own words, developing opinions, and personalizing the information. Many people find it helpful to reorganize information into the main idea and "Who, What, When, Where, and How" details. Finally, as you review your highlights and notes, it may be beneficial to discuss the information with another person. The goal is to involve as many language modalities as possible (seeing, saying, hearing, and writing it) in order to improve your reading ability. It may take extra time to process information in this fashion, but the likelihood of recalling it later is much greater.

Recently I'm finding that it takes me a very long time to do routine tasks like paying the bills and balancing my checkbook. I even make errors on simple calculations. I don't want to have to ask my husband to do this for me. Is there a solution to this problem?

The skills required for effective money and checkbook management are more complex than most people realize. Not only are adequate vision and hand function important, but a whole host of cognitive skills are involved (e.g., attention to detail, calculation ability, calculator use, organization, sequencing, decision-making, problem-solving, and the ability to follow through and complete an activity). If independence in money and checkbook management is a realistic goal, the cognitive rehabilitation specialist can use treatment strategies such as: devising a monthly budget; developing a flow chart for bill-paying; and teaching you how to avoid checkbook errors by "talking your way through" checkbook entries, and double-checking your work with a calculator. If you are comfortable with the use of a computer, you may be instructed in the use of a money management software program.

If independent money and checkbook management is not a realistic goal, the cognitive rehabilitation specialist can work with you and a family member to develop ways for you to be involved in financial decision-making without the burden of maintaining a checkbook and paying bills. In some communities, banks and special agencies can provide automatic bill-paying services and assistance in reconciling your checkbook with the bank statement on a fee-for-service basis. As always, it is important to have a thorough evaluation of the problem in order to set realistic goals and develop appropriate solutions to problems such as these.

I've been having problems with my memory, managing the household, and keeping track of things I have to do. Would an electronic organizer or computer be helpful to me?

A variety of compensatory aids can help with memory and organizational problems. These include the day planner notebooks that have become so popular in recent years, pocket electronic organizers, and computers. Dictaphones and voice organizers can also be used if problems with hand coordination or weakness are making it too difficult to read or write. Taking time each day to make a "To Do" list, and to check off each task as it's completed, can help keep you organized and on track. Keeping a detailed log of important events, *soon after they happen*, can help you recall them later. Keeping a monthly calendar for appointments, and transferring those appointments to your daily "To Do" list, can help you avoid missing important engagements. Whatever system you choose to develop, keep in mind that it should be small enough to be with you always (so that you can consistently refer and add to it). It should also have all of your important information in it, in order to avoid slips of paper here, there, and everywhere.

The disadvantage of computers and electronic organizers is that learning how to use them can be somewhat complex. However, if you can master their operation, they are among the most powerful tools at your disposal. Pocket electronic organizers can keep track of names and addresses, appointments, and to-do lists. In their more expensive incarnations, they can even send faxes and do word processing. Computers do all these things and more, but are not as portable.

There are also many types of computer software that can assist your memory and organizational efforts. Personal information managers perform most of the functions that loose-leaf organizers can do, but generally also have a powerful database capability. You can type in notes on a given subject, such as "Christmas List," and later do what is called a "random search," in which all your notes on the subject are retrieved, sorted, and presented to you. Money management software can allow you to keep tabs on your checking account and reconcile your bank statement in a matter of minutes, with no need to do any arithmetical computations yourself. If you find that memory problems are requiring you to write yourself a lot of notes or lists, the computer can be invaluable. Large amounts of data can be managed and retrieved using database and/or word processing software. Sometimes relying exclusively on paper can become cumbersome as you begin to accumulate piles of notes, reminders, and other materials.

Electronic organizers and computers are not magic. Like all compensatory strategies, they require learning and practice to make best use of their potential. Working with a cognitive rehabilitation specialist can help you to develop skill and consistency in using these modern marvels. Ideally, your response to MS cognitive changes should involve a comprehensive program that includes individual, social, paper-and-pencil, and electronic strategies. A well-balanced combination of all of these approaches should enable you to deal effectively with many of the cognitive changes brought about by MS.

I have always been an organized person. Now I seem to be having a lot of trouble scheduling my time and estimating how long it will take me to get a job done. Even when I have figured out what I am going to do, I seem to have a lot of trouble getting started. Is there anything that I can do about this problem?

Organizational skills are extremely important for a person's independent functioning; these include goal setting, planning, scheduling, monitoring the progress of a task, and completing tasks in a timely fashion. MS can affect your ability to carry out activities efficiently, causing you to take "detours" along the way or to backtrack in order to take care of a step or two that you inadvertently left out. MS can also cause you to get "stuck" while trying to solve problems that come up in daily life. Problems with these types of executive functions are thought to be due to MS lesions in the white matter connecting the front portion of the brain (*frontal lobes*) with other important brain structures.

Cognitive rehabilitation for problems with executive functions typically has the dual focus of teaching compensatory strategies and identifying environmental modifications. Helpful compensatory strategies might include using structured approaches to analyzing tasks and activities, developing a checklist of steps to follow, setting realistic timetables, using an alarm on your wrist watch to signify when to begin a planned task, and using problem-solving flow sheets. Environmental approaches might include maintaining a consistent daily schedule and involving family members to guide you in planning and problem solving, or to cue you to begin an activity. Generally, the greater your problems with executive functions, the greater the likelihood that the cognitive rehabilitation specialist will emphasize environmental approaches to address them.

My friends and family have started to complain that I interrupt a lot and seem to have trouble waiting until they're finished before I start to speak. I've always disliked people who interrupt a lot and I don't know why I'm doing this. Can I learn to control it?

Conversational problems such as poor listening and interrupting others are referred to as "pragmatic communication deficits." These deficits are thought to be executive dysfunctions caused by MS lesions that affect connections to the frontal lobes. A person who has pragmatic communication problems may be unaware of them or of subtle negative feedback from the listener. Social isolation can be a significant consequence of these communication deficits, because people tend to avoid interacting with those who dominate conversations, interrupt them when they are talking, do not listen well, or do not take turns.

A speech/language pathologist is skilled at evaluating and treating deficits in the pragmatics of communication, using both individual and group therapy techniques. The first step in learning to control these problems is for you to become aware of behaviors that you or others exhibit that can disrupt communication. Watching a videotape of yourself in conversation, and getting feedback from the speech/language pathologist and others, are good starting points. The speech/language pathologist can then teach you ways of improving your listening skills through the use of eye contact, verbal and nonverbal acknowledgments (e.g., saying "that's interesting" or nodding), and minimizing interruptions. To improve your speaking skills, you may learn how to take turns in conversation, be concise, limit comments, ask questions, and solicit responses from others. The goal is to change from speaking in a monologue to participating in a dialogue that includes the other person more actively in the communication process. You may be videotaped practicing these skills so that you can monitor the reactions of others to these behaviors and chart your progress. Improving your pragmatic communication skills can make a major difference in the quality of your social interactions and the enjoyment you derive from social relationships.

I seem to have trouble coming to the point when I'm talking. Even though I know what I want to say, I can't find the right words, and I seem to go off on tangents and talk too long. Is there a solution to this problem?

People tend to become "wordy" and go off on tangents when they are having trouble retrieving specific words or find it difficult to organize the complex thoughts they wish to express. "My vocabulary seems to be shrinking," "It's on the tip of my tongue," or "My thoughts and speech are out of sync" are commonly-heard complaints from people with MS. While these word-finding difficulties can be quite frustrating, they are typically less noticeable to the listener than to the speaker. Evaluation and treatment by a speech/language pathologist or other cognitive rehabilitation specialist are recommended for these mild cognitive/language difficulties.

Therapy may include word association techniques and self-cueing strategies to improve specific word retrieval. Learning to "impose a delay" and quietly organize your thoughts before speaking often helps verbal expression. Concise, specific expression of ideas is possible when adequate time is allotted for preplanning.

Using a "Beginning, Middle, End" format can help you stay on the topic and teach you how to delete unnecessary, irrelevant comments. During therapy, it is also important to refine your self-evaluation skills to help guard against wordiness and tangential speech.

Recommended Readings

Erlich J, Sipes A. Group treatment for communication skills for head trauma patients. *Cognitive Rehabilitation* 1985;3:32–37.

Prutting C, Kirchner D. Applied pragmatics. In: Gallagher T, Prutting C (eds.). *Pragmatic Assessment and Intervention Issues in Language.* San Diego: College-Hill Press, 1983.

Rao S, Leo G, Bernardin L, Unverzagt F. Cognitive dysfunction in multiple sclerosis. I. Frequency, patterns, and prediction. *Neurology* 1991;41:685–91.

Rao S, Leo G, Ellington L, Nauertz T, Bernardin L, Unverzagt F. Cognitive dysfunction in multiple sclerosis. II. Impact on employment and social functioning. *Neurology* 1991:41:692–96.

Sohlberg M, Mateer C. *Introduction to Cognitive Rehabilitation: Theory and Practice.* New York: Guilford Press, 1989.

Booklet available from the National Multiple Sclerosis Society (Customer Service: 212-986-3240; Information: 800-344-4867):

◇ *Solving Cognitive Problems*—Nicholas G. LaRocca, Ph.D., with Martha King

Therapy Resources

American Speech-Language-Hearing Association. *Effective Communication Series: American with Disabilities Act Manuals.* Rockville, MD: American Speech-Language-Hearing Association, 1994.

Black, H and Black, S. *Building Thinking Skills: Book 3—Verbal.* Pacific Grove, CA: Midwest Publications, 1985.

Brubaker, SH. *Workbook for Cognitive Skills: Exercises for Thought Processing and Word Retrieval.* Detroit, MI: Wayne State University Press, 1987.

Brubaker, SH. *Workbook for Reasoning Skills: Exercises for Cognitive Facilitation*. Detroit, MI: Wayne State University Press, 1987.

Dohrmann, V. *Treating Memory Impairments: A Memory Book and Other Strategies*. Tucson, AZ: Communication Skill Builders, 1994.

Holloran, SM and Bressler, J. *Cognitive Reorganization: A Stimulus Handbook*. Austin, TX: Pro-Ed, 1983.

Kirkpatrick, K. *Putting the Pieces Together: A Linguistically Based Cognitive Retraining Manual*. Akron, OH: Visiting Nurse Service, Inc., 1985.

Marquis, MA and Addy Trout, ED. *The Question Collection: Teaching Questioning Strategies-A Pragmatic Approach*. Tucson, AZ: Communication Skill Builders, 1989.

Parker, VS and TenBroek, NL. *Problem Solving, Planning, and Organizational Tasks: Strategies for Retraining*. Tucson, AZ: Communication Skill Builders, 1987.

Sohlberg, MM, et al. *Improving Pragmatic Skills in Persons with Head Injury*. Tucson, AZ: Communication Skill Builders, 1992.

Sohlberg, MM and Mateer, CA. *Attention Process Training Programs I & II*. Tacoma, WA: Association For Neuropsychological Research and Development, 1989.

Selected publications available from your local chapter of the National MS Society

◇ *Solving Cognitive Problems* (ECS 6029)

10

Psychosocial Issues

Rosalind C. Kalb, Ph.D
Deborah M. Miller, Ph.D.

Multiple sclerosis has been compared to the unexpected visitor who arrives at your house, complete with bag and baggage, and never leaves (as described by Jaclyn Faffer, Ph.D.). This visitor has the tendency to spread his belongings through every room of the house, affecting the lifestyle and activities of all the members of the household. MS, with its varied symptoms and unpredictable course, is an intrusion that the whole family must learn to accommodate. While a relatively small number of people with MS experience severe disability, the uncertainty and variability of the disease create their own day-to-day stresses even for those with minimal impairment.

By necessity, the adjustment process is an ongoing one; as the symptoms of MS come and go, or come and stay, coping and adjustment ebb and flow as well. Since each family member will approach this challenge with his or her own particular coping style, effective communication will enhance the family's ability to work together to handle the day-to-day challenges of life with a chronic illness.

The questions in this chapter cover those aspects of a person's social and emotional life that are most often touched by MS, including self-esteem, coping efforts, and relationships with family members and friends. The answers also serve to highlight the role of ongoing education, effective coping strategies, and supportive counseling in each individual's and each family's efforts to live comfortably and productively with this intrusion in their lives.

Sense of Self

How do I begin to figure out who I am now that I have difficulty doing so many of the things I used to do?

Your self-image has been built up slowly over your lifetime. Your accumulated skills and life experiences all contributed to the picture you have of yourself. If MS interferes with your ability to do something that is important to you, that is a significant loss over which you'll need to grieve. Because MS can affect a person in so many different ways, you may find that you are grieving over one loss or another much of the time. At the same time, however, you are in the process of learning new things about yourself. As you confront the challenges of everyday life with MS and learn alternative ways to do things, you will begin to identify strengths and talents you never knew you had. If you are forced to give up one or another activity that has been important in your life, try to experiment with others that may turn out to be equally satisfying. Most importantly, look for that aspect of yourself that MS is unable to touch. For one person it may be her sense of humor, for another his religious beliefs, for yet another her love of music. By identifying this "MS-free zone" within yourself, you can retain a sense of who you are, even in the face of stressful changes.

I still can't bring myself to tell anyone about my diagnosis. I don't know how people will react and I'm not sure I'm ready to find out. What is the best way to talk about my MS with other people?

While it is never possible to predict exactly how another person will react to your MS, it is safe to assume that most people will take their cues from you. Be prepared to explain what MS is and to let the person know if you feel comfortable talking about it and answering questions. Some people will want to tell you about others they have known with MS; others will want to give you a lot of suggestions or advice. Most, however, will express shock and concern and then wait for you to tell them what you want or need from them. Since you will want or need different things from different people, think this through before you talk to a person. Try not to jump to conclusions about his or her reactions to you. Some people may seem to withdraw a bit; this is probably a reflection more of their own anxiety about how to talk to you about the MS than any lack of care or concern on their part. For more information about talking to your employer or colleagues about your MS, refer to Chapter 14.

Family, friends, and work are each important parts of my life. Now that I have MS, I don't have enough energy to deal with any of them as well as I would like. How can I learn to accept my limitations and feel less guilty?

Accepting personal limitations is always difficult, but everyone, with or without MS, experiences the frustration of overload at one time or another. Try to remember that the MS is not your fault and that doing the best you can is all that anyone can ask of you. Then take time to think through your priorities at home and at work and look at your weekly schedule to see if the way you actually spend time matches these priorities. Most people find that they spend too much time on activities that are not really necessary or important to them. Be sure to allow yourself enough time for brief rests if you need them. The time you invest in these rest periods will help you be more productive in all your activities. Talk with the significant people in your life about the ways in which MS affects you and share with them your concerns about limitations on your time and energy. They will be reassured to know that you care enough to discuss this with them, and you will be relieved of some of the worry about letting people down.

What is a support group and what kinds of groups are there for people with MS?

A support group is a form of self-help in which people with a common problem get together to share information, feelings, and ideas—or just to listen. Some of the larger groups (anywhere from twenty to two hundred people) are more educational in nature, with invited speakers coming to talk about various topics of interest. Other groups, usually with a smaller, more consistent membership (eight to ten people) from one meeting to the next, place greater emphasis on mutual support and shared problem-solving. Groups can be led by trained professionals, peer-led (by someone with MS who has taken on the leadership role), or have no leader at all. Some support groups are time-limited while others continue on a regular basis until the membership decides that it is time to stop.

At the present time the National Multiple Sclerosis Society sponsors more than 1,500 support groups. Among the most common are groups for the newly diagnosed, for those with more severe disability, and for couples, spouses, or children. There are also employment groups in which people discuss problems related to job stress, disclosure, reasonable accommodations, and retirement. There are singles groups for men and women who want to meet others with MS and share some of the problems and frustrations of life with the disease. The important thing to remember about groups is that they can vary in size, structure, focus, and quality. Consult your local MS Society chapter about the groups available in your area. Ask someone from the Chapter Programs staff to help you select the group that is most suitable for you. If you try one and it does not seem to meet your needs, try another. If you try several and cannot find what you are looking for, think about starting one of your own. The MS Society is interested in your suggestions and ideas and will be very helpful in your efforts to find a support group or start one in your area.

I'm embarrassed to be seen using a cane. If I ever get to the point of needing a walker, I'm afraid I'll just lock myself in the house. What can I do about this feeling?

Some people are reluctant to be seen using a cane or walker because they are worried that other people will think less of them. Others are afraid that people will feel pity. The first step in dealing with these concerns is to look at your own feelings about the cane or walker. If you believe that you are less of a person or that you have less to offer others because of these aids, try discussing this with your spouse, a close friend, or a colleague. Let them remind you of the qualities and talents they value in you, whether or not you need a mobility aid. You might also think about joining a support group with others who use mobility aids. As you get to like and respect others in the group, you will gradually learn to see beyond their canes, walkers, or wheelchairs; you will find that you notice the people and not their hardware. As you begin to see beyond their mobility aids, you will also begin to see beyond your own.

The second step in adjusting to a cane, walker, or any other mobility aid is to begin to see it as an important energy-saving tool in your life. Rather than interfering with your ability to do your chosen activities, the mobility aid makes it possible for you to do them more safely, quickly, and effectively. As you start to view the aid as a tool for getting things done, others around you will begin to view it in the same way.

Although there are many things I'm still able to do, all I can think about is ending up in a nursing home. How can I learn to stop anticipating the worst and get back to enjoying the life I have?

For most people, "ending up in a nursing home" means totally losing control over one's life. While a small percentage of people with MS do require residential care, the reality is that the vast majority does not. Therefore, the best way to deal with the fear of loss of control is to break it down into more manageable bits. Try to identify those areas of your life in which you feel most vulnerable and least in control and tackle them one by one. There are many resources available to help you with this problem-solving effort. Your physician can help you to manage MS symptoms as effectively as possible; an occupational and/or a physical therapist can recommend tools and strategies for dealing with many aspects of daily life; a lawyer and/or accountant can help you plan effectively for the future; a support group can help you learn how to live more comfortably with the uncertainties that MS brings to your life. As you begin to tackle some of the stressful problem areas, you will find that you feel less vulnerable and therefore more able to enjoy your daily life.

I have a lot of very supportive family and friends trying to help and encourage me. But no one really understands what I'm going through with my symptoms. I feel very alone and don't know what to do about it.

Perhaps the loneliest aspect of life with MS, or any other illness, is that even the most loving and supportive friend cannot "get in your shoes" and feel what you are feeling. Because so many of the symptoms of MS are invisible, e.g., fatigue, visual problems, and sensory changes, family and friends will often have a hard time understanding what is going on with you. Let them know when you are not feeling well, explain your symptoms, and offer reading materials about the illness to those who would like them. Do not expect people to be able to read your mind. Try to remember that a person does not have to be able to understand exactly what you are experiencing in order to offer you love and support.

Sometimes the best way to feel less alone is to spend some time with others who know firsthand what it feels like to live with this disease. There are a variety of ways to share experiences with others who have MS, including reading what others have written—in books or MS publications—posting messages on computerized bulletin boards, or joining a discussion group.

MS has taken away a lot of my independence. It has been many years since I needed anyone to help me with toileting, eating, and dressing. How can I hold on to my self-respect when I need so much help with everything?

We all spend many years learning to be self-sufficient, independent adults, and it is painful to lose any aspect of this hard-earned independence. Because the symptoms of MS make it impossible for you to perform routine activities of daily living in the usual way, you need to rely on special equipment and/or the help of other people to get the job done. Part of the process of learning to cope with this change in your life is recognizing that you are still getting the job done. In the same way that you developed self-respect as a child by learning to master the environment, you can and should take satisfaction in meeting the challenges of life with MS. Your self-respect will come from finding solutions, identifying useful tools, and availing yourself of whatever resources might enable you to lead your life in the fullest way possible.

Loss of self-esteem is a central focus of many MS support group discussions. As people deal with the changes and compromises that MS sometimes forces them to make in their lives, they find that sharing these experiences and problem-solving with other adults bolsters their sense of self-worth.

I get angry at colleagues and friends who tell me, "But you look so good. . . ." How can I explain to them that I almost never feel as good as I look?

Some people say that you look good because they are trying to be supportive and encouraging. Others are asking in a roundabout way why you are not being more active or more productive. Almost everybody who says it is trying to figure out what MS is and how it affects you. Try to remember that most people's experience with illness is that it makes you feel and look sick for a few days or weeks and then you get better. It will take them quite awhile to understand that MS does not go away like the flu or the measles, and that it affects how you feel and act even when they cannot see any signs of it. Be patient; answer people's questions about MS; and, whenever possible, try to explain how you are feeling in ways that others can relate to ("Because of my optic neuritis everything looks as though I'm seeing it through a dark mesh screen." "When I walk around it feels as though I'm slogging my way through thick mud." "I constantly feel as though I just stepped off the roller coaster and haven't got my balance back."). Additionally, there are several short, easy-to-read pamphlets about MS, which you can give people if they are interested.

I used to have a pretty active social life. Now I don't even try to meet people. Why would anyone be interested in a relationship with a person who has MS?

Before you can understand why others would be interested in having a relationship with you, it is important for you to reconnect with those parts of yourself that you value. In spite of the fact that you have MS, you are still a person—complete with interests, opinions, and feelings. You may have gotten so overwhelmed by MS-related stresses and changes that you have temporarily lost sight of the rest of you. Take some time to get to know yourself again. Whether you do this in an MS support group, in psychotherapy, or with a close friend, try to identify those aspects of yourself and your life that are independent of the MS. Then leave the rest up to others. You cannot decide for another person whether he or she will want a relationship with you. All you can do is be yourself. Some people will be put off by the MS, but many others will not.

I was diagnosed with MS about a year ago and most of my symptoms are not apparent to other people. Occasionally I need to use a cane when my walking is a bit unsteady. When should I tell someone I begin to date about my MS?

As with other interpersonal issues, there is no single correct answer to this question. You need to do whatever makes you feel most comfortable, given your sense of the situation and the person with whom you are dealing. The following guidelines may be helpful:

◇ First dates are a time for deciding whether you have any interest in pursuing the relationship further. There is no need to share any personal information with someone you do not like enough to see a second time.

◇ Once you have decided that the person is someone with whom you would like to develop a longer-term friendship/romance, keep in mind that half-truths and secrets make a very shaky foundation for a healthy, comfortable relationship.

◇ Revealing information about a chronic illness does not usually get easier as a relationship progresses; the more involved you are and the more you care about a person, the greater the potential loss.

◇ In deciding when to reveal significant information about yourself, think about when you would want to know similar kinds of information about the other person.

◇ Although some people will probably be frightened or put off by the MS, many others will not. You may be better off knowing the relationship's potential sooner rather than later.

Coping

If the doctor could just tell me what was going to happen with my MS, I think I could handle it. It's never knowing what's going to happen that upsets me. Is there any way to cope with all this uncertainty?

Unfortunately, unpredictability is one of the hallmarks of MS, and you are not alone in finding this so stressful. Most people find that they gradually adjust to taking life one day at a time, making the most of good days and putting up with the bad days. If you find yourself dwelling endlessly on "what if. . .?" (. . . I get worse, . . . I can't walk, . . . I can't see, . . . I can't do my job), it may be helpful and reassuring to do some advance problem-solving. Think through how you would deal with these changes, make contingency plans, and look into available resources. Some people find it very comforting to know that they have strategies in mind to deal with possible problems. Allowing yourself to think through the unthinkable can enable you to feel more prepared and more in control whatever the future brings.

Since my diagnosis, my husband has begun to hover over me all the time. I know he's worried about me, but I feel as though I've totally lost my independence. How can I explain to him that I need to learn how to live with my MS in my own way?

Each of you will need to learn to live with MS in your own way. At the same time that you are learning to cope with varied and unpredictable symptoms of MS, your husband will be adjusting to his own feelings about the illness and its impact on your daily life. Your husband's protectiveness is a sign of his anxiety about your health and safety as well as about your future together. Describe your symptoms to him so that he can understand how you are feeling. While explaining to your husband how much you value your independence, you can assure him that you will use caution and good sense and that you will ask him for help when you need it. Invite him to come with you to visit your physician so that he can hear what the physician has to say and ask any questions about the illness. Your physician will be able to offer reassurance and reinforce your need to be as independent as possible.

You and your husband may find it helpful to join a couples' support group. In this setting, each of you can learn from others how they have coped with the impact of MS on family life. Your husband might also enjoy a spouse group in which he can share his feelings and concerns with other husbands and wives whose partners have MS.

My wife was just diagnosed with MS. She keeps giving me articles to read and insists I go to the doctor with her. All her symptoms have gone away. Why can't we just forget about this for now and get on with our lives?

Being diagnosed with a chronic illness can be a very frightening and lonely experience. Your wife is trying to learn as much as she can about MS so that she will feel less afraid and more prepared to cope with it as time goes on. She may be asking you to share the learning process with her so that she does not feel so alone. Although MS is an unexpected intrusion in both of your lives, you may have very different styles of coping with it. While talking and reading a lot about MS helps her to feel better, the same strategies might make you feel worse! The more she tries to get you to talk or think about MS, the more you will struggle to put it out of your mind. It is important to talk to each other about your different coping styles. One style is not necessarily better than the other, but she may misinterpret your reluctance to read or talk about her MS as not caring about her or her feelings. Try to reassure her while at the same time explaining that you need to deal with her illness in your own way. Perhaps you can reach a compromise that satisfies both her need for your support and your need to focus on other things in your life.

I used to deal with life's frustrations by exercising and playing a lot of sports. Now that I'm not able to be as active as I used to be, I'm having trouble dealing with the pent-up feelings. How can I find other outlets that work for me?

Most people who play a lot of sports derive satisfaction from both the physical exertion and the competition. If your primary satisfaction from sports is the exertion itself, talk to your doctor about alternative forms of exercise that might be suitable for you, such as Tai-Chi, yoga, swimming, weight training, or a stationary bike (see Chapters 2 and 5). If what you miss most is the competitive aspect of sports, explore other forms of competition such as competitive bridge, chess, or computer games. Then remember that another way to release pent-up feelings is to talk about them. In the past it may never have been your style to talk about feelings, but you may find at this point in your life that talking—whether it be with a spouse, a friend, or in a support group—is a satisfying relief.

Since my husband was diagnosed with MS a few months ago, it's all he thinks and talks about. It seems as though our whole family has been taken over by this disease. Is this normal?

While each individual reacts to the MS diagnosis somewhat differently, it is not uncommon for a person to react initially by being quite preoccupied with the illness. One person might show this preoccupation by being totally unwilling to think or talk about any aspect of MS, as if ignoring it will make it go away. Another person shows the preoccupation by talking and thinking about MS to the exclusion of everything else. Whether or not they are currently experiencing symptoms, each is aware of a new and threatening problem over which he or she has very little control. Both of these individuals are trying to come to terms with a diagnosis that changes the way they think about themselves, their lives, and the future.

A newly-diagnosed person's preoccupation with MS can be very difficult for family members. Your husband may be experiencing a variety of strange and uncomfortable symptoms that you are unable to see or understand. At the same time that he is trying to deal with MS, you are trying to cope with your own feelings about it as well as everything else that is going on in the household. Although his feelings and concerns may be quite normal, it is still important for him to understand how his behavior affects other family members. Try to talk to him about your feelings. Ask him about going to a support group for the newly diagnosed. If, in another month or two, your husband still seems overly preoccupied with the MS, ask him if he would go with you to a therapist to talk about the impact of MS on the entire family.

I've been having a pretty hard time adjusting to the MS and all the changes it has caused in my life. My doctor suggested that I might want to get counseling to deal with some of my feelings but I've never needed therapy before and I don't see how it could help me now.

Your physician knows that being diagnosed with a chronic disease is a stressful and bewildering intrusion in any person's life. In short-term, problem-focused psychotherapy, a therapist who is knowledgeable about MS can help you understand and cope with your reactions to this intrusion. First, the therapist can help you work through the normal grief reaction that comes from having to alter your self-image to include a chronic illness. Second, he or she can provide you with a relaxed setting in which to ask questions and explore your options; most people find it very difficult to think of all their questions and concerns in the short time spent with the physician. The therapist can help you integrate the information you are receiving from your physician and sort through the advice and reactions of well-meaning friends and relatives. Coping with MS is an ongoing process that ebbs and flows with the changes that the disease causes in your life. As the MS follows its unpredictable course, you may find it useful to maintain intermittent contact with a therapist who can serve as a familiar resource whenever new symptoms add further stress and challenge at home or at work.

I was diagnosed a year and a half ago with MS. Although I have had two exacerbations since then, the symptoms have mostly disappeared and I'm feeling pretty well. My doctor prescribed one of the injectable treatments for me, to slow disease progression, but I'm finding it difficult to continue on this medication. I'm doing well and am trying to focus on other things in my life. Giving myself an injection is a constant reminder of the MS and I find it depressing.

This is a situation that is very much influenced by how you think about it. Your current view is that the injections are a reminder about your MS, something that you would rather not think about. Developing a different approach to the injections could help you see them in a different light. If you can look on the injections as something very important you do for yourself to manage MS, they can become much more acceptable. Adapting this new attitude may be something that you can do on your own or you may benefit from working with a counselor or therapist to help you reformulate your thinking and get yourself into the habit of making the injection part of your usual routine. Many others with MS have faced the same issues that you are dealing with and have been successful in adjusting to self-injection. By participating in your NMSS chapter support group you have a ready-made information network of others who have adjusted to this kind of treatment. This is a great resource that you should utilize.

Also, keep in mind that you do have choices you can discuss with your physician in regard to injectable medications. The medicines vary in frequency and route of injection. Work with your doctor to select the one that is most acceptable to you.

Finally, keep in mind that there is the matter, in years to come, of how you feel about what you have done to take care of yourself. We do know that there are some people whose MS progresses even when they take the medicine. Most of those who experience progression tell us that they still feel good about taking the medicine because they know that they did everything they could to slow down their MS as much as possible.

My doctor has prescribed one of the injectable drugs for me, but I am finding it impossible to give myself the shots. I have been afraid of needles my whole life and this feels like my worst nightmare. Is there anything I can do about this fear of mine?

Please be assured that many people who have conditions that require injectable medication have been able to overcome the same kind of distress you are feeling. Medical personnel have worked with generations of people with diabetes, who may be required to take as many as three shots a day, overcome this needle phobia. The first thing you have to do is to tell your doctor or nurse about your fear and let them know that it is interfering with your ability to take the medicine. Based on that discussion, there are several different recommendations your health care provider may make to help you manage this. If the problem is your fear of needles in general, regardless of who is giving you the shot, it may be recommended that you work with a nurse or therapist who has specialized training to help people overcome their needle phobias. If your biggest difficulty is in giving yourself the injection you could explore other options. There are many people with MS who, because of hand tremor, vision problems or other symptoms, are not able to self-inject. In those situations, a family member or friend may give the shot. In other situations, the injections are administered in the doctor's office.

The important thing to remember is that there are many possible solutions to this. Do not feel embarrassed or ashamed to discuss your fears with your health care providers. They can help develop a solution that matches your situation.

I'm feeling overwhelmed and confused by the choices I need to be making in my life. Everyone's giving me different advice—which drug to take, what to do about work, whether to have a child or not—and I can't figure out what to do. All I know is, I don't want to make wrong choices.

The good news is that people with MS now have many options available to them that they never had before. It wasn't very many years ago that a person diagnosed with the disease was told that he or she would just have to go home and learn to live with it. There were no disease-modifying agents, women were told they should never have children, and both men and women were advised to quit their jobs and stay home and rest. In other words, people with MS had to live with the stress of having their choices and options taken away from them.

Today's stresses are different. Now, people are being told by their physicians to make the choices that feel right for them, and they are worried about making a mistake. Fortunately, there are no right or wrong answers here. The "right" choice for one person may be the "wrong" choice for someone else. Let your choices be guided by your personal priorities and goals, keeping in mind that no one else can tell you what those should or should not be. Your best strategy for any important life decision is to: 1) Think about what is important to you. 2) Gather as much information as you can from your physician, the National MS Society, and other resources such as those recommended in this book. 3) Seek counseling from people you trust and who have expertise in the field of MS. 4) Talk to others who have faced similar decisions—perhaps in an MS support group or via the Internet. Then choose the option that best meets your needs and fits with your lifestyle.

Whatever choices you make, keep in mind that there are many resources available to help you pursue your goals. There is no need to "go it alone."

Family Life

My boyfriend and I are talking about getting married next year. He knows that I have MS and he says it doesn't matter to him— he loves me anyway. He has never been to the doctor with me and seems reluctant to go. I think it's important for him to hear what the doctor has to say so that he knows what he's getting himself into. How can I explain this to him?

You might try suggesting to your boyfriend that marriage is challenging enough without going into it blindfolded. Although love is an important part of a successful marriage, the ability to talk, problem-solve, and make decisions as a couple is also essential—particularly when life involves a chronic illness. Explain to him that you would be more comfortable sharing your life with him if you were confident that he had some understanding of what that might entail. If you are concerned that your boyfriend might be frightened by what your physician has to say, tell him so and assure him that you would rather start dealing with his fears and doubts now than be overwhelmed by them later.

We have worked hard to save money for our daughter's education. Soon my husband, who is in a wheelchair, may need a van to drive himself to work. How can we possibly choose between a college education and a van my husband needs in order to get to his job?

The heavy expenses related to chronic illness can drain family resources and necessitate compromise on the part of every family member. Before you start trying to choose between a van and a college education, however, be sure to look into possible funding sources for each. Education loans and scholarships based on financial need are often available, and chronic illness in the family is a valid and recognized financial hardship. Contact your chapter of the National MS Society to ask if there are any local sources of aid toward the cost of a van. Some automobile companies also have programs to help people meet the cost of adaptive equipment. Once you have gathered all the financial information, sit down as a family to review your options and decide which choices make most sense for your family.

Our son recently told me that he didn't like to bring friends over any more because the whole house is starting to look like a surgical supply store. There's no space to "hang out" without tripping over one piece of equipment or another. How should we deal with this?

All members of the family need to feel "at home" in the house. When the needs of one person begin to crowd out everyone else, the balance is out of kilter and needs to be restored. Ideally, there should be space for all of you to relax, converse, and entertain without tripping over medical equipment or mobility devices. Have a family meeting to talk over the problem and see if together you can come up with any space-saving, organizational ideas for managing the assistive equipment and creating equipment-free areas. The essential point to share with the whole family is that it is important for each of you to feel comfortable in the home.

You may also want to discuss with your son his feelings about MS. Depending on his age, he may be feeling embarrassed or self-conscious about his parent's illness and the need for assistive devices. He may be concerned about what his friends will think and he may be uncomfortable with their questions. If he seems to have difficulty talking this over with you, you can offer him age-appropriate reading materials from the National MS Society and alert him to the possibility of talking or writing to youngsters his own age who also have a parent with MS. Your local National MS Society chapter can help him to make these kinds of connections.

Our family used to do a lot of hiking and camping. Since my wife got MS, she can't really hike for any distance and she's uncomfortable "roughing it." I don't know whether I should take the children camping without her or give up camping and try to find another kind of inexpensive family vacation.

Like many of the other questions in this chapter, there is no one correct answer. The solution lies in talking the options over with your wife (and children if they are old enough to understand and participate) and deciding what works best for all of you. Your goal should always be to try to balance the needs and wishes of all family members. One solution may be to compromise; go on occasional father-and-children camping excursions and at the same time begin investigating other, less physically strenuous, possibilities for the whole family. If you give up camping altogether, the less than desirable outcome may be that you and the children feel a bit resentful and your wife feels guilty. Consult a travel agent who is knowledgeable about vacation opportunities for the disabled (see Appendix D). There are even camping programs for mixed groups of disabled and able-bodied people.

I've had to move back in with my mother since I can no longer manage alone in my apartment. We got along fine when I was on my own, but now we're back to the old tensions from my teenage days. How do families handle this kind of problem?

Parents and children spend many years preparing to separate. By the time the children have grown up enough to leave home, they feel ready to take personal responsibility and make decisions for their own lives. Parents let them go, usually with some trepidation and a big sigh of relief. As time passes, parents and their adult children learn to relate to each other in a slightly different way, with gradually growing separateness and mutual respect. When an adult child returns home, the parent-child relationship may need to be negotiated all over again.

Your mother once again has one of her children living with her but her parenting role is different from what it was when you were younger. You have returned to your mother's house after having spent time on your own, running your own home, making your own decisions. Presumably, you want your mother to treat you like an independent adult, free to make your own decisions and come and go on your own schedule. She, on the other hand, wants to continue to feel that her home is her own, subject to her tastes and preferences. Additionally, she has always related to you as your mother and may not know how to interact with you in any other way. Particularly when illness and/or disability are part of the picture, parents often feel an increased need to help and protect. Your mother may need time to learn how to balance your needs for help and support with your needs for freedom and independence. You may need the same time to reconcile yourself to being back in your mother's home and sphere of influence.

This is not an easy situation for any parent and adult child. You and your mother need to talk about the conflicts you are having and try to renegotiate your relationship. If you and your mother find that this renegotiation process is too difficult or stressful, a family therapist can help you communicate your individual needs and mutual expectations more effectively.

My husband has had MS for several years. I know that things are very difficult for him, but the MS has made things tough for me and the children as well. How can I explain to my husband that we're all having trouble dealing with the changes and losses in our lives?

Some people have so much difficulty coming to terms with the impact of MS on their own lives that they have a hard time realizing how it affects other members of the family. Others feel so anxious and guilty about the impact of their disability on family members that they try not to think about it. Thus, there may be a variety of reasons why your husband seems insensitive to the feelings of other family members.

Presumably, you have tried to talk with him about the ways in which MS affects you and the children. If he feels that you are being selfish and unfeeling when you talk about your own needs, try communicating about them in a different way. For example, you might consult your local chapter of the National MS Society about family programs that you could attend together. Share with your husband some of the literature published by the National MS Society on families living with the disease. Perhaps he can hear your message more clearly if it comes from someone else. Knowing that all families living with MS find it stressful, and that family members cope best by helping one another, may enable him to feel less alone and more able to respond to you and the children.

Although I need to use a wheelchair most of the time, I have learned to be quite self-sufficient in my own apartment. My parents want me to live with them, but I really want to stay where I am, in a familiar neighborhood, close to my friends. How can I convince my parents that I'm fine right where I am?

Your parents are probably worrying about your physical safety and your ability to get help if and when you need it. One way to reassure them is to create a home "safety net" for yourself. This is a good idea for any disabled person living alone, whether or not Mom and Dad are worried!

A portable telephone can be carried in a pouch attached to your wheelchair. This will enable you to make and receive calls even if you cannot get to the regular phone. You might also wish to install a medical alert system that gives you immediate access to emergency help (see Appendix D). This kind of system comes in several varieties, but the general principle is that the push of a single button (worn around your neck or attached to the wheelchair) alerts a central office that you are in some kind of trouble. After determining the type of problem you are having, the central office calls one of the individuals on your emergency list: neighbor, family member, physician, police, fire department, and so on. If you were to take a bad fall, for example, and find yourself unable to get back up or reach a telephone, you could get immediate help simply by pressing the alert button.

The Medic-Alert identification bracelet is another useful safety precaution (see Appendix D). If you were unable for any reason to communicate clearly about your condition (following a serious fall, for example), the bracelet would indicate that you have MS and identify the medications you are taking. Any other important information about your health status would be available in your Medic-Alert file.

Knowing that this kind of safety net is in place may help your parents feel more comfortable with your independence. Knowing that you are looking out for your own welfare and safety may make them less inclined to feel that have to do it for you.

Parenting

Now that I've been diagnosed with MS, I don't know if I should have children. I'm afraid that I won't be able to do things for a child that a father is supposed to do. What if I can't even play catch or teach the child to ride a bicycle?

Most parents, with or without MS, will tell you that their experiences with raising children were very different from what they had expected. They will also tell you that there is no single or correct way to be a "good" parent. Your decision to have children should be based on your desire to have this experience in your life as well some assessment of your ability to provide the kind of love and security that all children need.

The diagnosis of MS should not necessarily interrupt your wishes or plans for parenthood in any way. Keep in mind that it is impossible to predict with any certainty how your MS will affect you; you might not have any of the difficulties you are anticipating. You might even have a child who has no interest in playing catch! It is certainly reasonable to expect that MS will have some impact on your future family. The best way to prepare for that is for you and your wife to educate yourselves about MS, talk to the doctor about your particular symptoms and the course they are likely to take, and talk to each other about how you plan to share the parenting and breadwinning responsibilities. Ultimately, the goal is for you and your wife to feel comfortable as an effective parenting team, with consistent ideas about raising children, mutual support, and flexible ideas about what are "father jobs" and "mother jobs."

My children don't bring their friends around the house any more. Now that I'm in a wheelchair, they seem embarrassed about me. What is the best way to discuss this with them?

It is important that families living with MS do not automatically relate all of the changes they experience to the disease. Otherwise, changes that occur because of normal maturation or because of some stress other than MS could be misinterpreted. For example, it is quite typical and normal for young teenagers to begin spending less time at home and more time with their friends. Or children may bring fewer friends around if they sense that Mom or Dad is very tired or cranky a lot of the time.

Begin the conversation with your children by letting them know that you have noticed a change. It is important to do this in a very neutral way so that your children feel free to respond to the observation you have made rather than to the tone of your voice. Ask them if they have noticed that their friends are not over at the house as much as they used to be, and, if they have, ask them what they think has changed. If they do not offer any explanation, or if they offer one that you do not quite believe, let them know that you are concerned this might be related in some way to your MS. Assure them that you want to know about any feelings or concerns that they might have because it is important to you that they and their friends are comfortable in the house. If they do voice concerns about the MS or anything else, work with them to develop strategies to make the situation more comfortable.

Now that my wife has become a bit more disabled, the children have a lot more chores to do around the house. Will this responsibility be too much for them?

Research has indicated that children who have a parent with MS are very much like children whose parents do not have any major health problems. They continue to develop and thrive in spite of the added stresses and responsibilities. Let your children know that you are aware that they have more responsibilities than their peers and that you appreciate their efforts. Offer your children choices about which chores they take on and give them some leeway in deciding when they will complete them. Reassure them with both words and actions that, in spite of their increased responsibility, you are there to parent, protect, and take charge. Try to make sure that your children have time in their lives to *be* children; they need some regular opportunities, however limited, to participate in a school activity or be with friends. If, in spite of these efforts, you notice a significant change in your children's school performance, usual moods, or social relationships, it would be best to have a consultation with a child or family therapist.

I went into the hospital for a four-day course of steroids. We told our seven- and nine-year-old children about the admission ahead of time and they seemed okay with it. But while I was away, the older one got really upset at school and my husband had to go pick him up. How should we handle this in the future if I have to be admitted again?

Children have a difficult time with the unknown, and you and your husband were right to try to prepare them in advance for your admission. In spite of parents' best efforts, however, children are often frightened by the idea of a hospital stay (since many people who go into hospitals are sick or dying) and worried that the parent will not come home again. Having you return safely from this initial hospitalization is the first step in preparing them for any future ones that you may need. Take the time now to describe what happened to you during this hospital stay and let them talk to you about what it was like for them while you were gone.

If and when you need to be hospitalized again, ask the hospital staff if the children can accompany you during the admission process. Find out if the hospital has child life workers on staff who can talk with them about the hospital and its procedures. Make plans with your children to talk with them by phone at a scheduled time each day—or to have a visit if that is allowed. The idea is to give your children an understanding of what happens during the admission and how it will help your MS, and assure them that you are okay and available by telephone while you are gone.

We have told our parents and a few of our closest friends about my MS. I've asked them not to talk about it because I don't want my children to know yet. My husband thinks I'm wrong to try to keep this from them. I think that eight- and ten-year-old children are too young to have to worry about this. What should we be telling them?

Eight- and ten-year-olds are very observant people who generally have a sixth sense when something is not right in the family. Your children are probably aware that you are having some sort of health problems, whether or not these problems are influencing your usual activities with them. The ideas that children conjure up for themselves are almost always more frightening than the reality, particularly if they get the idea that the "something" is so terrible that Mom and Dad cannot even talk about it. In short, not discussing your MS with the children can, in the long run, cause them more worry than talking about it would. Additionally, the longer you delay talking to them, the more you increase the risk that they will hear the news from someone other than yourselves. By openly discussing an important issue like this one in your life, you also lay the groundwork for good parent-child communication about issues that will come up in their lives.

I know that all children need to test and "see who's the boss" sometimes. But since I started to use a cane, it feels as though the children are testing all the time. How can I discipline my children when I can't even keep up with them?

There are many different styles of discipline. The better your negotiation and communications skills and the more consistent you are in using them, the less you will have to depend on being mobile to provide discipline. Different approaches to parenting and discipline are described in the parenting literature (see Recommended Readings). Additionally, many community centers and schools offer parent effectiveness programs that are designed to help you build confidence and consistency in using these techniques. Keep in mind that being a good parent does not mean doing it all on your own. Enlist your spouse or other adults to help you learn and use these different approaches. In the meantime, remember also that children sometimes "test" in order to reassure themselves that the adults in their lives are still in charge and can still take care of them. Your children may be expressing their fears about MS and whatever effects it is having on you. Be alert to their questions and worries, and read or talk with them about the MS whenever it seems appropriate.

I always used to enjoy doing things with my children after school or in the evening before their bedtime. Now I'm so exhausted by the time they get home that I am either asleep or so cranky that they wish I were asleep! Is there any way to deal with this problem?

Fatigue is a common MS symptom that is usually best managed by prioritizing your activities and budgeting your energy. In some cases fatigue may also be helped with medication (see Chapter 2). At your first opportunity, discuss the fatigue with your physician, who can help sort out its causes(s). The physician may also refer you to a physical or occupational therapist who can design a personalized exercise program to increase your energy, as well as work simplification and energy conservation strategies to help you make effective use of the energy you have (see Chapters 5 and 6). Your best day-to-day strategy is to find a time to recoup some energy before the children come home so that you can resume some of the activities that you and they are missing. Since MS-related fatigue is most noticeable in the late afternoon, try to work in a brief rest just before the children arrive home. You may want to rearrange your daily routine so that you do more of your physically demanding chores earlier in the day and then have a chance to rest. If you are returning from work late in the day, schedule a regular rest time for yourself and make a "date" with the children for some special time together before they go to bed. Brainstorm with the children about some new "quiet time" activities that you could enjoy doing together.

Since my wife began having difficulty getting around the house and doing things for herself, she's always after the rest of us to do, or get, or go. The children and I want to be helpful but we don't like being constantly on call. How can I make her understand how we feel?

There are two very difficult aspects to the situation you are describing in your family: how frustrated and out of control your wife must be feeling; and how unappreciated and burdened you and your children are feeling. One key to making home life more satisfying and comfortable for all of you is to develop some ways of talking about what is happening so that you can start building solutions together. The best way to start talking with others about your own feelings and needs is to show some understanding of theirs. This helps to facilitate open communication and cut down on everyone's tendency to become defensive. Then you can begin to tackle specific areas of stress and conflict one at a time. Let your wife know that the family wants to meet her various needs, but that you each have needs and commitments of your own to deal with as well. Family members should speak openly about how they would like requests to be made and how they feel when their own needs and activities are ignored. If you find that these conversations become too difficult because of all the issues that seem to emerge, keep in mind that there may be a lot of emotions in the situation that need to be sorted out. You may want to enlist the help of a family therapist who is knowledgeable about chronic illness to get you started on this process.

My 12-year-old has had to help me up from the floor a couple of times when I have fallen. Now he's afraid to be at home alone with me. How can I help him with these feelings?

Your son's feelings may be difficult for him to describe, but are probably related to a fear that he cannot do enough to help you, or that he is having to deal with a problem that is bigger and stronger than he is. For both your sakes, do everything you can to protect yourself from falls. Arrange for the two of you to have a session with an occupational therapist or physical therapist in your home. This professional can point out ways to maximize your stability and safety, perhaps by removing area rugs, installing bathroom safety equipment, or recommending a mobility aid. The therapist can also show you different ways of performing transfers and teach your son techniques for helping if you do fall. You might also consider having a medical alert system installed in your home that enables you to notify family, neighbors, or community safety officials that you need help. These steps will reduce your son's fears by demonstrating to him that you are doing everything you can to protect yourself and that you do not expect him to be solely responsible for your safety.

Our youngest daughter will graduate from high school next year. Recently she started talking about getting a job rather than applying to college. My husband and I are afraid that she feels worried about leaving me now that I've become so much more disabled. Should we push her to go to school?

Your daughter's second thoughts about college could be caused by any number of factors. As her parents, you should certainly discuss her plans with her and share your feelings about her going away to college. However, it would do little good to force her into a decision about leaving home; her reasons for deciding against college at this point could be very well thought out and unrelated to your illness. If her change in plans does seem to stem from anxiety or guilt about your MS, let her know what steps you and your husband have taken to manage your increasing disability. Remind her that just because she is the youngest child does not mean that her role in life is to take care of you. If finances are her major concern, share with her your plans for balancing medical costs and any help you plan to give her with her educational expenses. Be prepared to help her explore options for attending college away from home or locally. The goal of the conversation should be to let her know that her needs and priorities are important to you and that you can, as a family, come up with a plan that addresses the needs of all the members of the family.

Sometimes my son or daughter has to help me with getting dressed or going to the bathroom. I don't like this any more than they do and I'm worried about how this will affect them.

Your concern about having the children help with your personal care activities is very understandable and appropriate. Providing that kind of intimate assistance can be very confusing for youngsters who are developing their self-concepts and working to attain more independence from their parents. Additionally, your children's involvement in personal care sends a strong message that you would be "lost" without them—a message that could have a significant impact on their plans for the future.

Some of the tasks that you need help with happen at the same time each day. Try to develop a schedule with adults in your family to help with your morning routine. Ask to talk to a social worker about the possibility of getting help from a home health agency or, perhaps, the local chapter of the National Multiple

Sclerosis Society. If, in spite of your best efforts, you can find no other helpers, consider involving your children in individual or family counseling. An opportunity to sort out their feelings about their caregiving role could relieve some of the stress on all of you.

My husband has been very upset and angry about the way his MS is getting worse, and he seems to take a lot of it out on the children. They try so hard to please him but he yells a lot and criticizes everything they do. What is the best way to talk to him about this?

While your perception is that your husband's relationship with the children is very strongly affected by his MS, he may not recognize the ways in which his reactions to the disease are spilling over onto the family. The sooner you begin to talk this over with him, the better it will be for all of you. He needs to begin to understand the impact of his behavior on the children. It is best to start this process by talking about a particular situation rather than about his general attitude or the way he is coping with MS. Discussing how to improve on the outcome of a specific, recent event will be less threatening. Undoubtedly, one conversation will not reverse the pattern that has developed; it will, however, lay the groundwork for future conversations.

It is not unusual for people to take out their uncomfortable feelings on those closest to them. As MS interferes with a person's sense of independence and personal control, the natural tendency is often to try to take control in other ways—perhaps by bossing people around or "trying to organize the raindrops." Children often feel that they get the brunt of this type of behavior. The most effective way to deal with this problem is often to help the person talk about the loss of control and brainstorm about more effective ways to restore a sense of order and independence in daily life.

Keep in mind, as well, that mood swings, irritability, and depressive feelings are also fairly common in MS (see Chapter 11). While the exact relationship between these emotional changes and the illness is not well known and can certainly vary from one individual to another, the resulting behaviors can have a significant impact on family life. If you feel that your husband is behaving very differently from his "usual self," you could ask him to go with you to a psychotherapist *who is familiar with MS* to talk over these changes.

Most of my MS problems don't show on the outside; fatigue and vertigo are my worst problems. How can I help my children understand how I am feeling? They are angry about things I can't do any more and don't seem to appreciate the things I still manage to do for them.

It is difficult to describe to children symptoms that they cannot see and have probably never experienced. Try to describe your symptoms in terms that they can readily understand. For example, you might have your children experiment with ankle and wrist weights to learn how your body feels when you are fatigued. Or you might tell them to spin themselves around a bit and then try to walk from one room to another. Reading together about MS will let them see that other parents experience very similar symptoms. The National Multiple Sclerosis Society has several excellent booklets written for children in different age groups. Many chapters of the National Multiple Sclerosis Society also offer special programs to help children learn about the disease and its symptoms and provide ways for them to get in touch with other children who have a parent with MS. Contact your local chapter (see Appendix D) to learn more about these services. Your physician can also be a valuable resource. For example, the children might sit in during one of your office visits to learn about the neurologic exam and the ways in which your physician tests those "invisible" symptoms. He can also refer you to a child or family therapist who can help your family develop more effective ways to talk about MS and the ways it is affecting each of you.

As you try various strategies for teaching your children about MS, keep in mind that no two children learn in exactly the same way. What seems to work with one of your children may be of no interest to the other(s). One child might be interested in reading or talking with you about MS, while another might want to attend a meeting and talk with other children who have a parent with MS. Some children want simply to be reassured that you will continue to be able to take care of them.

Should I let my children's teachers know about my MS?

Under most circumstances it is very helpful to let your children's teachers know about your diagnosis. School can be a very important source of stability and self-confidence, and the teacher is a primary player in any child's day-to-day experiences. If they are aware of the MS, teachers can be very helpful to you in gauging how your children are responding to your illness and the changes it is causing in your family. Additionally, awareness of your situation will enable the teachers to be attentive to any changes in your children's school performance and social relationships and prepared to provide help and support as needed.

The Caregiving Experience

Everyone is always asking how my husband is. How do I let them know that my life has changed almost as much as his and that I need them to ask about me too?

Your feelings are shared by many well spouses. There is no reason to feel embarrassed, selfish, or in any way inadequate because you have needs of your own. Over the course of the illness, you will need support just as much as your husband does, but you may have to look for it from different sources. Having one special friend or relative with whom you are comfortable sharing your feelings can be much more meaningful than expressions of concern from people with whom you have a more casual relationship. Many chapters of the National Multiple Sclerosis Society sponsor spouse groups that provide the opportunity to meet with others who are sharing your experiences. The National Well-Spouse Foundation (see Appendix D) is another organization that provides support to care-giving spouses through newsletters, local support groups, and annual national meetings. An increasing amount of reading matter is available to inform, support, and empower you in your role as the spouse of someone with a chronic illness (see Appendix C).

My wife can't play tennis anymore. She gets upset when I go and play and I feel guilty about wanting to play. Should I give up the active things that I like to do because she can no longer do them with me?

There are likely to be a variety of changes that you and your wife will have to face together in dealing with MS, and responding to changes in her level of disability is a very significant one. Before making any decisions about continuing to play tennis, try to talk the situation over with her. Your wife's distress may stem from feelings of loss and envy; she may simply find it very painful to know that you are doing something that she loves but can no longer do. Or she may be concerned that the two of you will have less time together if you continue to play without her. She may also worry that she will miss out on the social contacts the two of you had with other players. Identifying the sources of her distress will help the two of you decide the best way to deal with the situation. Make sure that your wife understands how important it is for you to keep playing tennis while reassuring her that you are interested in finding other activities that you can do together. Support her own efforts to find satisfying and enjoyable hobbies to replace those that she can no longer do. It is important that family members not rush to give up any and all activities that the person with MS is unable to do. The eventual cost in resentment and guilt is too great.

I've started to feel more like a caregiver than a husband. I am committed to my wife and have no wish to leave her, but I really miss the companion who shared so much with me. How do other people cope with the loneliness and loss of companionship?

The feelings of loss you are describing are particularly common for couples who have always shared many interests and activities but now increasingly spend time simply managing the consequences of MS. In the same way you have partnered each other in other aspects of your life, try to become partners in the management of MS. An important goal of this partnership is to be able to communicate effectively about ways to integrate MS-related care activities into your lives in such a way that there is still time and energy left for other enjoyable activities. This will help both of you to feel that you are managing the MS rather than the other way around. It will also help you regain your feelings of togetherness so that each feels less alone with the burdens imposed by MS. Discussing your concerns at a couples' support group could benefit you and your wife in several ways: You will be reassured to learn that other couples are living with, and finding solutions to, the kinds of stresses and strains you are describing. The group can brainstorm together on ways to solve commonly shared problems and find substitute activities for ones that you can no longer do because of the MS. You may also find that the group becomes a social outlet as well.

I feel as though my whole life is controlled by MS and I don't even have the disease. How can I regain my life and still make sure my husband has the care he needs?

When life with MS becomes so overwhelming that you feel you are losing yourself in the disease, it is time to take a step back from the situation and find ways that it can be made more manageable. The first step in this process is to begin to think of yourself as your husband's care *partner* rather than care*giver*; the responsibility for managing the MS and the needs that it generates rests on both of you.

In as objective a way as possible, the two of you should make a list of his needs and yours. Try to identify the specific ways in which the MS-related needs have infringed on yours, paying particular attention to those times when you feel especially burdened or overwhelmed. Finally, write down those activities that you personally are missing and want to regain in your life. The goal of this process is to help you think in more specific terms than "MS" and "my whole life." The more specific you are able to be, the more likely it is that you and he will be able to identify strategies for regaining a sense of independence and control in your lives.

While it will not be possible for you to free your lives totally of MS, you will be able to adopt strategies and identify resources to help both of you meet your needs. This kind of problem-solving requires good communication and a lot of creativity. Working with a family therapist can help with the process if you find that, individually or together, you are feeling too overwhelmed or emotionally overloaded to be able to discuss the issues. Also keep in mind that MS support groups can be a particularly helpful resource, particularly those designed for couples.

My wife is desperate to find a cure for her MS. Every time a new treatment is mentioned in the newspaper, she is ready to fly around the world to get it. I get angry when she is ready to spend our retirement money on every quack gimmick that comes along. How can I get her to understand that the money we saved is for both of us and that we need to agree on how to spend it?

This commitment to trying every publicized MS "cure" can be especially frustrating to family members. In addition to making them feel as if their own needs have become unimportant, it tends to keep the entire family on an uncomfortable emotional roller coaster as hope is repeatedly replaced with disappointment. Your wife may be responding more with emotion than with reason to these reported "cures." In order to give her some background on the great number of these that have turned out to have no real value, you may want to read together a book entitled *Therapeutic Claims in Multiple Sclerosis* (see Appendix D). This book describes most of the proclaimed treatments and cures, the reported ways that each was thought to work, and the quality of the scientific research done to evaluate their effectiveness. Another way to help your wife feel satisfied that she is doing everything possible to treat her MS is to encourage her participation in a clinical trial of one of the very promising drugs that are now being scientifically tested (see Chapter 3). If your wife continues to want to use your retirement savings to pursue untested "cures," the two of you might consider a consultation with an accountant or tax attorney to determine how her spending will affect your retirement and how to establish a financial plan that will protect your retirement funds.

My husband has become quite disabled by his MS and doesn't get out of the house much any more. Friends have stopped inviting us to do things because he is no longer able. How can I let them know that I still need to see people and have a social life even though he can't come with me?

You are wise to take the initiative with your friends rather than waiting for them to take the initiative with you. Your friends may simply need to hear from you that you want to maintain your social relationships and continue to be active. You may start by inviting one friend or couple over for dinner and saying that your husband will join you for part of the evening but excuse himself if and when he becomes too tired. Or, invite them to join you at a restaurant for dinner and let them know that although your husband won't be coming, he is pleased that you are arranging an evening out. During the evening, after you have had a chance to catch up with one another, ask your friends to tell other members of your circle that you are still looking to socialize with them. You may want to let them know, if it is indeed the case, that you and your husband have talked this over and are both comfortable with the idea that you will continue to make plans even if he is not always able to be with you. It is by your own example that your friends will become comfortable seeking you out for social engagements even if your husband cannot always participate.

I've been able to deal relatively well with my wife's physical problems but the cognitive changes and mood swings have been much more difficult for me. At times she seems like a different person and I begin to feel as though I have lost my life partner. How can I learn to accept this loss?

As painful as it is to recognize the cognitive changes that your wife is experiencing, it is fortunate that you understand their possible relationship to her disease. Many spouses and family members, who don't know that MS can directly cause these memory and behavioral changes, tend to misinterpret the problems and believe that the person with MS is being deliberately difficult or forgetful. With a more complete understanding of the situation, you can begin to deal with it more realistically. Chapters 9 and 11 provide an orientation to the cognitive problems and emotional changes that can occur in MS, and describe how these problems are assessed and managed.

The changes your wife is experiencing are undoubtedly having a major impact on you and your relationship. First, you are probably assuming more of those household responsibilities your wife used to manage, as well as providing more care and supervision for her. Finding the time and energy for this can be a challenge given the many responsibilities you already have at work and at home. Even more importantly, the changes your wife is experiencing are literally taking her away from you. You may be missing her sense of humor, her intellect, her interest in your work and the comings and goings of your children, or her ability to participate with you at social gatherings with family and friends. She is not, in very fundamental ways, the person you married.

This idea of having "lost" your spouse while she remains in your home and under your care can be very difficult to accept, and requires a unique kind of grieving process. It is important that you begin to think of your relationship as being very different than most marriages. This grieving process will help you acknowledge the help your wife needs, while allowing you to let go of the woman you married and accept the wife who is now so dependent on your care. The grieving process will also help you shift your expectations for the relationship and prepare for your new responsibilities.

Although family, friends and support group members can be helpful and sympathetic, few of them will have any experience with the loss you are experiencing in your marriage. For that reason, it is very useful to work with a mental health professional experienced in dealing with the grief of your ever-changing relationship with your wife. The therapist can help you deal with the losses you are experiencing, the paradox of having to care for that person who is in many ways no longer your spouse, and in sorting out how you and the rest of your family can continue with your lives.

There is no one correct way to manage this situation that suspends you between being partner and nurse. A mental health professional can be an important ally as you find your way in managing this very difficult situation. This can include exploring ways to maintain relationships and activities that you used to share with your wife, or developing new ones. Just as importantly, working with a therapist can help you identify and hold on to the parts of your relationship with your wife that remain intact.

My husband insists on driving a car even though some of his MS symptoms are making him an unsafe driver. We added hand controls to the car two years ago, when leg weakness was his major problem. But now his vision is very bad and I'm afraid that his concentration is just too poor for him to be safe. He has already had one accident and I'm afraid that someone will be hurt the next time.

People find it very difficult to give up driving because it represents a tremendous loss of independence. However, as you have indicated, the consequences of severely impaired driving skills can be life-threatening. Trying to convince your husband by yourself that he should stop driving might be difficult. If you are uncertain about his driving competence, or if you believe that your husband will resent your suggestions, you might accompany him to his next medical appointment and raise the issue with his physician. Explain your concerns to the doctor and ask about the availability of a driving evaluation. This kind of evaluation, which should test both physical and cognitive skills, is often available at rehabilitation facilities. With your husband present, ask about the doctor's responsibility for reporting unsafe drivers to the state bureau of motor vehicles (this responsibility varies from state to state). If your husband insists on continuing to drive, and you are certain in your own mind that he is an unsafe driver, let him know that you and your other family members will not ride in the car when he is driving. Help him to make arrangements for rides to those places he is accustomed to going on his own. Many communities have door-to-door transportation services that can help him remain independent. You might also encourage him to consult a psychotherapist for help with the feelings of loss and helplessness that accompany this kind of major life adjustment.

My husband wants our sexual relationship to be the way it used to be. But I am exhausted after a full day of work and taking care of him. It's hard for me to feel romantic after helping him with his other personal needs. How can I discuss this without hurting his feelings?

A couple's sexual relationship is important because of both the physical pleasure it provides and the emotional intimacy that it expresses. At different times over the course of every marriage, the sexual relationship is influenced by how the couple is getting along, their family responsibilities, and their physical and emotional health. Remaining close and intimate with each other during these times is an important part of sustaining a good marriage. Before discussing your sexual relationship with your husband, you may want to spend some time sorting out your own feelings. As you have described, your sexual feelings for your husband have been affected by your own physical exhaustion as well as changes in how you feel emotionally. It is also possible that some of your husband's MS-related physical changes are interfering with your sexual activities or your sexual response to him. It will probably make your conversation easier if you have sorted through some of these feelings in advance and perhaps talked them over with a therapist.

The next time your husband talks about your sexual relationship, try sharing some of your feelings with him. As with any important conversation, be sure to put as much effort into hearing him as in expressing yourself. By being honest with him about the way you are feeling and open to his response, you are initiating an important and satisfying form of intimacy. The two of you might also consider talking with a therapist who specializes in sexual relationships. That person can help you talk about your feelings and concerns, explore ways of being sexual that accommodate your husband's disability, and otherwise enhance the intimacy in your relationship. The sexual relationship in MS is discussed in detail in Chapter 12.

I have always loved my wife, and until her MS came along, we seldom even argued. I would never have believed that I could intentionally be hurtful to her. But now that she is at her most vulnerable, my temper is becoming shorter and shorter. Last night she woke me three times to help her to the bathroom. The second time, at 3:00 in the morning, I found myself shouting at her that I had to be up at 5:30 and she could wait until then. When she called me again a half-hour later, it was because she had had an accident. Even though I knew it was a bowel accident, I let her lay in the soiled bedclothes while I tried to "cool down" and get control before going to help her. I was afraid I might hurt her. These bad feelings and reactions are very frightening to both of us, and they are coming more often and more powerfully. I am frightened for her and for me. What can I do?

Fortunately, you have begun to recognize your need for help in managing the reactions you are having to your wife and her care needs. We know from research and clinical practice that couples who have no history of domestic violence can become hurtful to each other in the course of living with a chronic disease like MS. This hurtfulness is often a reaction to the physical stress and emotional strain of living with the illness. We also know that this kind of aggressive behavior is more likely to occur when the illness involves personality and behavioral changes or bowel or bladder incontinence. This is by no means an excuse for becoming either emotionally or physically abusive. It is an alert that anyone can become abusive and that income, gender, and level of disability are no protection when the stress of the situation becomes too much.

You are right to be worried about your reactions. This is the kind of situation that will only become more stressful and dangerous if you try to manage it on your own. Counseling with a mental health professional is a useful and essential strategy for dealing with emotions that are beginning to feel out of control. The professional can help you and your wife to develop a short-term plan to relieve the immediate pressure related to her care, and a long-term strategy to prevent future occurrences. If you do not know a therapist, ask for a referral from your physician or the local chapter of the National MS Society.

It is important to let your wife's doctor know immediately that the caregiving has become too much for you, and that you need help in caring for her. You can also ask the National MS Society for information about local options for respite care, in-home nursing care, and a variety of other strategies (see Chapter 15). It is fortunate that you have had the courage to recognize the danger that you and your wife are facing. It is now essential that you find the strength to get professional help to correct the situation.

I know that elderly couples have to face the possibility of nursing home placement when they can no longer care for each other any more, but my husband and I are in our 40s and facing that possibility now. How can we begin to talk about this frightening topic?

One of the most difficult aspects of facing nursing home placement at this time in your lives is that it is such an unanticipated event. Few if any people in your immediate circle can appreciate the practical, emotional and financial issues you are facing. You may be feeling guilty that your husband's care needs have become overwhelming in spite of any assistance you have been able to enlist from friends, relatives, or professionals. In addition, you are probably concerned about the likelihood of finding a facility that has other young adults. You may also be concerned that your family and friends will think you are "abandoning" your husband.

To deal with these issues, it is important to step back from the jumble of overwhelming thoughts and feelings, and take an objective look at your situation. The fact that you and your husband are considering residential care for him means that you feel you have exhausted all the other long-term care options. You can refer to Chapter 16 for a detailed discussion of long-term care to determine if this is indeed the case.

As you and he examine the positive and negative aspects of each long-term care strategy, you can choose the one that best meets the needs of everyone in the family.

Your husband's ability to participate in this discussion, and the subsequent planning involved, will depend on his cognitive abilities—in particular, his ability to recognize and appreciate his care needs. As this is a decision that will significantly affect both of your lives, it is important that he be included in this decision to the greatest extent possible.

The starting point for this kind of planning and decision-making is the acknowledgement that you, your husband, and your children each have needs that need to be met, and each person's needs are just as real and valid as everyone else's. Much of the anxiety and guilt surrounding this difficult issue results from the mistaken belief that family members *ought* to be able to care for a loved one at home *no matter what*. However, research has demonstrated that the physical and emotional health of caregivers can be severely compromised by the extraordinary demands of caregiving. The goal is to arrive at a plan that ensures the health and well-being of the entire family, and allows family members to love and care for one another in the most comfortable way possible.

If your husband is not able to participate meaningfully in this decision because of cognitive impairment, you may want to discuss your options with members of his family. Family members, friends, a clergyman, and a caregivers' support group can all be valuable sources of help and support during this difficult time. It may also be helpful to work with a mental health professional who can provide a "reality check" concerning the options you are considering, guide your efforts to select a facility and arrange placement and, be a source of support as you advise family and friends about your decision.

Recommended Readings

Garee B (ed.). *Parenting: Tips from Parents (Who Happen to Have a Disability) on Raising Children*. Bloomington, IL: Accent Press, 1989.

Halligan F. *The Art of Coping*. New York: Crossroad, 1995.

James J. *One Particular Harbor*. Chicago: Noble Press, 1993

Kalb R. *Families Affected by Multiple Sclerosis: Disease Impacts and Coping Strategies*. New York: National Multiple Sclerosis Society, 1995.

Kalb, R. *Multiple Sclerosis: A Guide for Families*. New York: Demos Medical Publishing, 1998.

LaRocca N, Kalb R, Foley F, McGann C. Psychosocial, affective, and behavioral consequences of multiple sclerosis: treatment of the "whole" patient. *J Neuro Rehab* 1993;3(4):30–38.

Pitzele S. *We Are Not Alone: Learning to Live with Chronic Illness.* New York: Workman Publishing, 1986.

Selected publications available from your local chapter of the National Multiple Sclerosis Society (800-FIGHT-MS):

- ◇ *Living with MS* (ES 0087)
- ◇ *What Everyone Should Know About Multiple Sclerosis* (ER 100)
- ◇ *Things I Wish Someone Had Told Me: Practical Thoughts for People Newly Diagnosed with Multiple Sclerosis* (ES 6028)
- ◇ *PLAINTALK: A Booklet About MS for Families* (ECS 55)
- ◇ *Someone You Know Has MS: A Book for Families* (ES 0045)
- ◇ *When a Parent Has MS: A Teenager's Guide* (ECS 6024)
- ◇ *At Our House* (a coloring book for ages 3–5) (ECS 6033)
- ◇ *Multiple Sclerosis and Your Emotions* (ES 6007)
- ◇ *Taming Stress in Multiple Sclerosis* (ES 6034)
- ◇ *Knowledge is Power*—Rosalind Kalb, Ph.D. and Marla Shawaryn, Ph.D. A series of articles for individuals newly diagnosed with MS.
- ◇ *Living Well with MS*—a series of workbook written for, and by, people who have been living with MS for some time (including *Coping with Change, Considering Assistive Devices, Working with MS,* and *MS and Wellness)*
- ◇ *A Guide for Caregivers* (ES 6010)

11

Stress and Emotional Issues

Nicholas G. LaRocca, Ph.D.
Jill Fischer, Ph.D.

Stress is no stranger to MS. In fact, many people living with the disease believe that stress may be one of the precipitating factors in the onset of MS and its progression. While research has provided little evidence to support this belief, there is no doubt that MS *creates* significant stress in people's lives.

Life's stresses are primarily of two types. The first is caused by major events or changes that require significant adjustment. Such stressful life events might include the loss of one's job, the birth of a new child, or the diagnosis of a disabling illness. The other type of stress, aptly termed "hassles" by some, consists of the pressures of everyday life. While these daily hassles do not call upon us to make major changes in our lives, they are still emotionally taxing. Examples of this type of stress might include fighting rush hour traffic, paying bills, or dealing with children's homework. While everyone is subject to both types of stress, having MS seems to worsen the effects of both.

Since stress is so much a part of life with MS, it is not surprising that people report all sorts of emotional *dis*-stress. It is safe to say that adjusting to something as unpredictable and potentially disabling as MS may entail quite a bit of emotional turmoil. To experience such distress and turmoil from time to time is therefore a natural and normal reaction. It is important to keep this in mind because at one time it was believed that MS was the result of an emotionally weak and immature personality. Such notions have long since been abandoned, but one occasionally encounters the idea that people with MS should respond without complaint to the changes and losses imposed by this disease. Not only would such a reaction be unnatural, but it would also interfere with the normal and necessary adjustment process.

People often look for a road map to guide them in their adjustment to MS and are disappointed to find that there is none. Unlike terminal illness, in which a person's adjustment may follow a fairly consistent set of emotional "stages," adapting to life with MS follows no fixed pattern. It is impossible to map out predictable "stages" of adjustment because the disease can vary so much in the types of symptoms it presents and its speed of progression. However, significant emotional issues are likely to arise intermittently over the course of the illness:

◇ *Uncertainty* may be the first emotional challenge facing people with MS. It begins with the initial mysterious symptom of MS, be it fleeting optic neuritis, intermittent numbness, or a fall. When symptoms first appear, the person believes that something is wrong but is uncertain what it might be. Months or years may go by before a diagnosis is established, during which time uncertainty breeds a lingering feeling of anxiety. Uncertainty remains even after the diagnosis has been made. Will the symptoms get worse? Will new symptoms appear? How long will walking be possible? Will working become impossible? Creating a sense of security in one's life in the face of such uncertainty is a significant and lifelong challenge.

◇ *Accepting* the reality of having a chronic, disabling illness is not a simple matter. Most people with MS will say that they have never really "accepted" it, any more than they would "accept" living in the middle of a battlefield. People sometimes feel a sense of relief when the diagnosis is first pronounced, simply because some of the uncertainty is resolved and many of their questions have finally been answered. However, a sense of shock and disbelief often follows—a state that may be prolonged by a person's inability or unwillingness to acknowledge what has happened.

For most, this reaction is short-lived, and the reality of the diagnosis is eventually recognized even though it may never be "accepted."

◇ *Grief* often ensues as the reality of the diagnosis sinks in. The person grieves for his or her lost sense of self. Most people think of themselves as invulnerable to disease and take for granted their physical and intellectual abilities. A chronic, disabling illness robs people of this old sense of self and may also compromise many of those physical and intellectual abilities. As people mourn these losses, they are forced to reformulate their expectations for themselves and the future.

◇ *Self-image* is likely to go through a transition. The person slowly and painfully lets go of the old sense of self and works gradually to build a new one that incorporates the limitations and constraints brought about by the MS.

◇ *Accommodation* occurs as people with MS and their families make specific changes in their life patterns in response to the disease. Such accommodations may involve changing jobs, swapping roles within the household, making alterations in the house, and giving up certain physical activities.

◇ *Re-emergence* eventually occurs as people make the necessary changes in their lives. The disease may occupy a great deal of attention and effort at the time of diagnosis and during subsequent exacerbations. As it stabilizes somewhat, people may find that they can pay less attention to the disease and more to the business of living.

Adjustment to MS takes time. Moreover, since the disease can wax and wane, many people find that they have to adjust over and over again. They may go through a grieving process each time new disabilities appear. Because of the changeable nature of MS, people may experience dramatic fluctuations in their emotional state. They may plunge into a severe depression when a bad exacerbation begins and experience joy and relief with the onset of remission. Living through this emotional roller coaster is one of the most significant challenges of MS.

Adjustment to MS is as complex as it is slow. Many factors may influence how a person copes with the illness, including disease course, personality and coping style, the availability of social supports and financial resources, and other concurrent life stresses. A very important factor influencing adjustment is one's self-appraisal. People who view themselves as ineffectual and powerless are likely to adjust differently than those who view themselves as effective and able to manage what life brings them.

Emotional Aspects of MS

How common is depression in MS?

The answer to this question depends in part on what you mean by "depression." People tend to use the term to describe many different feelings. Everyone feels distressed, demoralized, and "down in the dumps" from time to time. When we feel that way, we say we are "depressed." However, technically, we are simply experiencing the generalized psychological distress that is a standard part of living.

If this generalized state of sadness and distress is fairly constant and continues for years, it is known as chronic dysphoria (or dysthymic disorder) and probably warrants professional treatment. A third form of "depression" is really grief, which comes about as the result of the loss of someone or something that is important to us. MS can bring about significant losses in people's lives, including the loss of certain abilities, expectations for the future, and employment. As a result, most people with MS go through a grieving process that may be repeated many times over the course of the illness as new losses occur.

The most serious form of depression is a "major depressive episode," characterized by sadness that is severe and unremitting, and accompanied by a variety of other symptoms such as low self-esteem, sleep disturbance, changes in appetite, hopelessness, and sometimes suicidal thoughts. Some people experience recurrent major depressive episodes, and others seem to alternate between episodes of major depression and periods of unusually good or "high" moods (manic episodes). Alternating episodes of depression and mania are known as "bipolar disorder" (formerly referred to as manic depression).

There is ample evidence that people with MS are at greater risk for depression in all its guises than the general population. It has been estimated that at any given point in time, one out of every seven people with MS is experiencing a major depression. Approximately 50 percent of people with MS will experience a major depressive episode during the course of their illness, compared to 5 percent to 15 percent in the general population. Bipolar disorder is less common than major depression, occurring in about 15 percent of people with MS.

The estimated frequency of severe depression in MS is quite controversial. The diagnosis of depression is highly technical and requires a very specific set of symptoms along with an equally specific time frame. Additionally, many of the symptoms of depression can easily be confused with MS symptoms and effects. For example, the symptoms of depression include fatigue, sleep disturbance, difficulty concentrating, and feelings of worthlessness. These symptoms are often part of the MS picture as well. It can thus be very tricky to diagnose a major depressive episode in a person with MS.

Keeping the above in mind, it is important to remember that MS is a psychologically challenging condition. People with MS are at greater risk than the general population for a variety of emotional complications. Those who deal with MS, either their own or someone else's, need to be alert to the potential need for help, especially professional help. For the sake of clarity in the remainder of the chapter, the term *depression* will be used to distinguish the more severe major depressive episode or chronic dysphoria from the relatively common, episodic feelings of distress and discouragement that most people experience from time to time.

Why do some people with MS get severely depressed while others do not?

The intensity of a person's reactions seems to depend on a variety of factors in addition to the severity of the disease itself, including personality style and coping skills, availability of social supports, financial security, and genetic predisposition to depression. Additionally, there has been some speculation among researchers that MS may cause demyelination in certain parts of the brain that play a role in the experience or expression of emotions. Therefore, disease severity is by no means the most reliable predictor of a person's emotional response. A person with less disabling disease may develop a severe depression while one with greater disability does not.

If depression in MS is caused by demyelination in the brain, what would be the point of psychotherapy or antidepressant drugs?

The idea that demyelination causes depression in MS is at present hypothetical. Studies that have looked at total lesion area on MRI or lesions in specific parts of the brain, have not generally supported the concept. Other types of studies have been tantalizing but inconclusive. For example, there is tentative evidence that some persons with MS show a dysfunction in the brain mechanisms that play a role in regulating certain of the hormones involved in mood, called **glucocorticoids**. One study found that both affective disturbances and **neuroendocrine** abnormalities were related to white cell counts in the **cerebrospinal fluid** and to **gadolinium-enhancing lesions** on MRI. Another study found that improvement in self-reported depression was related to a drop in levels of **interferon-gamma** (a naturally appearing substance that is thought by some to be associated with exacerbations of MS).

MS has wide-ranging effects on the brain. It would therefore not be surprising if future research confirmed that MS-related changes in the brain play a major role in depression. Even if MS does involve such a 'direct' or 'biological' influence on mood, however, it is unlikely to be the only factor involved. Depression is a complex phenomenon and in any given person there are probably many factors at work in determining the type and severity of depressive symptoms. Some of these factors might include one's appraisal of altered life circumstances, the availability of social support, inherited pre-disposition to affective disturbances, and life stress. Since it is a complex problem, depression demands a sophisticated response. Even if the causes of depression involve biological changes in the brain, psychotherapy and medication can still help to alter mood and assist people in dealing with these and other MS-related changes. Research to date has shown that both psychotherapy and medication are effective in treating MS-related depression. As we refine our understanding of this problem we will be able to develop increasingly effective, multi-faceted treatments.

How can I tell if I'm having a normal reaction to being diagnosed with a chronic illness or if I have a serious depression?

Almost everyone reacts negatively to being diagnosed with a disabling illness. Reactions may include shock, disbelief, anger, anxiety, sadness, grief, pessimism about the future, and loss of self-esteem. These reactions can at times become fairly intense and may be difficult to distinguish from depression.

However, depression does have some distinguishing characteristics. Serious clinical depression consists of more than just feeling down in the dumps. The feeling of sadness tends to be constant, with little or no relief. People who are depressed may lose interest in most of the things that used to be enjoyable, such as hobbies, visiting friends, reading, work-related projects, and sexual activity. They may experience loss of appetite or gradually begin eating much more than usual. Sleep may be disturbed by early morning awakening or they may begin wanting to sleep longer or more frequently. Depression can include feelings of worthlessness and self-blame for everything that seems to be going wrong. Individuals who are depressed may also feel guilty without knowing why, as if they had done something horrible that must be punished. A depressed person's thoughts and actions may be slowed, and behavior may appear listless. However, unlike those who are simply suffering from MS fatigue, people who are depressed do not really care about feeling listless because they are not interested in doing anything. The person who is depressed may also be plagued by thoughts of death and even suicide.

In contrast to this devastating picture of clinical depression, the reaction to having a chronic illness tends to be less severe and not as broad in its effects. For example, individuals who are reacting to MS may also feel downhearted, blue, and pessimistic, but can still be interested in life activities and forget their troubles long enough to take care of their responsibilities and engage in enjoyable activities. The person who is learning to live with MS may struggle with an altered self-image that includes newly acquired limitations, without necessarily feeling useless or worthless. Thoughts of suicide are less likely to arise.

It is important to keep in mind that there can at times be considerable overlap between the "ordinary reaction" to chronic illness and a serious depression. Most people are likely to experience something in-between—a reaction to MS that occasionally has some of the characteristics of depression. Consultation with a psychologist or a psychiatrist can help you to clarify the issues involved and identify the most useful form of treatment.

I was diagnosed with MS about a year ago and so far I seem to have done pretty well compared to some. I can't run anymore and my endurance is low, but otherwise I have few problems. I think that I should be grateful that my MS is so mild but instead I feel depressed. Why should I feel depressed if I'm doing so well?

There is no simple relationship between how well one does physically with MS and how one feels emotionally. MS is generally progressive and can lead to increasing disability. Even though you say you are doing "pretty well," you still have lost some physical abilities. For many people, this initial loss, no matter how mild it may seem, can be the most emotionally challenging. Everyone reacts differently to the physical changes brought on by MS. However, it has been consistently observed that the first few years right after the diagnosis are often the toughest. During those early years people are still processing the sudden shift that has taken place in their expectations for the years ahead. Most of us anticipate good health and intact physical abilities for the foreseeable future. A diagnosis of MS undermines these expectations, even if the changes have not as yet taken place. An added burden for many is a sense of guilt because they are doing well but still feel upset about having MS. For most people, these feelings slowly subside as they get used to having MS in their lives. Moreover, many find that having gone through this initial distress helps to prepare them should the MS lead to other changes in their lives.

I can't tell if I'm tired all the time because I'm depressed or depressed because I'm always tired. Who can help me find the answer to this question?

Depression is often accompanied by a feeling of listlessness and/or a lack of interest in everyday activities. On the other hand, people who experience MS fatigue often feel "down" because they are not able to do the things they would like to do. It is not always easy to separate depression from an intense feeling of fatigue; however, people who have experienced both usually report that they feel quite different. You are probably not depressed if you are frustrated because your fatigue prevents you from getting your chores done and enjoying your hobbies and social life. However, you could well be clinically depressed if you wake up in the morning feeling tired, and find you don't really care if you get anything done or not.

The difference between depression and fatigue is not just academic. It is important to have an accurate assessment because the treatments for clinical depression and fatigue are quite different. Consultation with your neurologist in conjunction with a psychiatrist or psychologist can help you to identify the exact nature of your problem. Depression should be treated with psychotherapy and/or medication. Fatigue is usually treated with drugs such as pemoline (Cylert®) or amantadine (see Appendix B) and by energy conservation measures such as schedule changes, naps, and the use of adaptive equipment. Keep in mind, however, that depression and fatigue can occur in the same person and may both need to be addressed.

What is the best treatment for depression in a person who has MS?

Appropriate treatment requires identification of the exact nature and severity of the depression. The two major approaches to the treatment of depression are psychotherapy and medication. Psychotherapy is generally conducted individually (although it can be done in groups) by a qualified psychiatrist, psychologist, or social worker. Support groups and peer counseling may be a useful addition to treatment but are not a substitute for psychotherapy (see Chapter 10). Research has shown that psychotherapy can improve depression in MS, sometimes in just a few weeks. However, psychotherapy generally requires several months to achieve substantial results. While there are many different approaches to psychotherapy, the important factor seems to be the ability of the therapist.

Many people find that a combination of psychotherapy and medication works well; the medication helps to elevate mood while the therapy provides a supportive setting in which to explore feelings and learn more effective coping strategies.

A variety of medications have been used successfully to treat depression in MS. For many years, tricyclics were the treatment of choice, e.g., imipramine (Tofranil®), amitriptyline (Elavil®), nortriptyline (Pamelor®). In recent years, however, the seratonergic antidepressants, e.g. fluoxetine (Prozac®) sertraline, (Zoloft®), paroxetine (Paxil®), and venlafaxine (Effexor®) have become more widely used (see Appendix B). There are a number of other anti-depressants that have been used less frequently in MS and which are neither tricyclics nor seratonergic. These include Bupropion HCL (Welbutrin®), nefazodone (Serzone®), and trazadone (Desyrel®). Each of these medications has a slightly different side-effect profile. Since no two people are exactly alike in the side-effects they experience, one or another of these drugs may be preferable for a given person. These medications should be administered under the supervision of a psychiatrist who can monitor your progress and adjust the dosage as needed. In some instances, electroshock therapy can be very effective and extremely safe. In rare instances in which episodes of depression alternate with periods of elevated mood and hyperactivity, a mood stabilizing drug such as divalproex sodium (Depakote®), lithium carbonate (Eskalith®), or carbamazepine (Tegretol®) may be used in addition to or instead of an antidepressant. Whatever you are experiencing, you need not suffer alone. Getting help is a constructive and active coping strategy. It does not imply weakness or giving up. Quite the contrary, it means that you are determined to confront the emotional challenges of life with MS.

I have had MS for seven years. I think that I have been depressed on and off much of that time. My doctor never asked me about my mood and I never thought I needed any treatment. Recently, at my wife's urging, I saw a social worker who referred me to a psychiatrist. I have been taking an antidepressant for about two months now and seeing the social worker once a week. I feel like a new person. Is my experience common?

Unfortunately, your experience is all too common. One study found that in a sample of persons moderately disabled by MS, 80 percent had experienced a psychiatric disorder during the past year but only 60 percent had received any form of psychiatric treatment. There seem to be several reasons for this. People with MS are followed by neurologists, whose primary focus may be on the physical aspects of the disease. In addition, many neurologists tend to assume that a person's more general medical needs (e.g., mood disorders, gynecological problems, high blood pressure, etc.) are being addressed by a primary care physician. People with MS may also assume that feeling a little depressed is simply their lot in life, to be endured with the rest of their symptoms or problems. As you have seen, however, one does not necessarily have to go through life feeling chronically depressed. Help is available. If the doctor doesn't ask about mood, the person with MS should bring up the subject.

Some of my friends without MS have been taking St. John's Wort for depression and tell me that it works well and has no side effects. I have mild bouts of depression that often last for a few weeks. Should I consider St. John's Wort?

St. John's Wort is an extract of a flower that grows wild in many countries, and has been used medicinally for centuries. The active ingredient is thought to be hypericum. Hypericum has been tested in a number of European studies of mild to moderate depression. Most of these studies have shown hypericum to be about equal in effectiveness to the tricyclic antidepressants in treating mild to moderate depression, with few side effects. No comparisons were made to the serotonergic antidepressants (e.g., Prozac and Zoloft) in the European studies. Hypericum is not considered to be appropriate for the treatment of severe clinical depression. Here in the United States, the National Institutes of Health have funded a large clinical trial of hypericum, but the results will not be available for some time. To date, there are no clinical trials of hypericum in multiple sclerosis.

St. John's Wort is widely available in drug and health food stores in the form of capsules, tea, and even St. John's Wort tortilla chips. These products vary widely in purity, consistency, and the amount of hypericum they contain. This has created an unusual situation in which utilization of a new drug has leaped ahead of the normal regulatory process. If the positive results of the European studies are confirmed by the American studies, use of hypericum will probably increase because it seems to have few side effects. At present, its safety and efficacy in MS are unknown and product quality varies widely. Before you take any medication, whether prescription or over-the-counter, you should discuss it with your physician. Moreover, if the problem is depression, you should speak with a psychiatrist, psychologist, or social worker. There is more involved in the treatment of depression than just finding the right medicine.

My friends and relatives have begun to notice how nervous I am lately. I don't remember ever feeling this anxious before in my life. What is the best treatment for anxiety in MS?

There are a number of anti-anxiety medications classified as benzodiazepines, e.g., diazepam (Valium®) and alprazolam (Xanax®). However, because these medications (particularly Xanax®) can be associated with physical and psychological dependence, they should generally be used on a short-term basis and only if other strategies such as psychotherapy have not completely resolved the problem. There is a newer drug, buspirone (Buspar®), that has been used to some extent in MS and which has less potential for dependence. There have not been controlled clinical trials of these drugs in MS, so their use in this disease is based on clinical experience and studies done in other populations.

Anxiety almost always can be traced back to life circumstances. Everyday stresses, worry about the future, and financial strain can all precipitate or worsen anxiety. It may be helpful to try to identify the sources of your anxiety and evaluate your current way of handling these difficult circumstances. This can best be done through psychotherapy, counseling, or stress management with a professional. It is often possible to reduce anxiety through a better understanding of its sources and by altering one's approach to dealing with it. Medication can at times facilitate this process by reducing anxiety to a more manageable level. However, the long-term goal is to be able to deal with the sources of anxiety without having to rely on medication.

Can any of the medications I'm taking for my MS affect my mood?

Yes, many of the medications used in MS can affect your mood. Space does not permit a discussion of all of them, but here are some of the more important ones.

◇ Antidepressants are sometimes used to treat bladder problems and unpleasant sensory symptoms, generally in doses lower than those used to treat depression. However, some people find that the antidepressants may improve their mood even in these low doses.

◇ Pemoline (Cylert®) is used to treat fatigue in MS. It is a stimulant and may in some cases make you feel more optimistic or slightly irritable.

◇ Valium® is a benzodiazepine (a class of tranquilizers) that is sometimes used to treat spasticity (see Chapter 2). Valium® may make you feel more relaxed both physically and psychologically.

◇ Baclofen (Lioresal®) is the drug most commonly used to treat spasticity. When treatment is started, many people feel drowsy until their bodies get used to the drug. However, a more dramatic side effect may occur if you abruptly stop taking it, especially if you are on a very high dose. Stopping a high dose of baclofen abruptly may cause you to experience extreme symptoms such as hallucinations (seeing or hearing things while awake that are not there), agitation or restlessness, convulsions, or mood changes. It is therefore important not to cease taking this medication abruptly, but to taper the dosage.

◇ Steroids that are used to treat MS exacerbations can produce a variety of mood alterations. Some people become depressed on steroids while others become happy, euphoric, irritable, or hyperactive. This steroid "high" is often followed by a "low" when treatment ends. Individuals react differently to steroids. Moreover, the same person may have different reactions at different times. In other words, just because steroids gave you a "high" the last time you had them does not necessarily mean that you will have the same experience the next time. People who have a history of extreme reactions to steroids are sometimes treated in advance with mood-stabilizing drugs such as lithium carbonate (Eskalith®), divalproex sodium (Depakote®), or carbamazepine (Tegretol®) to prevent these wide and upsetting swings. It is important to work closely with your physician when you are treated with steroids and to report promptly any unusual reactions (see Appendix B).

Will I ever stop feeling angry and sad all the time?

Many people with MS go through periods when they feel acutely and persistently distressed. This often happens when the disease is first diagnosed and when symptom flare-ups cause greater disability. At times like these, the disease (and your feelings about it) seems to fill your life, crowding out other thoughts and feelings. Most people find this to be a temporary experience. You will probably find your distress becoming less acute as you begin to get used to having MS and learn how to make a place for it in your life. This will gradually allow more space for other emotions to return. MS will no longer occupy your total attention and you will once again become interested in your work, family, social life, and hobbies.

If you remain persistently sad and angry, despite the passage of time and despite improvement or stability in your symptoms, you probably need to seek professional help. A psychiatrist, psychologist, or social worker can help you determine whether you need some psychotherapy or medication to help you get through these feelings. If and when the MS flares up, you may find that the disease once again becomes an all-encompassing emotional preoccupation. These periods of intense distress followed by relative calm are not uncommon in MS. Because of this, many people with MS find that they benefit from brief psychotherapy at several points in the course of their lives. When things get tough, they may return to therapy for a "tune-up." *Adjustment to MS is an ongoing and evolving experience, not a one-time happening.*

I have read that suicide is very common in MS. Is this true?

Although precise estimates vary, suicide is at least twice as common in MS as it is in the general population; indeed, it is one of the major causes of death among people with MS. This frequency probably stems from many roots. Suicide is most often associated with depression, and depression is more common in MS. However, suicide is generally more common among people with chronic, "incurable," debilitating illnesses. Many of the so-called "assisted suicides" that have been in the news recently have been individuals with MS. The disease can create the sorts of conditions (e.g., financial strain, family stress, isolation, overall deterioration in quality of life, and a bleak outlook for the future) in which suicide occurs. Suicide tends to result from feelings of hopelessness rather than depression per se.

At present a great ethical debate is raging in the United States concerning suicide, particularly assisted suicide. Many believe that one has the right to choose to end one's life. Others believe that the desire to take one's own life is by definition a psychiatric condition against which the person needs to be protected by society. Tragically, many individuals take their own lives while in a state of depression and hopelessness that could have been successfully treated with psychotherapy and/or medication. Depression can make a person perceive the life situation as more hopeless than it really is. However, there are people who seem to choose suicide not as a result of the distortions attending depression, but as rational adults in full command of their faculties who see clearly what they want for themselves. The debate over suicide will continue and expand during the next few years. For a variety of reasons, MS will occupy an important place in that debate.

Since my husband quit working because of MS, he seems to have lost interest in most of the things that he used to enjoy. Now he just sits in front of the TV all day doing nothing. Why is this and what can I do to help him?

Lack of motivation and failure to initiate activities can be symptoms of depression, but they can also occur when there has been extensive demyelination in important brain regions responsible for planning and initiating activities. Oftentimes, the family member is more distressed by this behavior than the person with MS. If your husband left work because of MS-related physical problems but his mind is still "sharp," he could well be depressed. Depression is fairly common following a major life change such as leaving the workforce. If, on the other hand, he was having trouble performing his job due to changes in his cognitive function, or if you know that he has had an MRI that showed a lot of MS plaques in the front part of his brain, his difficulty initiating activities may be due to structural changes in his brain rather than just a result of feeling discouraged.

In either case, you should discuss your concerns with both your husband and his neurologist. The neurologist can refer you to a neuropsychologist or neuropsychiatrist who, through a diagnostic interview and appropriate testing, can identify the likely cause of your husband's problem. If the cause is depression, treatment may involve psychotherapy, medications, or a combination of these. If the cause is demyelination, recommendations may include setting up a daily schedule with activities appropriate to his level of function and making sure that he has the help he needs to get started and continue working on activities. Depending on your situation, this could be carried out at home, or you might want to look into having your husband get involved in a structured activity program at a clinic or community center. You will have a clearer idea of which solutions are likely to work best for both of you once you have a better sense of the cause of the problem.

My husband seems to go through a lot of mood swings lately, which make him pretty difficult to live with. Are these mood swings caused by the MS and is there anything to do about them?

The issue of mood swings is one of the most common mentioned by MS families. The disease causes structural changes in the brain that may increase the risk of abrupt changes in mood and emotional expression that can occur within minutes. This type of mood swing is often referred to as "emotional lability" to distinguish it from the longer lasting periods of depression and mania that typically alternate in bipolar disorder. Some mood swings may be caused by medications, especially high-dose steroids. Many people also use the term *mood swings* to refer to the anger and frustration felt by people who have had their lives turned upside down by MS. Regardless of the cause, abrupt changes in mood can make family life stressful and unpleasant for all concerned. It is important to seek professional consultation and treatment for this problem.

Depending on the cause, mood swings can be handled in different ways. Emotional lability may respond to low doses of tricyclic antidepressants such as amitriptyline (Elavil®). Mood swings caused by high-dose steroids should abate once the steroid treatment has ended. For someone who has reacted strongly to steroids in the past, the physician may prescribe some preventive treatment such as lithium, divalproex sodium (Depakote®), or carbamazepine (Tegretol®) to diminish the reaction (see Chapter 3). Mood swings related to frustration may be helped by psychotherapy and/or medication. Family therapy is often extremely useful, both to help family members understand the problem and to ensure that they are not inadvertently contributing to the deteriorating emotional climate within the family. Finally, if the mood swings last significantly longer (two weeks or more) and are part of a bipolar disorder, treatment typically involves a combination of medication (usually lithium or Depakote®) and psychotherapy.

I find that I cry at the drop of a hat. Any time I feel the least bit emotional I start crying and can't stop. I never used to be like this and it's very embarrassing when I'm trying to talk to a colleague or have a simple disagreement with my husband. Is there anything to do about this problem?

Many people with MS find that they cry easily and have trouble stopping once they have begun. The crying is likely to be precipitated by any type of heightened emotional tension. The first step in handling this problem is to be aware that it is something that happens to you in times of tension or distress. With enhanced awareness, you are less likely to let your reactions run away with you.

For example, if you are trying to discuss something with a colleague or family member and suddenly find yourself becoming "choked up" and tearful, try to stop and take a few deep breaths. Remind yourself that you need to take the strength of your reaction with a grain of salt. You should not discount what you are feeling, just realize that the *strength* of that reaction may be out of proportion to the situation. Many people find that they can forestall the worst effects of this problem by slowing down a bit and reflecting. Self-awareness and deep breathing can help you to regain at least some of the control that has been lost. Working on this problem with a psychotherapist can be extremely helpful. In therapy you can identify those situations most likely to set you off and experiment with different types of strategies.

Sometimes my wife starts laughing or crying for no reason. Sometimes she even seems to be doing both at the same time even when there is nothing funny or sad going on. She thinks her "wires are crossed." Why is this happening to her?

Your wife is probably experiencing what is known as *affective release* (or *pseudobulbar affect*), a condition in which fits of laughing and crying can occur with no obvious precipitating event. This condition was formerly thought to be caused by damage to some of the nerves passing through the medulla oblongata (a structure in the **brainstem**). The current thinking is that affective release is associated with lesions in the limbic system, a group of brain structures involved in emotional feeling and expression and structures connected with it. Recent attention has also focused on the possible role of lesions in the frontal lobes. To date, research on this question has been inconclusive.

In contrast to the mood swings discussed earlier, the person's actual mood may be totally unrelated to the emotion that is released. A fit of crying may thus begin even when the person is feeling rather content. Once these laughing or crying episodes begin, the person is often unable to stop them. This symptom requires patience and understanding on the part of family and friends. The bouts of laughing and crying can be misunderstood by others, who may be offended by what they consider to be inappropriate or embarrassing behavior. Some types of antidepressant medications may help. One small study found some benefit from the use of amitriptyline (Elavil®). Although there are no studies to date, there are anecdotal reports that the selective serotonin reuptake inhibitors, e.g., fluoxetine (Prozac®), may be helpful for this symptom. Many people find that the experience becomes somewhat less frightening once they get used to the fact that these uncontrolled bouts are going to happen from time to time. Again, the understanding of others is a key part of dealing with this problem.

My husband has gotten depressed about all the changes in our lives since the MS got worse. I've asked him to see a psychiatrist but he says he's not crazy and adamantly refuses to go. What should I do? I'm really worried about him and about our relationship.

Going to a psychiatrist or other mental health professional still carries an unjustified stigma for many. You might try pointing out to your husband that depression is one aspect of life with MS that can be effectively managed. If it's OK to seek help for problems with walking or vision, why not for the emotions? Using psychotherapy and/or medication, it is possible to come to grips with depression, feel more optimistic about things, and thus put more enjoyment back into life.

Going for psychotherapy does not mean that someone is crazy. Quite the contrary, it indicates that he or she is sharp enough to know when some assistance is needed to get through a difficult life situation. You might suggest that your husband see a therapist on a trial basis. Many people resist this sort of help until they meet a therapist who makes talking seem comfortable and enjoyable.

Since you are having a hard time with your husband's depression, you might also want to tell him about your own feelings. Ask him to see a therapist for the sake of your relationship and offer to go with him. Treatment cannot be sustained over a long period of time if it is being done only for the sake of another person, but this may be a way to get him started. If all else fails, you should consider going to see a therapist yourself for assistance in dealing with the situation. Individual therapy for the non-MS partner can be quite helpful, and in many instances the MS partner eventually agrees to join the therapeutic effort. Some adamant spouses grudgingly show up for the first session, determined never to return, and wind up staying for the duration of treatment. For you, the important thing is to get help for all who are willing to use it, even if that means only you.

I've read some older books about MS that talk about the "MS personality." What type of personality does this refer to?

At one time it was thought that certain medical conditions were caused, at least in part, by specific personality types. MS was supposed to be more likely to develop in people with emotionally immature and dependent personalities. Such archaic notions of disease were abandoned long ago. Some people still believe that MS can "produce" a specific type of personality after the disease develops, but this is not the case. People with MS may find that they share similar problems, experiences, and concerns, and so have a lot in common. However, they do not have the same personality. The personality characteristics one had before getting MS are likely (for better or worse!) to be the same ones the person has after getting MS.

What is euphoria and is this a common phenomenon in MS?

MS euphoria is an exaggerated and unrealistic state of happiness or well-being that, to the observer, seems out of keeping with an individual's life situation. People with MS are said to be euphoric when they appear blasé and lighthearted in the face of serious or life-threatening problems. Someone who is euphoric may tend to giggle inappropriately, even when nothing funny has happened. This inappropriate giggling almost always occurs in people with severe intellectual loss. The combination of cognitive dysfunction and unrealistic optimism can lead to the neglect of important self-management issues, such as medical care, nutrition, and personal safety. Euphoria is thought to be the result of damage to parts of the brain involved in judgment and the control of emotions. It is sometimes confused with the uncontrollable laughing and crying that can affect people with MS, but these are more often precipitated by something that is emotionally charged and can occur even in the absence of significant intellectual loss.

My sister has had MS for 10 years. She walks with a cane and has some visual loss and bladder problems. Three times during the past two years we have had to call the police because she had had violent rages during which she threw things, yelled, and tried to attack members of the family. The last time this happened she punched a neighbor and is now up on charges. Can MS cause this type of extreme behavior and if so, what can be done about it?

Just because a person has MS does not mean that every physical and psychological problem is due to the disease. There are people without MS who have rages and become violent. However, the behavior you describe can be one of the more unusual manifestations of MS. Although some of your sister's anger may arise from frustration related to her illness, it is more likely due to changes in those areas of the brain concerned with the expression and control of emotions. We all get angry from time to time but in most cases we manage to control the expression of those emotions so that we do not physically assault other people. Your sister may have lost some of the ability to control these strong emotions. She should be evaluated by a neuropsychiatrist, a psychiatrist who specializes in conditions having both neurologic and psychiatric aspects. The type of problems your sister is experiencing can sometimes be helped with a regimen of medication and psychotherapy. Very often, the neuropsychiatrist will also teach the family to recognize the warning signs of an impending blow-up so that it can be avoided. You may never know for certain whether these symptoms are due in whole or in part to MS. Whatever the cause, the treatment is much the same.

Stress and MS

Can stress cause MS or make it worse?

There is perhaps no more controversial question in MS than this one. Many investigators have attempted to show that stress can precipitate the onset of MS, trigger exacerbations, or hasten progression. Although some studies have found limited evidence to support one or more of these ideas, the relationship between stress and MS remains uncertain. Most of the studies used methods that were of poor quality, thus rendering their findings suspect.

Recent studies have begun to focus on different questions. Some studies have attempted to determine how stress might affect the immune system, and through the immune system, affect MS. Research in a variety of medical conditions and in healthy controls has shown that the immune system is sensitive to stress in a variety of ways. By understanding the links between immune function and stress, we may shed light on the possible links between stress and MS. Other studies have looked at the relationship between stress and changes on MRI. In one such study, it was found that persons with MS reporting higher amounts of stress and depression tended to show more gadolinium-enhancing lesions on MRI eight weeks later. While the findings from all of these studies are suggestive, they need to be confirmed in larger samples.

In the meantime, we should be very cautious about attributing changes in the disease to stress. Family members sometimes feel guilty in the belief that they caused stress that worsened a loved one's MS. Such beliefs are unfounded. People with MS occasionally quit their jobs in the mistaken belief that they can slow the progression of their MS by reducing "occupational stress." Nothing is gained by such actions, and the individual loses the stimulation and satisfaction that working can provide.

Everyone is searching for explanations for this mysterious disease, and stress is one explanation that is readily available because we encounter it every day. MS adds a lot of stress to most people's lives. Thus the real issue is not whether stress is altering the course of the MS, but how one can most effectively deal with the stresses that life and MS produce.

What should I do about the stresses in my life? I don't think I can make them all go away.

Sometimes people with MS are told by well-meaning people to try to "reduce the stress in your life." Nice trick if you can do it! Most sources of stress in our lives are not under our control. Moreover, many times when people set out to "reduce stress" they do so by bailing out of important life activities such as work or family responsibilities. These activities provide much of the stimulation and inspiration that make life worth living. Do not withdraw from life on the basis of the mistaken notion that this will reduce stress. The key is to learn how to cope with stress rather than to avoid it. You can learn to deal with this problem in a variety of ways, including stress management programs, psychotherapy, counseling, support groups, peer counseling, self-help books, exercise, and developing better organizational skills. The first step is to identify the sources of stress in your life and evaluate your present coping style. Next you need to experiment with more effective coping strategies. Learning to deal more effectively with stress is probably best done with a professional who is trained in the requisite skills. Once you have mastered these skills, you should be able to cope on your own, perhaps returning from time to time for a "tune-up" to sharpen your skills or learn how to deal with new situations that have arisen.

Recommended Readings

Burnfield A. *Multiple Sclerosis: A Personal Exploration.* New York: Demos, 1985.

James J. *One Particular Harbor.* Chicago: Noble Press, 1993.

Pitzele S. *We Are Not Alone: Learning to Live with Chronic Illness.* New York: Workman Publishing, 1986.

Selected publications available from your local chapter of the National Multiple Sclerosis Society (800-FIGHT-MS):

◇ *Multiple Sclerosis and Your Emotions* (ES 6007)
◇ *Taming Stress in Multiple Sclerosis* (ES 6034)

12

Sexuality

Frederick W. Foley, Ph.D.
Michael A. Werner, M.D.

Multiple sclerosis can affect the experience of sexuality in a variety of ways. People sometimes report feeling less sexually interested or aroused, either as a direct result of neurologic changes or because of their efforts to cope with the impact of these changes on their lives. Partners often misinterpret the sexual changes they observe in the person with MS, and may also experience their own changes in sexual responsiveness in the face of the illness. Both members of the couple often find it difficult to communicate with one another about their changing sexual and intimacy needs.

The few studies on the *prevalence* of sexual problems in MS have relied primarily on the survey or questionnaire method. Up to 85 percent of men with MS report at least occasional sexual problems, with erectile difficulties being the most commonly reported symptom. The proportion of women reporting sexual problems ranges from 56 percent to 74 percent, with loss of libido (sexual desire), changes in vaginal sensation and lubrication being the most commonly cited problems. Although these statistics may seem disturbing, it should be noted that the prevalence of at least occasional sexual dysfunction in the general US population ranges from 34 percent for men to 41 percent for women.

The best prevalence study to date utilized a case-control method, in which a group of persons with MS was compared to a group with other chronic diseases and a healthy group with no illness. This study found that 73.1 percent of the people with MS, 39.2 percent of those with other chronic disease, and 12.7 percent of healthy controls reported sexual dysfunction (Zorzon et al, 1999).

The ways in which MS can affect sexuality and expressions of intimacy have been divided into primary, secondary, and tertiary sexual dysfunction. "Primary sexual dysfunction" is a direct result of neurologic changes that affect the sexual response. In both men and women, this can include a decrease or loss of sex drive, decreased or unpleasant genital sensations, and diminished capacity for orgasm. Men may experience difficulty achieving or maintaining an erection and a decrease in or loss of ejaculatory force or frequency. Women may experience decreased vaginal lubrication, loss of vaginal muscle tone and/or diminished clitoral engorgement.

"Secondary sexual dysfunction" stems from symptoms that do not directly involve nervous pathways to the genital system, such as bladder and bowel problems, fatigue, **spasticity**, muscle weakness, body or hand tremors, impairments in attention and concentration, and non-genital sensory changes.

"Tertiary sexual dysfunction" results from disability-related psychosocial and cultural issues that can interfere with one's sexual feelings and experiences. For example, some people find it difficult to reconcile the idea of being disabled with being fully sexually expressive. Changes in self-esteem—including the way one feels about one's body, demoralization, depression, or mood swings—can all interfere with intimacy and sexuality. The sexual partnership can be severely challenged by changes within a relationship, such as one person becoming the other's caregiver. Similarly, changes in employment status or role performance within the household are often associated with emotional adjustments that can temporarily interfere with sexual expression. The strain of coping with MS challenges a couple's efforts to communicate openly about their respective experiences and their changing needs for sexual expression and fulfillment.

I've noticed a lot of changes in my body and my sexual feelings in the past few years. My doctor has never brought up the subject of sex and neither have I. Where is the best place to get information about sexual problems in MS?

Changes in sexual feelings normally occur throughout the life span. However, the experience of MS can complicate the typical changes that occur. MS affects sexual feelings both directly and indirectly, as discussed previously. Neurologists and other health care providers often do not spontaneously bring up the subject of sexuality. Physicians and nurses may ignore sexuality because they perceive this line of questioning as an unwelcome intrusion into the private lives of their patients, because of personal discomfort in asking about sexuality, or because of lack of professional training in this area. Although it can be difficult and potentially embarrassing, your sexuality is important enough to bring up with your primary MS physician. Discuss your changes in sexual feelings and ask directly about treatments that are available to enhance sexuality. Talk over with your physician the ways in which your MS symptoms, and the medications used to treat them, may be affecting your sexual responses. Although the burden of opening the door to communication about sexuality may initially fall on you, taking this step with your health care team will ensure that this frequently untreated problem gets the attention it deserves.

To get information about literature on sexual problems in MS, begin by contacting your local chapter of the National Multiple Sclerosis Society. Refer also to the Recommended Readings and Resources at the end of this chapter.

My wife still seems to enjoy having sex as much as she always did, but she doesn't have an orgasm any more. She says it's not my fault, but I don't understand what the problem is.

MS can interfere directly or indirectly with orgasm. "Primary orgasmic dysfunction" stems from MS lesions in the spinal cord or brain that directly interfere with orgasm. Orgasm depends on nervous system pathways originating in the brain (the center of emotion and fantasy during masturbation or intercourse) and pathways in the upper, middle, and lower parts of the spinal cord (which control sensations from erogenous zones such as lips, nipples, clitoris, and so on). Sensation and orgasmic response can be diminished or absent if these pathways are disrupted by plaques. Orgasm can also be inhibited by secondary or indirect symptoms, such as sensory **paresthesias**, cognitive problems, and other MS-related changes. In addition, anxiety, depression, and loss of sexual self-confidence or sexual self-esteem represent tertiary symptoms that can interfere with one's ability to enjoy the sexual experience and thus inhibit orgasm.

Treatment of orgasmic loss in MS depends on developing an understanding of what factors are contributing to the loss. If sensation is disturbed in the clitoris and lower body areas, the orgasmic response can sometimes be enhanced by increasing stimulation to other erogenous zones, such as breasts, ears, and lips. Sometimes, stimulating the edges of body zones that are experiencing numbness or diminished sensation can feel sensually or erotically pleasing. Similarly, increasing cerebral stimulation by watching sexually oriented videos, exploring fantasies, and introducing new kinds of sexual play into sexual activities can help trigger orgasms.

It can be both intimate and informative for the person with MS to develop a sensory "body map" by exploring the exact locations of pleasant, decreased, or altered sensations on his or her own body. In order to develop a "body map," the person begins by systematically touching him- or herself from head to toe (or all those places that are within comfortable reach), varying the rate, rhythm, and pressure of touch. It is helpful to allow approximately 15–20 minutes for the exercise, paying attention to areas of sensual pleasure, discomfort, or sensory change, and altering the pattern of touch to maximize the pleasure. The next step is for the person to share the "body map" information with his or her partner, instructing the partner in how to touch in similar fashion. This information can set the stage for the rediscovery of sensual and erotic pleasure.

Increasing stimulation through vigorous oral stimulation or via mechanical vibrators can help if decreased sensation in the genitals is a factor. Strap-on clitoral vibrators (available by mail order) do not interfere with intercourse and require little manipulation once in place. Vibrators that attach to the base of the penis provide direct clitoral stimulation when vaginal penetration is complete and can help stimulate erections in some men as well. In general, AC electric plug-in vibrators have more powerful motors and are more stimulating than DC powered battery-operated ones. However, some electric vibrators are quite powerful and can irritate vaginal or clitoral tissue if applied too vigorously.

My skin feels very tingly all the time. It used to feel good when my husband hugged me or rubbed my back, but now just being touched can feel uncomfortable. I even get pins and needles in my vaginal area. I need to do something about this problem before he gives up trying.

Painful or irritating genital or body sensations can sometimes be managed successfully with medications such as amitriptyline (Elavil®), carbamazepine (Tegretol®), and phenytoin (Dilantin®) (see Chapter 2 and Appendix B). Even with pharmacologic management, however, conducting a variant of the sensory body mapping exercises described above, *with one's partner*, is helpful for retaining a sensually pleasing relationship. Agree to do only the mapping exercise during this time and *not* to engage in sexual activities. Be in a comfortable location where you can be undressed. Have your partner begin by gently stroking the top of your head, and slowly moving down your body from head to toe. Your partner should vary the rhythm and pressure of touch while you give frequent verbal and nonverbal feedback about the kinds of sensations produced in each area. Mutually exploring alternative touches in the context of good communication can set the stage for sensual pleasure both during and independent of sexual activity. As with the treatment of all sexual symptoms in MS, sexual experimentation and communication are the keys to enhancing sexuality.

I love my husband very much but I seem to have lost all interest in having sex. He's worried that I don't love him any more but I keep telling him that I wouldn't be interested in sex with anybody right now. What's happening to my body? Will my sexual feelings ever come back?

The brain does not appear to have a specific, localized sexual center; rather, sexual interest and pleasure seem to be influenced by several different areas of the brain. Sexual interest normally waxes and wanes throughout the life span. We know that "libido," or sexual drive and interest, can be directly affected by MS lesions. Changes in libido can also occur as secondary or tertiary symptoms. For example, a person who is experiencing severe fatigue as a result of MS, or is depressed or demoralized, is less likely to feel interested in sexual activity. The reduced libido can then be a cause for misunderstanding by the partner and anxiety for the person with MS. The misunderstandings and anxiety associated with this problem will further reduce the person's sexual feelings and interest. Therefore, assessing and treating secondary and tertiary sexual symptoms are important components to restoring libido.

Increasing sexual drive that has been directly reduced by central nervous system changes is somewhat challenging. The man or woman with MS who is involved in a sexual or intimate relationship with another person can begin by focusing on the "sensual" and the "special person" aspects of the relationship. Sensual aspects include all physically and emotionally pleasing, nonerotic contact, such as backrubs, handholding, and gentle stroking of the face, arms, and other nongenital body zones. Sex partners often neglect these sensual, non-sexual aspects of their physical relationship during periods of diminished sexual drive, in part because of the difficult emotions that may accompany loss of libido. Making a date for a nonsexual but sensual evening can enable partners to enjoy each other physically and to engage in enjoyable sensual exploration of their bodies, without the pressure of working toward sexual intercourse. In essence, experiencing sexual pleasure has to be "relearned" when the central nervous system has compromised libido, since sexual desire is most often linked to sexual behavior. Relearning one's *sensual* nature is a critical first step in the process. The "body mapping" exercise described earlier in the chapter can help to reestablish the relationship between sexual pleasure and sexual behavior, even in the absence of libido.

The "special person" aspects of a relationship include all those behaviors that one engages in to show the other person that he or she is special and important. Loving gestures from an earlier, "romantic" phase of a relationship, such as unexpected flowers, a surprise note in a lunch bag, or a spontaneous, affectionate hug, tend to be forgotten amidst the pressures of raising children, developing careers, and coping with MS symptoms and disabilities. Restoring or increasing these special acts toward one another can set the stage for increasing intimacy which, can, in turn, stimulate new libido or set the stage for sexual pleasure without libido.

Exploration of one's sensual and erotic body zones is an important step in restoring libido for the person without a current sexual partner. Combining enjoyable cerebral sexual stimulation (achieved via fantasy, sexually explicit videos, books, and so on) with masturbation or sensual, physical self-exploration is sometimes helpful. Using vibrators or other sexual toys may complement these efforts. Although beginning to work on restoring libido may feel like an unrewarding "chore" when there is little or no intrinsic sex drive, working toward rekindling this vital aspect of "self" can be an important aspect of coping with MS.

Kegal exercises (also called pelvic floor exercises) are sometimes prescribed to enhance female sexual responsiveness, although they have not been tested in a clinical trial to determine whether or not they are helpful in MS. To perform the Kegal exercise, a woman alternately tightens and releases the pubococcygeus muscle (identifiable as the muscle that starts and stops the urine flow in midstream). Exercising this muscle several times when you urinate is recommended to help you identify which muscles are involved. After you identify the relevant muscle groups, flex them 10 times a day *when you are not urinating,* since incomplete emptying of the bladder may occur in MS. The rationale for these exercises is that sensation from the muscles around the vagina is an important part of erotic sensation, and female orgasm consists of contractions in several of them. Kegal exercises are directed at strengthening their tone and responsiveness.

Sometimes I have trouble getting an erection even though I feel sexually excited. Other times, I get an erection but then lose it partially or completely while my partner and I are trying to have intercourse. Why is this happening?

The first step in understanding MS-related erectile problems and their treatment is to understand the normal erectile mechanism. Getting an erection is like filling a balloon. Two things have to happen: one has to fill the balloon with air, and then tie the balloon to prevent the air from coming out. The arteries that lead to the penis are lined with smooth muscle. When a man is excited, either psychologically or physically, his body releases transmitting substances that cause relaxation of the smooth muscle. As the smooth muscle relaxes, the arteries become enlarged, allowing an increased blood flow into the penis. This increased blood flow into the penis is what causes an erection. As the penis becomes erect, the veins in the penis (that normally return penile blood to the body) become compressed, causing the blood to remain in the penis. This "trapping mechanism" allows an erection to be maintained until orgasm occurs.

Normal erectile function depends on an intact nervous system. A complex series of nerve impulses must travel between the brain, spinal cord, and penis in order for an erection to be initiated and maintained. When nerve transmission is impaired at any point along the way, a man's ability to achieve or maintain an erection can be affected. The lower area of the spinal cord has nerve pathways traveling to and from the genitals, which allow for reflex erections. If these pathways are intact, reflex erections (that do not involve the middle or upper parts of the spinal cord or brain) can usually be triggered by stimulating the penis directly. Therefore, some men with impaired erectile function can obtain reflex erections by vigorously stimulating the penis with a vibrator. Reflex erections can also result from "stuffing." To engage in stuffing, the woman sits astride her partner and *gently* inserts the flaccid penis into the (well-lubricated) vagina. It is important that the stuffing be done with some care because the flaccid penis can fold back on itself and be squeezed or injured by the pressure of the partner's weight. Internal damage to the penis could go undetected in the presence of reduced sensation.

Are there oral medications I can take for erection problems?

In March of 1998, sildenafil citrate (Viagra®), an oral medication for the treatment of erectile dysfunction, became available in the United States. Sildenafil works by blocking the action of an enzyme called PDE (type 5 phosphodiesterase enzyme). When PDE is blocked, another chemical compound called cGMP (cyclic guanosine monophosphate) remains at higher concentrations in the erectile tissues of the penis. Since cGMP mediates the erection response, blocking PDE allows for enhanced erections. In controlled clinical trials, Viagra® was associated with significantly improved erectile function and greater frequency of intercourse among men with impotence related to both physical and psychological causes. It is important to note, however, that the studies published to date on Viagra® have not included a large group of men with MS. In a recent, placebo-controlled clinical trial of Viagra® in men with MS Viagra was shown to have a positive impact on quality of life including sexual life, partnership relation, family life, social contacts, and overall satisfaction.

Viagra® has its maximum effect one hour after it is taken. It is broken down slowly in the body, and many men report the ability to get improved erections the morning after having taken a dose. It is available in doses of 25 mg, 50 mg, and 100 mg tablets, with the lowest effective dose suggested for use. The medication is relatively expensive (approximately $10 per pill in U.S. dollars), and some insurance companies in the United States will not reimburse for the costs of this medication.

Viagra® is the first oral medication that has been scientifically shown to be successful in enhancing erectile function in men with organic or psychogenic (emotional in origin) erectile disturbance. However, Viagra® is not associated with improvement in sexual desire. When there is significant conflict or distress in a relationship, counseling is necessary to restore intimacy and improve communication.

What are the side effects of Viagra®?

Viagra® is not to be used by men who are taking nitrate-based medications, such as ISMO®, Imdur®, Nitro-Dur®, Nitro-Paste®, Nitrostat®, Nitro-Bid®, et cetera. Men taking these or other nitrate medications in conjunction with Viagra® may experience a sudden and potentially dangerous reduction in blood pressure, *even if they only take the nitrate medications occasionally.*

Viagra® causes a small transient decrease in blood pressure in most men. Coupled with the cardiovascular stress of intercourse, this side effect can cause heart attacks or strokes in men with preexisting vascular disease. Men with recent heart attacks, significant high blood pressure, and/or heart disease should have a cardiology evaluation prior to being started on Viagra®.

It is important to take Viagra® only when prescribed by a doctor who knows all of the treatments and medications you are taking. Side effects of Viagra® in the clinical trials were relatively infrequent, with headache, facial flushing, indigestion, dizziness, and blue-green visual aura being reported. Although priapism (overly prolonged erection) was not reported in the clinical trials, it has been reported as a rare side effect since then. In a normal erection, the penis remains rigid because the trapping mechanism keeps blood from flowing out of the penis until ejaculation occurs. Since oxygen is delivered to body tissues via the circulating blood, the penis does not receive fresh oxygen for the period of time that the penis remains erect. Therefore, a man whose penis remains erect for too long a period of time risks irrevocable damage to the erectile mechanism and to the penis itself. *If a man's erection lasts longer than four hours, he must seek immediate medical treatment, since an erection lasting longer than 24 hours will permanently damage penile tissue.*

In the original Viagra® clinical trials, only 15 percent of men reported any side effects. Because the "blue-green aura" effect can interfere with the visual demands of operating an aircraft, the U.S. Federal Aviation Administration has advised pilots not to take Viagra® during the 24 hours prior to flight time.

Is Viagra® effective with women?

Women have erectile tissue in the clitoris that has recently been found to function in a similar biochemical manner to penile erectile tissue. It is therefore possible that Viagra® may help to sustain or enhance blood flow to the genitals in women, which may be associated with increased vaginal lubrication and/or clitoral engorgement. To date, studies of Viagra® in women with multiple sclerosis have not been conducted. Clinical trials of women with sexual dysfunction (but without MS) are under way in the United States and Europe. One small study in the United States of 33 postmenopausal women with sexual dysfunction found that 18 percent had a significant improvement in sexual function scores. Vaginal lubrication and clitoral sensation improved more than orgasmic response, and side effects were similar to those reported by men who have taken Viagra®. Since Viagra® does not enhance sexual desire in men, it is not expected to impact this sexual symptom in women with MS. Large well-controlled trials in women with MS are still needed to determine the potential usefulness of this drug for women.

Are there other oral medications or herbal alternatives available for dealing with sexual problems?

There are other oral medications that are sometimes used for certain types of sexual problems, but their efficacy from a scientific standpoint is generally poor. Testosterone is a sex hormone that is associated with libido in both men and women. Testosterone supplements have been prescribed for men and women with testosterone deficiency to improve impaired libido or arousal. Since testosterone deficiency is not associated with MS, however, there is no theoretical reason why this supplement should be useful for people with MS. Yohimbine is a chemical compound derived from the bark of an African tree that has been used for hundreds of years as an herbal tonic for enhancing general health, longevity, and sexual function. The herbal formulation has not been well standardized or studied. Standardized pharmaceutical preparations have been developed (yohimbine HCl), and studied in a few small, poorly designed studies, with mixed results. Yohimbine HCl and herbal yohimbine have been compounded with other drugs and/or herbals such as testosterone, strychnine, atropine, ginseng, thioridazine (Mellaril®), pemoline, and ephedrine. The safety and efficacy of these combination remedies remain uncertain. Large, well-designed trials of testosterone, yohimbine HCl, and combination compounds are needed.

Two oral agents undergoing clinical trials for erectile dysfunction are apomorphine, which stimulates a neurotransmitter system in the brain related to sexual function, and phentolamine (Vasomax®), which blocks a mechanism in the erect penis that causes it to become flaccid. Small study results on both of these agents suggest modest efficacy, although larger, well-controlled trials will yield more definitive answers. Largely driven by consumer demand, there are other oral agents in the development phase by several pharmaceutical companies.

Are there other options for dealing with erectile problems?

Several other options are available to treat erectile problems caused by MS. One noninvasive device that readily aids in erections is the vacuum tube and constriction band, which can be purchased with a prescription from a urologist or other physician. With this method, a plastic tube is fitted over the flaccid penis, and air is pumped out of the tube to create a vacuum around the penis. The pumping process may be done mechanically (via hand pump or squeeze bulb) or with a battery-operated, push-button mechanism. The vacuum draws blood into the erectile tissues and produces an erection. Once engorgement of the penis is achieved, a latex band is slipped from the base of the cylinder onto the base of the penis. Air is returned to the cylinder and the tube is removed. The band maintains engorgement of the penis by restricting venous return of blood to the body, thus allowing for intercourse or other sexual activity. However, the use of the band must be limited to 30 minutes or less to avoid any medical complications. Moderate hand sensation and dexterity are required for placing and removing the band in some models. Other models have assistor sleeves that permit hands-free placement of the constriction band. The constriction band alone can be used with satisfactory results by persons who can attain erections readily, but have difficulty maintaining them.

To date, the best-studied treatment for erectile dysfunction in MS involves the injection into the penis of medications that activate the engorgement and trapping mechanisms. The medication stimulates relaxation of the smooth muscle of the arteries so that the penis can become erect, and similarly activates the necessary trapping mechanism that keeps the penis rigid until ejaculation.

Men who have not responded to either oral or injectable therapies, and have been unsuccessful with sexual counseling may find the surgically implanted penile prosthesis to be a better alternative. Following a careful evaluation of your history and presenting symptoms (medical, psychological, neurologic, and sexual), your physician will work with you to determine which type of treatment would be most beneficial for you.

How would I use the penile injections to help me with my erectile problems?

Once you and your doctor have decided that penile injections are a reasonable treatment option, the doctor will teach you the injection techniques so that you can self-inject at those times when you wish to have an erection. The injection is done with a very fine needle into an area at the base of the penis, which, although somewhat sensitive to pleasure, is relatively insensitive to pain. The doctor may recommend an "auto-injector" that works with a simple push-button mechanism. Most men report very little, if any, pain from this injection. The sensation is best described as similar to being flicked by a rubber band. Some men with neurologic impotence of the type caused by MS report a slight achiness caused by one of the medications that is sometimes used in these injections. If this occurs, different medications can be substituted.

When you wish to achieve an erection, you can give yourself an injection (or be given one by your partner if you are unable to do it yourself). After the injection has been given, pressure needs to be applied to the penis for three to five minutes in order to stop any bleeding from within the penis. As you initiate foreplay or self-stimulation, you will develop an erection that will last for approximately an hour. Depending on your state of sexual arousal and the amount of medication you have been given, the erection may subside when you ejaculate or continue for some period of time beyond ejaculation. *The penile injections can be used no more than once in every 24-hour period.*

What medications are used most commonly in penile injections?

Injections for the management of erectile dysfunction have been available for over 15 years. Three different medications are currently prescribed (see Appendix B). Alprostadil (also called prostaglandin E1—Prostin VR®), which was introduced nine years ago, is both the newest and the most commonly used drug in individuals with MS. Alprostadil is the natural substance released by the smooth muscle cells when a man is sexually excited. This medication has been found to have the best treatment outcome with the fewest side effects. It has been approved by the Food and Drug Administration (FDA) for the management of erectile problems and is therefore paid for by most prescription plans.

Alprostadil is also available in pellet form for insertion into the urethra of the penis (Muse®), if penile injections are not desirable. In this form, the medication is inserted into the urethral opening with an applicator. Side effects may include urethral discomfort and burning. The medication may also cause a systemic drop in blood pressure. Muse® comes in doses of 250, 500, and 1,000 micrograms.

The original drug used for injections is a smooth muscle relaxant called papaverine. Its use is almost never associated with any pain, making it a good alternative for anyone who has a problem with alprostadil. Papaverine has a slightly greater tendency to cause scarring at the injection site and is associated with a greater risk of priapism (prolonged erection) because it remains active in the body for a somewhat longer period of time. Papaverine has not been approved by the FDA for the treatment of erectile dysfunction.

Phentolamine (Regitine®—United States; Rogitine®—Canada) is often used in combination with papaverine, or in conjunction with both alprostadil and papaverine, to heighten their effectiveness. Phentolamine is not active by itself and is therefore never used independently. Like papaverine, phentolamine has not been approved for this purpose by the FDA.

If the only FDA-approved, self-injection drug for the management of erectile dysfunction is alprostadil, does this mean that the other two drugs are not safe?

Medications are approved by the FDA for specific functions. They may be used for other purposes at the discretion of the physician. The fact that a drug is not FDA-approved does not mean that it is not safe; it means simply that a drug company has not gone through the costly and time-consuming licensing and testing of the drug for a specific purpose. The three drugs that are currently being used in penile injections are all safe and efficacious when used properly.

What side effects are associated with the use of these medications?

One possible side effect of these medications is priapism (see pp. 289–290). *Priapism almost never occurs in individuals who adhere to the prescribed dose of medication and who are properly trained in the injection procedures.* As rare as it is, priapism does occur with greater frequency with the injectable medications than with Viagra®.

A second potential side effect of penile injections is scarring at the injection site, experienced by approximately 7 percent to 10 percent of individuals. This problem seldom occurs in men who have been properly trained in the techniques of injection and compression of the injection site. When scarring does occur, it takes the form of a small nodule in the subcutaneous tissue of the penis. These nodules typically disappear once the injections are stopped. It is important to be medically monitored and treated so the scarring does not progress, as it may lead to penile curvature and cause difficulty maintaining an erection. Any man who is self-injecting should be examined by a physician every three months for possible scarring.

Will I become dependent on oral or injectable medications that are used for erectile dysfunction?

Sildenafil citrate (Viagra®), alprostadil, papaverine, and phentolamine are used only to potentiate the process of having an erection. No chemical dependency is associated with their use. Depending on the status of your MS symptoms, you may find that you need to use the oral or injectable medications at some times but not others. They can be a helpful adjunct when you are unable to achieve or maintain an adequate erection.

What is a penile prosthesis and how does it work?

A penile prosthesis is a mechanical device designed to give a man with erectile dysfunction the option of having an erection. There are two types of penile prostheses, semirigid and inflatable. With the semirigid type, a flexible rod is surgically implanted in each of the erection chambers (corpus cavernosa) of the penis. These rods can be bent upward when an erection is desired and bent downward at other times. Following insertion of the rods, the penis remains somewhat enlarged, with a permanent semierection.

With the inflatable type of prosthesis, a saline fluid is pumped from a reservoir behind the abdominal wall into expandable cylinders inserted into the erection chambers of the penis. The fluid causes the balloons to inflate, resulting in an erection. The man pumps the fluid into the chambers when he desires an erection and transfers the fluid back into the reservoir when he no longer wants the erection. The reservoir is surgically implanted behind the abdominal wall and the pump is implanted in the scrotum. Silicon tubing is used to connect the reservoir, pump, and balloons. Since the entire device is inserted through a single, relatively invisible incision in the scrotum, this type of prosthesis is barely noticeable. However, operating the pump through the scrotum wall can be difficult for individuals with reduced hand sensation or strength.

A spouse or long-term sexual partner should be included in the decision to get an implant, as well as in the selection of the type of prosthesis to be used. Extensive presurgery consultation with a urologist or physician familiar with MS will help to ensure that the man and his partner have realistic expectations after the surgery. Approximately 80 percent of men using these types of prostheses find them quite satisfactory. Many experience normal erectile sensations and normal orgasm. Additionally, they are able to have an erection for as long as they choose to do so.

What complications are associated with penile prostheses?

As with any surgery, there are possible complications related to anesthesia and bleeding. Infection occurs in approximately 3 percent of men receiving prostheses and can be quite serious. The entire device must be removed if an infection occurs. Replacement of the implant following treatment of the infection is usually feasible, but often more complicated.

How would I know if I am a suitable candidate for a penile prosthesis?

A penile prosthesis is only recommended when all other efforts to manage erectile dysfunction are not feasible or are unsuccessful. In other words, you would be considered a candidate for a prosthesis only if noninvasive measures were unsuccessful, oral and self-injection therapies failed, or an effective dose level or combination of medications could not be found.

Are there any nonmedical sexual aids available to help with erectile problems?

A number of sexual aids are available by mail order that do not require a physician's prescription (see mail order catalogues listed). Some people prefer strap-on latex penises, some of which are hollow and can hold a flaccid or semierect penis. Strap-on, battery-operated vibrators in the shape of a penis are also available.

Choosing a sexual device to aid with erections is best done with the advice of a urologist or sex therapist familiar with MS. If you have a long-term sex partner, it is important to include this person in the discussion. This will decrease anxiety and uncertainty when the devices are used and enhance intimacy by allowing both sex partners to explore them together. Counseling with a mental health professional who is knowledgeable about MS can facilitate the process if you have problems communicating or feel inhibited about talking through these issues.

Recently it has started to be painful for me when we have sex. My husband says I feel tight and dry. What is the best way to deal with this problem?

Similar to the erectile response in men, vaginal lubrication is controlled by two different pathways in the brain and spinal cord. "Psychogenic" lubrication typically originates in the brain and occurs through fantasy, reading erotic novels, or exposure to sexually related stimuli. Reflexogenic lubrication occurs through direct stimulation of the genitals or anus via a reflex response in the sacral (lower) part of the spinal cord. MS can affect nerve pathways that control either or both types of lubrication. Additionally, some medications used to treat bladder symptoms in MS can reduce vaginal lubrication. Psychogenic lubrication can sometimes be enhanced by establishing a relaxing, romantic, and/or sexually stimulating setting for sexual activity, incorporating relaxing massage into foreplay activities, and prolonging foreplay before intercourse.

"Reflexogenic" lubrication can sometimes be increased by manually or orally stimulating the genitals prior to attempting intercourse. Vaginal dryness can also be dealt with by applying generous amounts of water-soluble lubricants such as Replens® or K-Y Jelly® that are available over-the-counter in most pharmacies and drug stores. If condoms are used for birth control or disease prevention purposes, it is recommended that you use those that are lubricated and apply additional lubricant to the vaginal area as needed. Water-soluble lubricants that are marketed for sexual activity purposes can also be purchased by mail order via the catalogue services listed at the end of the chapter.

Health care professionals do not recommend the use of petroleum (oil)-based jellies (e.g., Vaseline®) for vaginal lubrication since they are not water-soluble. Petroleum-based jellies can leave residues in and around the vaginal and urethral openings that could set the stage for bacterial infections to develop.

Spasticity in my legs sometimes makes sexual activity very uncomfortable. Is there anything I can do about this problem?

Spasticity can make straightening the legs or changing leg positions for sexual activity uncomfortable or even painful. Active symptomatic management of spasticity will minimize its impact on sexuality (see Chapter 2, Appendix B). Range of motion and other physical therapy exercises are commonly employed, as

well as antispasticity medications such as baclofen (Lioresal®) or
tizanidine (Zanaflex®). Administering antispasticity medication
prior to anticipated sexual activity can be helpful. Be sure, however, to discuss any medication changes with your physician.

Exploring alternative sexual positions for intercourse is sometimes helpful when spasticity is a problem. Women who have
spasticity of the **adductor muscles** may find it difficult or
painful to separate their legs. The impact of adductor spasms
can be minimized by lying on your side, with your partner
approaching you from behind. Placing a towel between your legs
while lying in this position might help you feel more comfortable. You may find that lying on your back, perpendicular to the
bed, with both legs (from the knees down) hanging off the edge
of the bed, makes intercourse easier and more comfortable.

A man who has difficulty straightening his legs may find that
sitting upright in an armless chair allows his partner to mount
his erect penis in either a face-to-face or face-to-back position.
However, everyone's body is different, and the key to finding
alternative sexual positions is open exploration and communication between partners.

**My wife's MS makes her so tired that by the time we get the
children to bed she's too worn out to want to have sex. Is there
anything we can do about all this fatigue?**

Energy conservation and fatigue management are important
interventions to promote sexual activity and enjoyment. Fatigue
is managed from physical therapy, occupational therapy, and
pharmacologic perspectives. It can be helpful to have consultations at an MS center that offers comprehensive care or to obtain
referrals to MS experts in these areas. If stimulants such as
pemoline (Cylert®) or amantadine are prescribed for fatigue
management, administration prior to anticipated sexual activity
may be helpful (see Appendix B).

Even with effective symptom management, you and your wife
may still want to explore other strategies to enhance your sex life
and reduce the impact of her fatigue. Couples frequently engage
in sexual activity in the evening, when energy is at its lowest
ebb. Talk over the possibility of having sex in the morning, when
fatigue is at a minimum. Although making a "date" to awaken
earlier for sexual activity may initially seem undesirable, this
kind of adaptation may be necessary for retaining an enjoyable

sex life. Some couples are fortunate to have the flexibility in their schedules to make a periodic "lunch date" for intimate play.

Some sexual positions require less energy than others, and alternative positions that minimize weight bearing or tiring movements can minimize fatigue. As you try to initiate some of these changes in your sexual life, be aware that they require open communication and the willingness to engage in some trial-and-error exploration. Counseling may be helpful if you and your wife find it difficult to communicate about alternatives.

I've been having a lot of difficulty controlling my urine lately. I'm so worried about having an accident during sex that I keep making excuses to my husband. I want to have sex but I'm afraid that if I wet myself—or him—he'll never want to have sex again!

Fortunately, successful bladder management is attainable for most people (see Chapter 4). A critical first step in this process is careful bladder assessment, guided by your MS health care team or a urologist who is familiar with MS.

Try discussing your concerns about incontinence openly with your husband. Most partners are willing to "take the chance" once they are informed of the issues and assured that everything is being done to manage the bladder problems. Discussing your fears with him, and strategizing together with your health care team to minimize the risk of incontinence during sexual activity, will also give you more confidence. You may need to tailor your symptomatic management strategies a bit to allow for anticipated sexual activity. If, for example, you are taking ***anticholinergic*** medications, e.g., oxybutynin (Ditropan®) or tolterodine (Detrol®) for bladder storage dysfunction, you might try taking the medication 30 minutes before anticipated sexual activity in order to minimize bothersome bladder contractions. These medicines increase vaginal dryness, so you may need to compensate by using water-soluble lubricants. You can also minimize incontinence by restricting fluid intake for an hour or two before sex and doing intermittent catheterization just before sexual activity. Wearing a condom during sex is advised for men who are concerned with small amounts of urinary leakage.

A woman who has an ***indwelling catheter*** can manage by taping the catheter securely to the stomach, emptying the collecting bag before sexual activity, and putting additional tape around the top ring to minimize the chances of leaks. You can avoid putting pressure on the catheter or the collecting bag by lying in a "nestled spoons" position, with the woman in front and using rear-entry intercourse. An alternative position for a woman with a catheter is to lie on her back with her legs over the man's shoulders. He can support himself on his arms in order to reduce the weight on her. A variation of this position is for the man to sit on his knees, between the woman's legs, and position her legs over his shoulders. The latter position allows for less vigorous, more gentle "rocking" movements and allows a woman with spasticity to keep her legs closer together. These are examples of ways in which sexual activity can be modified in order to compensate for MS-related changes. Each couple will need to find the solutions that best meet their needs. Some couples will find these solutions through patient trial-and-error exploration. Others will find it useful to consult with an experienced sex therapist.

Trying new sexual positions that will compensate for MS symptoms and disabilities can be anxiety-provoking for many people. Taking the time to acquire information, explore, discuss, and obtain frequent feedback during sexual experimentation will help alleviate fears. Able-bodied partners may be fearful of causing pain, or they may feel insecure about knowing what to do and how to do it. Setting aside regular time to talk about sex gives it more importance in the relationship and sets the stage for the couple to air their fears and concerns and improve their communication.

My wife has difficulty moving very much during sex since she lost so much strength in her arms and legs. Will I hurt her if we try some different positions?

Weakness is a common MS symptom that frequently requires finding new positions for satisfactory sexual activities. Reclining positions do not place as much strain on muscles and are therefore less tiring. Pillows can be used to improve positioning and reduce muscle strain. Inflatable pillows, specifically designed to provide back support during sexual activity, can help minimize back strain. These wedge-shaped pillows have individually inflatable sections that allow for firmness adjustment and do not restrict movement. Oral sex requires less movement than intercourse, and using hand-held or strap-on vibrators can help compensate for hand weakness while providing sexual stimulation.

Anxiety about hurting your sex partner is fairly common when significant changes in physical functioning have occurred. Open discussions with each other before attempting new positions or sexual activities will allow your wife to educate you about her MS symptoms and enable you both to air your concerns while planning for sexual encounters. Conducting a "positioning" exercise before sex is attempted will help you both determine if the new positions are comfortable without introducing anxiety *during* sexual activity. If your wife has a physical therapist who knows her body strengths and weaknesses well, he or she may be able to advise you both about positions for sexual activity that take into account your wife's vulnerabilities.

I find that I lose my train of thought when I have sex. My interest and desire start out fine, but then my mind drifts and I lose interest. This is very frustrating for me, and my partner frequently feels like he's not doing something right. Is there anything I can do about this problem?

Changes in attention and concentration are common in MS and may derail the ability to sustain sexual interest and excitement. Partners sometimes misinterpret this symptom to mean that they are deficient or uninteresting as lovers. The person with MS sometimes feels guilty or inadequate. These negative feelings can increase the distractibility or lead the person to avoid sex altogether. Accepting distractibility as a valid MS symptom and discussing ways to help compensate for it are crucial steps to finding a solution. Attention/concentration problems tend to be worse when a person is fatigued, so it is vitally important to evaluate fatigue level and compensate accordingly. In general, *minimizing nonromantic or nonsexual stimuli and maximizing sensual and sexual stimulation during sex is the strategy for compensating.* You can help minimize this problem by creating a romantic mood/environment, using multisensory stimulation (e.g., talking in sexy ways, engaging in sensual and erotic touching, and playing music that has strong romantic associations). Developing an atmosphere of acceptance and permission for the person to "reenter the sexual experience" after losing focus can help. Sometimes, switching briefly from erotic to sensual (but nongenital) touching can facilitate interest when attention wanders. Refer to Chapter 9 for suggestions on the general management of attention/concentration problems.

My husband has changed a lot since he got MS. He grabs me a lot, even in front of other people, and seems to want to have sex all the time. We always had a comfortable sex life, but now it almost feels like he's a stranger in some ways and I'm not comfortable any more.

"Behavioral disinhibition," or acting on one's sexual impulses in an uncontrolled way, is occasionally (but rarely) reported in MS. It may be associated with MS-related cognitive impairments (see Chapter 9) or a separate and distinct type of depression that has both manic (hyperactive) and depressive features called bipolar disorder (formerly called manic depression). In general, referral to a psychiatrist who is familiar with MS is important so that an accurate understanding of the symptom can be reached. Medications can sometimes manage this symptom if the impulsive hypersexuality is part of the manic phase of bipolar disorder. Regardless of the origin of the disinhibition, counseling is important to help the person with MS and the sexual partner cope with the impulsivity. If the symptom is associated with cognitive changes or other changes in judgment, the appropriateness of cognitive rehabilitation could be explored.

I've become so discouraged lately. Nothing seems worth the effort. My wife wants to have sex with me and it's the furthest thing from my mind. I'm too angry and sad all the time to even think about sex. I know it's not fair to her but I can't seem to shake this mood.

MS is frequently associated with emotional challenges that include grief, demoralization, changes in self-esteem and body image, and clinical depression (see Chapter 11). These emotional states can temporarily dampen interest in sex or the ability to give and receive sexual pleasure. Addressing these emotional challenges in an effort to enhance sexuality has several aspects: education, assessment, professional treatment, and coping interventions.

Education about emotional challenges in MS is available through the National MS Society. Additionally, groups in which people with MS and their partners can share information about MS are widely available. These resources can help you and your wife to understand the feelings you are experiencing and recognize the ways these feelings can affect your sexual relationship.

Assessment of a person's emotional responses to the stresses imposed by MS can be done by a mental health professional who is familiar with the disease. Correctly identifying the type of emotional distress a person is experiencing is a prerequisite to providing the appropriate treatment. In other words, it is necessary to find out what is causing your distress in order for you to be able to "shake this mood." A normal grief reaction to the stresses and losses imposed by the illness might be dealt with very effectively in a support group or short-term, individual psychotherapy. A more acute clinical depression, however, might best be treated with some combination of psychotherapy and antidepressant medication.

Sometimes antidepressant medications can cause sexual problems, such as delayed orgasm or loss of libido. Talking with your doctor about possible sexual side effects, if they occur, can set the stage for managing them effectively. For example, coadministering other medications, or altering the timing of taking antidepressants can frequently alleviate the sexual side effects.

As you begin to experience some relief from these distressing feelings, you and your wife may find it easier to talk about the ways in which MS and your feelings about the disease have affected your sexual relationship. One of the most important coping strategies for dealing with emotional and body image changes is ongoing, intimate communication with your long-term sexual partner. It may be particularly difficult to explore new options, discuss disappointments, and express what both of you feel and want in the face of coping with all the other changes associated with MS. MS peer groups, couples groups, and/or individual or couples counseling can facilitate this process.

My husband has become quite disabled and I am his primary caregiver. It's hard for me to think of him as my husband and my lover when I also dress, bathe, and clean him. I know he wants me to have sex with him but I just don't feel like it any more.

Changes in former sexual patterns and roles represent significant challenges to intimacy and sexuality. Perceptions of being ill or disabled may be incompatible with an image of being sexually active and vigorous. Role changes that involve the "well" partner assuming many caregiving functions may challenge that person's ability to view his or her partner as a source of sexual excitement. When caregiving becomes an extensive part of a relationship, it is difficult to relax and have sexual fun. If possible, nursing activities should be done by someone other than the sexual partner so the person with MS does not assume the role of "patient" in the intimate relationship. To the extent possible, the bedroom should be preserved as a private place for closeness and intimacy; medical equipment and other illness-related paraphernalia should be kept to one side or in another room. Ideally, time for intimate talk, cuddling, or sexual activity should be set aside, separate from the times for caregiving.

Obviously, these suggestions are not always viable. Finding "substitute" caregivers to provide nursing care is not always possible. Families do not always have the luxury of keeping medical equipment in a separate space. Additionally, some couples are unwilling to give up the caregiving and care-receiving roles since much of the closeness that remains in the relationship may be in the context of these caregiving activities.

For someone who is attempting to juggle the dual roles of nurse/caregiver and sexual partner, it is very important to be able to discuss this challenge to intimacy. You may be hesitant to discuss your feelings with your husband because you do not want to upset him. In turn, he may find it difficult to express his frustration and resentment over the change in the sexual relationship because he does not want to risk hurting or angering you—his primary caregiver. Yet this reluctance to share these difficult and painful feelings represents a further loss of intimacy. You and your husband may find it helpful to talk over these issues with a family therapist experienced in chronic illness and sexuality.

Since my wife was diagnosed with MS, it feels as though we are drifting apart. Initially we worked together to cope with the uncertainties of the diagnosis and the aftermath of her first few exacerbations. Yet we seem to be feeling less and less close over time even though she is not that physically disabled. It's harder for us to be sexual with each other and to feel close.

There is a heavy emphasis in present-day Western culture on youth, beauty, health, and physical vigor. Men and women in our culture often feel burdened by the pressure to be eternally young and vigorously sexual. The experience of MS, with its associated changes in body functions, can trigger a dramatic sense of sexual or sensual inadequacy in the face of these cultural pressures. It is difficult to feel sexual with another person when one's sexual feelings and performance are being threatened. Men and women with MS may have difficulty enjoying and expressing their sensual/sexual nature because of the widening gap between culturally based ideals and their own illness experience.

Pressures also exist for the sexual partner of someone with MS. The partner may begin to think of the person with MS as too fragile to engage in sexual activity or as a "patient" who is too ill to be sexually expressive. The physical, cognitive, and emotional changes sometimes associated with MS can also strain the intimacy between two people; a partner can begin to feel as though he or she is trying to relate to a person who is somehow different or unfamiliar. Similarly, the role changes that are sometimes required in the face of MS, such as one partner becoming the other's caregiver, can drastically alter the mutual feelings and expectations within a relationship.

All of these changes can lead to an increasing sense of personal isolation within a relationship. Each partner may feel less and less able to understand the other's experience, feelings, and needs. In turn, a diminishing capacity to understand and work through these differences can create greater isolation and misunderstanding. Mutual resentment can begin to fester and grow.

Throughout this chapter we have emphasized effective communication between partners (and between partners and health care providers) as a necessary step toward restoring sexual enjoyment and intimacy. However, there are many barriers to effective communication. Images of sexuality and sensuality are rampant in Western society, yet they are not depicted in a way that provides an open and acceptable means of discussion and problem solving. Most sexual language is either too "medicalized" or technical or considered "dirty" or unacceptable to allow for easy conversation between lovers.

Part of the solution to these barriers involves developing a more comfortable vocabulary about sexuality and intimacy. Education about MS symptoms and the anatomy and physiology of sexuality can help to provide a basis for mutual understanding and problem solving. The organizations listed at the end of this chapter can add to the information provided here. There also are many self-help books available at most bookstores that are designed to enhance communication, sexuality, and intimacy. Reading these materials together can help you become comfortable with the vocabulary you need in order to be able to discuss personal and intimate subjects. Talk to each other about what you are reading and how it might be applied to your relationship.

Another approach involves setting aside time each week to devote exclusively to restoring intimacy and talking about sexuality. This can set the stage for a couple to begin talking more easily about their intimate needs, wants, and differences. A helpful but more challenging adjunct to this process is to make regular "dates" when you are free from caregiving, child rearing, or household tasks. This kind of opportunity to focus exclusively on one another recalls the early romantic phase of most long-term intimate relationships, which has all too often been sacrificed to the pressures of careers, parenting, and coping with MS-related tasks. Partners need to rediscover each other as their roles and expectations are updated or reconciled with the changing MS situation. Many couples, however, become anxious or frustrated with their efforts to reconnect with one another. If you and your wife find the process to be too difficult on your own, you may find that couple's counseling can provide a safe atmosphere in which to begin exploring these aspects of your relationship.

I am gay and have MS, and find it difficult to talk to my doctor about my sexual concerns. What resources are available for gay and lesbian people with MS?

The experience of having MS frequently causes one to become "marginalized" in society. For example, social circles may become narrower, and/or job opportunities may become more constricted. MS Societies and other MS organizations around the world combat this disabling tendency toward isolation by providing a variety of outreach services, education, training, and research funding. This marginalization is compounded greatly if one is gay or lesbian and has MS. Many people with MS who are not gay or lesbian have found that it is very difficult to discuss intimacy and/or sexuality issues with their health care team or National MS Society staff/volunteers because of fears that they will be misunderstood, rejected, or judged negatively. If one is gay or lesbian with MS, the possibility of receiving rejection or disapproval in the context of reaching out for help is even greater. An important ingredient in combating the social isolation and lack of professional support entails networking and reaching out to other gay and lesbian people with MS in order to receive support and validation. Although the very nature of marginalization makes this difficult to accomplish, the Internet has been quite helpful for some in this regard. The Multiple Sclerosis Society of Great Britain and Northern Ireland, based in London, England (see Recommended Resources at end of chapter), can provide information for people with MS regarding gay or lesbian issues and Internet information.

Getting through each day has gotten very hard for me. Nothing is easy any more and nothing can ever be spontaneous. We used to have sex whenever we wanted to—just because we felt like it. Now we have to plan it all so I'll be comfortable and not too tired.

One of our common Western cultural expectations is that sex should be spontaneous and passionate, with the lovers becoming "swept away" in a torrent of romantic and intimate urges. Couples may feel disappointed if this or other internalized visions of what sex "should be" are not met—so disappointed, in fact, that they may fail to explore other sexual possibilities or even stop having sex altogether.

Additionally, the changes imposed by MS frequently make it necessary for there to be some preparation for sexual encounters, possibly including changing the timing of certain medications, altering the time of day for sexual activity, and learning new sexual activities that compensate for disabilities. In the face of these adjustments, some couples may decide that sex—that day, that week, or even that month—is just not worth all the trouble. When there is a major symptom flare-up or any other life situation that interferes with sexual expression, it is important to communicate with your partner about the changes and feelings you are experiencing. This will allow you to retain a sense of closeness and intimacy even in the absence of sexual activity. You can use this period of time to focus on other pleasurable aspects of the relationship, such as the sensual or "special person" aspects discussed earlier.

Failing to communicate, either verbally or nonverbally, about those times when sex "isn't worth all the effort" will put you at risk for withdrawing from each other even further. Joining together in the decision "not to have sex right now" will also enable you to ask each other "what *do* we want right now?" and "how can we go about achieving it for ourselves?"

Recommended Reading

Foley, FW. (1998). Sexuality and Intimacy in Multiple Sclerosis. In: R. Kalb (ed.) *Multiple Sclerosis: A Guide for Families.* New York: Demos Medical Publishing.

Foley, FW, & Sanders, A. (1998). Sexuality and Multiple Sclerosis. In: J. Halper and N. Holland (Eds). *The Multiple Sclerosis Self-Care Guide.* Washington, D.C.: Paralyzed Veterans of America.

Foley, FW, & Symonds, S. (1999). The impact of MS on sexuality and loving. London, England: Burnett Publications. (Booklet available from the Multiple Sclerosis Society of Great Britain and Northern Ireland, 25 Effie Road, Fulham, London, SW61EE, England).

Kaplan HS. *The Illustrated Manual of Sex Therapy (2nd edition).* New York: Brunner Mazel Publishers, 1987.

Kroll K, Klein EL. *Enabling Romance: A Guide to Love, Sex, and Relationships for the Disabled.* New York: Harmony Books, 1992.

Mooney TO, Cole TM, Chilgren RA. *Sexual Options for Paraplegics and Quadriplegics.* Boston: Little, Brown, 1975.

Neistadt ME, Freda M. *Choices: A Guide to Sex Counseling with Physically Disabled Adults.* Malabar, FL: Robert E. Krieger Publishing, 1987.

Yaffe M, Fenwick E, Rosen R, Kellett J. *Sexual Happiness for Women: A Practical Approach.* New York: Henry Holt, 1992.

Yaffe M, Fenwick E, Rosen R, Kellett J. *Sexual Happiness for Men: A Practical Approach.* New York: Henry Holt, 1992.

Selected pamphlets from the National Multiple Sclerosis Society (1-800-FIGHT MS; 800-344-4867):

◇ *Sexuality and Multiple Sclerosis (3rd edition)*—Michael Barrett Ph.D. (available from Multiple Sclerosis Society of Canada, 250 Bloor Street East, Suite 820, Toronto, Ontario M4W 3P9, Phone: 416-922-6065)

Recommended Resources

◇ The Sexuality Information and Education Council of the United States (SIECUS) has a Resource Center and Library located at 130 W. 42nd Street, Suite 350, N.Y., N.Y. 10036 (Phone: 212-819-9770). SIECUS publishes an annotated bibliography on sexuality and disability, which was updated in 1994. They also run database searches for more specific topics, utilizing their own extensive reference library.

◇ *Sexuality and Disability* is a quarterly journal that publishes scholarly articles on rehabilitation, disability, and sexuality. It also publishes guidelines for professional clinical practice, case studies, and information for consumers. The journal is available from Human Sciences Press, Inc., 233 Spring Street, New York, N.Y. 10013-1578 (Phone: 212-620-8000).

◇ The American Association of Sex Educators, Counselors, and Therapists (AASECT) certifies professional sex therapists who can document that they have met their criteria for minimum educational and clinical experience standards. AASECT-certified therapists also must agree to adhere to a code of ethics. Although many highly qualified sex therapists do not choose to join AASECT, you can obtain a list of AASECT-certified sex therapists by writing to AASECT, P.O. Box 238, Mount Vernon, IA 52314.

◇ Planned Parenthood is a national organization that provides information on abortion and birth control. However, some chapters conduct sex counseling, and the chapters can provide competent local referrals for sex therapy and counseling. The national office is located at 810 Seventh Ave., New York, NY 10019 (Phone number: 212-541-7800; 800-829-7732).

◇ The Multiple Sclerosis Society of Great Britain and Northern Ireland has a collection of articles and pamphlets on sexuality that are reviewed by a professional panel, and annotated for the consumer. They also can provide information on gay/lesbian issues in MS. The Society can be contacted by writing to them at 25 Effie Road, Fulham, London, SW6 1EE, England (Phone: 011- 44-171-610-7171).

There are a number of discreet catalogue services available that sell sexually oriented materials. Most of these are not targeted toward people with disabilities, but they contain products that may be helpful to both disabled and nondisabled people. Some include:

◇ Eve's Garden International, Ltd. sells books, videos, and sexual aids/toys. Their catalogue can be ordered from their offices at 119 W. 57th Street, Suite 420, New York, N.Y. 10019-2383. (Phone: 800-848-3837).

◇ Good Vibrations, Inc. offers similar fare. Their catalogue can be ordered from 938 Howard Street, San Francisco, CA 94103 (Phone: 415-974-8990; 800-289-8423).

◇ Lawrence Research offers a catalogue full of sexual novelties and aids, videos, and books, called the Xandria Collection catalogue. They also have a small catalogue that targets those with disabilities (cost $4.00) and can be reached by mail at P.O. Box 31039, San Francisco, CA 94131 (Phone: 800-242-2823; call extension 39 for additional information).

References

Zorzon, M, Zivadinov, R, Boxco, A, Monti-Bradadin, L, Moretti, R, Bonfigli, L, Morassi, P, Iona, L, & Cazzato, G.. Sexual dysfunction in multiple sclerosis: A case-control study. I. Frequency and comparison of groups. *Multiple Sclerosis* 1999; 5(6):418–427.

13

Fertility, Pregnancy, Childbirth, and Gynecologic Care

Kathy Birk, M.D.
Michael A. Werner, M.D.

A person might be symptom-free and feeling fine following the diagnosis of multiple sclerosis, but he or she now has a new piece of bewildering information to add to those factors that all adults must think about when considering parenthood, such as the stability of the marriage, financial security, and the commitment to raising children. Couples in which one partner has become somewhat disabled may also be facing decisions about starting a family or adding another child.

Regardless of the level of disability, a joint decision by prospective parents is vital. Specific questions about conception, pregnancy, and delivery are only the beginning; parenthood's bigger picture stretches many years into the future. Important long-range considerations include the possibility of increasing physical disability, the threat to financial security if income were to be lost due to that disability, the availability of adequate support from friends and extended family, and the ease or comfort with which the mother and father could share parenting and wage earning roles if needed. No single decision is "right" for everyone, and a couple may find that agreement on family planning decisions does not come quickly or easily. Proactive ways to become more comfortable with these decisions might include: working together as a couple to make an honest assessment of your family situation—including the emotional, financial, and medical aspects of your daily life; asking your doctor to participate in a thorough discussion of present disease activity and possible disease progression; talking to other families in which one of the parents has MS; and seeking information from the MS Society.

Included in this chapter are answers to some of the most commonly asked questions about family planning, fertility, pregnancy, childbirth, and nursing, as well as suggestions for well-woman care. So often, those with a chronic condition do not receive basic screening tests, medication options, and health care practices that are routinely offered to those without an illness.

Family Planning and Fertility

I am a 25-year-old woman with MS. What types of contraception are safe for me to use until my husband and I decide that it's time to start a family?

Contraceptive choices should be made after considering such factors as personal preference, manual dexterity and coordination, other medications being used, and the possible risk of infection.

The use of barrier contraceptives, such as the diaphragm, spermicides, and condoms, requires manual dexterity and control, or a partner who is willing and able to provide assistance. Using a diaphragm may increase your risk of bladder infections. Additionally, the diaphragm requires application of a spermicide prior to each act of intercourse and should be removed eight hours after insertion. For maximum reliability, it is recommended that a condom be used in conjunction with the diaphragm. Some women find it easier to use a spermicidal suppository that is inserted ten minutes prior to intercourse. Used in combination with a condom, the spermicide is just as reliable as a diaphragm. The condom, alone or in combination with another birth control method, reduces the risk of sexually transmitted diseases.

Birth control pills are generally a safe and highly effective means of birth control. *However, the use of certain drugs, such as antibiotics, Dilantin® (phenytoin), and Tegretol® (carba-mazepine), may reduce the pill's effectiveness* (see Appendix B). Women who are taking any of these medications should discuss with their physician the need for additional protection, e.g., a condom or other barrier-type contraceptive. Birth control pills should not be used by any woman with high blood pressure or by women over the age of 35 who smoke, due to the increased risk of heart disease.

The long-acting progesterone shot (Depo-Provera®) is effective for 12 weeks and is not known to be affected by those drugs that may alter the pill's effectiveness. Depo-Provera® is also a safer method of birth control for women who are unable to stop smoking. The long-acting, implantable progesterone (Norplant®) is effective for five years and requires no ongoing attention. Each of these methods may be associated with side effects (including weight gain and irregular bleeding) and must be carefully reviewed and understood before opting to use them.

The intrauterine device (IUD) currently in use in the United States (Paraguard®) is a safe, effective, and convenient form of birth control for women with a mutually monogamous relationship who are not planning to have any more children. Its insertion is a simple, reversible office procedure. Some concern exists that the use of antibiotics or immunosuppressive medications could decrease the effectiveness of the IUD. Women who are taking any of these medications should discuss with their physician the possible need for additional birth control protection.

Vasectomy, a safe, effective sterilization procedure for men, is usually performed in a physician's office. Since reversal of a vasectomy requires delicate microsurgery that is only sometimes successful, it should be undertaken only after careful deliberation. Tubal ligation, a sterilization procedure for women, is typically done in the hospital under general anesthesia. This procedure must also be considered irreversible.

Will my MS make it difficult for me to get pregnant?

The disease itself does not cause infertility. The lower pregnancy rates that have been reported among women with MS result from a variety of factors: some of the medications used to treat MS may lead to problems with regular ovulation; women sometimes delay becoming pregnant because they are reluctant to stop taking medications that are important in the management of their MS but are not safe for use during pregnancy; and some couples decide not to have children, or to have fewer children, because of the illness.

My husband has recently been diagnosed with MS. Will this disease make him sterile?

MS does not affect sperm production. Unless your husband had a preexisting and unrelated problem with sperm production, there is no reason why he would become sterile in the future as a result of the disease. Some medications may contribute to a compromise of sperm quality. Any woman who is trying to become pregnant should discuss with her physician all of the medications her husband is taking. Additionally, some men with MS experience difficulties with intercourse and ejaculation that can interfere with conception, despite having normal sperm counts.

Sometimes I have difficulty getting or keeping an erection during intercourse. Will this problem prevent me from being able to father a child?

It is important to distinguish between the ability to have intercourse and the ability to ejaculate sperm and ultimately father a child. Many men who have difficulty maintaining an adequate erection for neurologic or nonneurologic reasons are still able to ejaculate. If you are able to ejaculate, even though you sometimes have difficulty maintaining an erection that is firm enough for intercourse, your doctor can teach you how to use a syringe to collect your ejaculate and place it directly into your wife's vagina. There is no truth to the commonly held belief that ejaculation outside the woman's vagina in any way affects the quality of the sperm or their ability to fertilize an egg. Refer to Chapter 12 for a discussion of MS-related erectile problems and available treatments.

I am a 28-year-old man with MS. For the past several months I have had difficulty ejaculating during intercourse. My wife and I have been trying to have a baby for several months without any luck. How will we be able to have a child if I can't ejaculate?

If you are able to ejaculate on some occasions but not others, you have the option of banking your sperm for insemination during your wife's fertile period. The disadvantage of this type of banking is that the quality of the sperm does deteriorate somewhat when frozen and thawed. If you are unable to ejaculate even intermittently, there are medications that can be used to try to stimulate you to ejaculate. The most commonly used drugs are pseudoephedrine and imipramine. These are prescribed by a fertility specialist who will closely monitor your ejaculation in order to adjust dosage levels. Some men who seem to have no ejaculation actually experience a "retrograde" or backward ejaculation. These same medications can convert a backward ejaculation to a forward ejaculation.

If you are unable to ejaculate even with the use of these medications, a reflex ejaculation can sometimes be induced through vibratory stimulation of the underside of the penis. This technique is effective for those individuals whose ejaculatory mechanism is impaired because of faulty nerve transmissions between the brain and spinal cord. Your doctor can show you how to use a vibrator effectively to achieve a sufficient level of stimulation. The ejaculate can be placed in your wife's vagina for attempted fertilization if the timing is appropriate, or stored for insemination at a later time.

Some men are unable to ejaculate with either medications or vibratory stimulation. A third technique, which completely bypasses the spinal cord and directly stimulates the nerves that release the ejaculate, is called electroejaculation. During a day hospital admission, under general anesthesia, the man is given a brief series of electric shocks through a probe placed into the rectum. The electric stimulation produces an ejaculation that can then be used for insemination. This technique has been used for some time in men with spinal cord injury, but has also been used successfully in individuals with MS.

My doctor has told me that there are various kinds of treatments for impotence caused by MS, including medications and surgical implants. Would I be able to father a child using any of these treatments?

Impotence does not lead to infertility. As long as you are able to ejaculate, at least intermittently (with or without the medical interventions described in the previous answer), none of the treatments for erectile dysfunction will interfere with your ability to conceive (see Chapter 12).

Pregnancy, Labor, and Delivery

Do I need to stop the medications I am taking before I start trying to get pregnant? I'm worried that my MS will get worse if I'm off the medications for too long.

As a general rule, *the use of any medications while a woman is pregnant or trying to become pregnant, including ones that are bought over-the-counter, must be done with caution and under the advice of a physician who is familiar with their use during pregnancy.*

Medications used to treat MS fall into two groups—those that treat symptoms and those that are used to reduce disease activity. In many cases, the medications used to treat symptoms or occasional medical problems (such as bladder infections) are safe to continue. This is not the case for most of the drugs used to treat the disease itself. Many of the latter are immunosuppressive drugs, most of which have not been studied sufficiently during pregnancy to show whether or not they cause problems for the baby. None of the newer drugs, including Betaseron®, Avonex®, Copaxone®, or Rebif® (not available in the United States), have been studied in pregnancy. While you might wish to continue taking a drug that holds promise for slowing the progression of MS, the health of your unborn baby must be a primary concern. It is important to stop these medications as soon as you begin trying to conceive because the fertilized egg will begin to develop a few weeks before you know that you are pregnant. You can resume your medications immediately after delivery if you choose not to breast-feed your baby.

I am afraid to tell my gynecologist that I have MS. I don't want anyone to tell me that I shouldn't have a baby. What should I do?

There is now ample evidence that a woman should not be discouraged from becoming pregnant simply because she has been diagnosed with MS. The major factors in the decision to become pregnant for couples affected by the disease are the same as for most other couples: how will adding a child to their lives work for them, and is this the right time?

Historically (and occasionally even now), couples have found that some members of the medical profession discourage pregnancy, and even parenting, for a woman who has MS. It was often suggested to women who became pregnant that they abort. These women were even encouraged to be sterilized. We now know that there is no medical reason for women with MS to avoid pregnancy. There is less risk of relapse during pregnancy itself, followed by an increased possibility of relapse in the immediate postpartum months. Most importantly, research has shown that women who do choose to become pregnant and deliver a child do not develop more disability over their lifetime than women who never become pregnant.

In spite of these changes in medical opinion about pregnancy in women with MS, many couples find that they are discouraged from becoming pregnant by their physicians or well-meaning friends and family members. Women who are considering becoming pregnant should seek information and support from the MS Society and consult a physician who is knowledgeable and willing to discuss their questions and concerns in a supportive manner. The decision to start a family or add additional children is a very personal one that needs to be made with careful attention to current and future emotional, medical, and financial factors. If you do not feel that you can discuss this subject comfortably with your present physician, perhaps you should find another with whom you are more at ease. An open and trusting relationship with your doctor is vital to your pregnancy and childbirth experience.

I recently found out that I am pregnant. My husband thinks we should terminate the pregnancy because of my MS. I can't make him understand how much I want this baby. How do I decide what is the right thing to do?

As discussed previously, pregnancy itself will not contribute to long-term disability in most women. The strength of the desire to raise and share life with a child should be the major factor in the decision for both you and your husband. As a couple, you need to weigh your feelings about parenting against a thoughtful assessment of your existing disability and possible future limitations that the disease might impose. Encourage your husband to think about his own desire for fatherhood and perhaps contact the MS Society to talk with others who have faced the fear of future parenting when MS is part of the picture.

The decision to have a child, as well as the lifetime of parenting that follows, should be a team effort. You and your husband both need to be comfortable with the decisions that you make. If the two of you are finding it difficult to communicate openly and effectively about this important life decision, you might consider talking together with your physician or with a knowledgeable psychotherapist.

Can a woman who has MS have a normal pregnancy?

MS does not appear to affect the course of pregnancy, labor, or delivery. Studies reviewing hundreds of pregnancies have found no evidence of an MS-related threat to the fetus. For many women, the risk of relapse or worsening of MS is lower during pregnancy, with the result that many women feel particularly well during this period. Problems with weakness or *flexor spasms* in the legs are manageable with assisted deliveries (forceps or with a vacuum device) and with an epidural type of anesthesia during the labor and delivery.

I recently had a miscarriage in my second month. Will this make my MS worse?

Some disease worsening may occur in the months following any pregnancy, whether the pregnancy ends in delivery or earlier because of spontaneous abortion (miscarriage) or elective termination. This possible disease worsening is likely to be temporary; studies have found no differences in long-term disability in women having no pregnancies, one pregnancy, or two or more pregnancies. Miscarriage during the first trimester of pregnancy is more common than most realize (occurring in up to 15 percent to 20 percent of all pregnancies) and is not caused by MS.

My MS symptoms seem to get so much better when I'm pregnant that I wish I could just stay pregnant all the time. What is the reason for this?

There is something about the condition of pregnancy that causes a woman's body to be in a mildly immunosuppressed state. During pregnancy, you experience naturally the *immunosuppression* that certain medications can provide artificially for people with MS and some other *autoimmune diseases* (e.g., rheumatoid arthritis). This natural immunosuppression is probably the cause of reduced disease activity during pregnancy. The most recent research indicates that a woman's relapse rate decreases progressively over the course of a pregnancy, hitting its lowest point in the third trimester.

The precise reason for this helpful reduction in **immune system** activity is not clear. Recent research in **experimental allergic encephalomyelitis** (EAE), the animal model of MS, suggests that estriol, a form of estrogen with anti-inflammatory properties that is only present during pregnancy, may be responsible for the decreased disease activity in pregnant women. As a result of these findings, a small clinical trial is currently underway with 12 non-pregnant women with relapsing-remitting or secondary progressive MS to see if estriol might be a safe and effective treatment for women with MS. If the results of this trial are positive, a larger clinical trial will follow.

What drugs are safe for me to take while I am pregnant?

As discussed, *one should assume that all drugs could affect the fetus*. Notable exceptions include certain antibiotics used to treat bladder infections. This is important because bladder infections are fairly common in individuals with MS and are also more likely to occur during pregnancy. Ampicillin is commonly used to treat these infections and is very safe during pregnancy and for nursing mothers. Increasingly, however, some of the infections are found to be resistant to ampicillin, as well as to some of the commonly used sulfa drugs, so other, safe alternatives will be utilized by the doctor.

Steroid medications are often used during acute **exacerbations** of MS. Fortunately, as noted previously, such disease activity is decreased during pregnancy. Prednisone is a steroid that has been used fairly commonly in pregnant women with a variety of illnesses, including MS, asthma, and arthritis. Women with a history of steroid use (particularly within the past 12 months) need to be provided with a fairly high dose of steroids (called a "boost") during labor because the labor process may stress the adrenal gland beyond its ability to respond.

If new drugs for MS become available while I am trying to get pregnant, is it safe for me to take them?

No. Extreme caution is necessary when new drugs are approved before any research has been done on their use during pregnancy. The impact of a new drug on the newborn is often learned gradually, as women who are using the medication become pregnant and choose not to terminate the pregnancy. The long-term effect on an infant's development, function, and cancer risk are not clear at the time of birth or for many years to come.

This is an increasingly important question as greater numbers of women diagnosed with MS are prescribed one of the disease-modifying drugs, Betaseron®, Avonex®, Copaxone®, or Rebif® (not available in the United States). The standard approach has been to encourage them to stop the drugs as soon they begin trying to become pregnant. Since it may take several months for a woman to conceive, she will be without the protection of the medication for an extended period of time. Fortunately, the hormones activated during pregnancy seem to provide approximately the same degree of protection as the new immunomodulating agents.

How will my labor and delivery be affected by my MS? Is there anything specific my doctor needs to know to help me have a safe delivery?

Your labor is unlikely to be significantly different from what other women experience. Although MS does not increase the chance of having your delivery by cesarean section, you should be aware that all women face a 15 percent to 20 percent possibility of delivery by C section. Take advantage of available prenatal classes that will teach you and your partner about the stages of labor, delivery routes, and pain management strategies, and acquaint you with birthing alternatives available at the hospital.

Try to meet with someone from the anesthesia department to discuss your MS and the options (e.g., epidural) for pain control during labor. An epidural can also be beneficial for women who have difficulty with leg control and spasms caused by *spasticity*. If fatigue or muscle weakness occurs after two hours of pushing to deliver the baby, the delivery may be assisted using forceps or a suction cup on the baby's head.

As mentioned previously, be sure to let your doctor know your history of steroid use, particularly during the past 12 months. If you have taken steroids during that time, you will need an extra "boost" of steroid medication during labor.

Which types of anesthesia are recommended for labor and delivery in a woman with MS?

The use of epidural anesthesia for pain relief during labor has become increasingly popular. An epidural during labor or for a cesarean section is acceptable for those who have MS, particularly when it is provided by a skilled, experienced person. An epidural is different from spinal anesthesia, which has traditionally been avoided in patients with neurologic diseases, including MS. General anesthesia is also considered safe for patients having cesarean sections.

Postpartum and Beyond

What is the likelihood that the MS will get worse after my baby is born? Is there anything that I can do to decrease this likelihood?

While virtually all the studies have found that women with MS are less likely to experience relapse or worsening during the nine months of pregnancy, the disease does tend to be more active following delivery. About 10 percent of women experience relapses during the nine months of pregnancy, while 29 percent may have an exacerbation during the first six months after delivery.

For many women, a more significant concern than the experience they might have during pregnancy or postpartum is whether the decision to have a child will increase their long-term disability. Most research has found no difference in long-term disability between women with MS who had pregnancies and those who chose to remain childless. A recent, long-term study in Sweden even suggests that women who become pregnant after being diagnosed with MS may be less likely to develop a progressive course than women who do not become pregnant after the diagnosis.

No specific treatment has been advocated to reduce the risk of postpartum relapse. Given the increased risk of disease activity in the postpartum period, you and your doctor may decide to start or restart one of the immunomodulating treatments (Avonex®, Betaseron®, Copaxone®, or Rebif® [not available in the United States]) as soon as you have delivered.

While the extreme exhaustion that characterizes new motherhood may mimic the fatigue so common in MS, that symptom alone should not warrant new medication use. Your postpartum lifestyle should allow you to focus on caring for yourself, resting, and feeding the infant. This will require that other household tasks be attended to by others, including some of the infant care, shopping, and social events. If you are employed, find out now how much maternity leave your employer will allow. Six to eight weeks of leave time is typical in the United States. Ideally, women with MS should have a longer leave since any disease relapse that occurs is likely to have its onset in the fourth to eighth week post partum.

I always hoped to breast-feed my babies. Now that I have MS, would nursing be safe for me and the baby?

Historically, neurologists have discouraged women with MS from nursing, feeling that it posed an additional physical burden to a woman already at increased risk for an *exacerbation*. However, nursing is now widely encouraged if you have adequate dexterity, strength, and stamina. It eliminates the effort involved in bottle preparations and provides your baby with the best possible food.

Certain medications are absolutely unsafe for a nursing infant because they are secreted into the breast milk. Because of the increased risk of relapse postpartum, some women may consider using one of the disease-modifying medications (Avonex®, Betaseron®, Copaxone®, or Rebif® [not available in the United States]) to reduce the likelihood of an attack. Since these medications may be secreted into the breast milk, you should not take any of these medications if you plan to nurse your infant.

The high doses of prednisone that are prescribed for exacerbations of MS do result in significant concentrations of the steroid being present in breast milk. Since any postpartum relapse is likely to resolve spontaneously, any decision you make to use steroids must include the possible risk to the nursing baby. Because the immunodulating drugs and the high doses of steroids prescribed for exacerbations do raise concerns about suppression of the newborn's immune system (as well as the mother's), nursing should be stopped if these drugs become necessary.

The new mother's postpartum lifestyle, as well as the care and support available to her, may help to avoid disease worsening. Caring for a newborn is an exhausting experience for all new parents. In an effort to assure yourself adequate, uninterrupted sleep, try to have someone else do at least one of the night feedings. If you are breast-feeding, do all of the feedings yourself during the first two weeks in order to build up steady and sufficient milk production. After that initial two-week period, someone else can take over the nighttime feedings with formula or pumped and stored breast milk.

Can I start taking my regular MS medications as soon as my baby is born?

As discussed previously, the only limitation to medication use is whether a woman is nursing. If you are not planning to breast-feed, you may resume whatever medications you and your physician feel are best.

What is the likelihood that I will pass my MS on to my children?

The lifetime risk of MS in a child born to a person with MS has been estimated to be as high as 5 percent, much higher than the lifetime risk for the general population of 0.1 percent. While there is some increase in the risk to children with a family history of the disease, the actual risk is small (95 percent chance that MS will not occur). At the present time there is no way to diagnose MS or assess the MS risk in a particular infant before or after birth.

I was able to get pregnant with no difficulty. Now I'm worried about how I'll be able to take care of my baby once it's born. I'm exhausted all the time as it is. What should I do?

Planning ahead is essential to a successful start at parenting. If you are employed, start by trying to arrange time off from work after your delivery. Maternity leave for at least eight weeks is in your best interest and your child's. The new father should also look into the possibility of family-leave time under the Family Medical Leave Act (see Chapter 14) or temporarily arranging his schedule to be home somewhat earlier in the day. The exhaustion of new motherhood will gradually increase throughout the day. This, coupled with the possible worsening of MS symptoms postpartum, means that you will be needing a significant amount of help and support. Good parental teamwork will make these early days go more enjoyably and comfortably.

As you shop for baby furniture and equipment, look for things that are easy and convenient to manipulate. Choose such items as a highchair, car seat, and bath equipment with an eye to both safety for your baby and energy conservation for yourself. Create child-friendly play areas in your home where you can watch and interact with your baby as easily and comfortably as possible. Try to arrange for some hours of babycare each day so that you can get uninterrupted rest.

Of course, couples who are planning a family can never know for sure what might happen to impact their parenting abilities. To the extent that you can brainstorm ahead of time about possible problems that might arise, you will feel more confident of your ability to manage in the days ahead.

Gynecologic Care

Do I need any special care from my gynecologist when I am not pregnant?

All women, including those with MS, need to be educated about their contraceptive options and knowledgeable about sexually transmitted diseases. Women who are managing the problems associated with a chronic illness sometimes neglect their routine medical care; regular checkups, Pap tests, and mammograms are as essential for those with MS as they are for anyone else.

Women who have used any immunosuppressive medications (including prednisone, beta-interferon, and glatiramer acetate) should have a Pap test every six months. Abnormal results on tests that screen for precancerous changes in the cervix are more common when the immune system is less able to discourage the formation of abnormal cells in general, including those on the cervix. All women should have a mammogram on the schedule recommended by the American Cancer Society: an initial screening mammogram between 35 and 40 years of age; every one to two years until the age of 50; annually after age 50.

My friends who do not have MS are all talking about taking hormones now that we are at menopause. I have just had a few hot flashes and I know that feeling warm sometimes makes my symptoms of weakness and numbness worse. Is it advisable for me to use the hormones?

Yes. Hormone replacement therapy (HRT) not only relieves hot flashes, but also has been shown to be of significant benefit to a woman's overall health, whether she has MS or not. Studies indicate that HRT may help with incontinence, decrease vaginal dryness, reduce the risk of colon cancer and Alzheimer's disease, have a favorable impact on cholesterol and heart disease risk, and improve hormone-related memory loss and cognitive dysfunction.

HRT is particularly important for any women who are at risk of falling because of impaired balance or walking, since estrogen dramatically reduces the risk of *osteoporosis* and the fractures of the hip, wrist, and spine that can result (see Chapter 2).

A very significant predictor of risk for osteoporosis and osteoporotic fracture is reduced bone mass. Women with MS have been found to have lower than average bone density of the hips and spine, probably due to their reduced mobility and increased use of steroids. The amount of reduction in bone density found in women with MS can be expected to increase their risk of fracture by two to seven times that of a person with normal bone density. A simple bone density test can alert you and your doctor if you are at risk for osteoporosis.

The disadvantages of hormone replacement include the addition of another drug for women who are already taking several, the possible continuation of (hopefully light and predictable) periods—depending on how the hormone is prescribed—and some unresolved questions about the degree to which hormone replacement might increase the risk of breast cancer. You will need to discuss with your own physician the relative benefits and risks of hormone replacement so that you can make an informed decision. Having made the decision to start hormone replacement therapy, you will want to educate yourself about the many options that are now available, including new and different drugs, lower effective dosage levels, vaginal creams, and skin patches.

Besides using hormone replacement therapy, are there any other strategies I can use to reduce my risk of osteoporosis?

All women, starting when they are very young, should be certain they are getting at least 1000 mg. of calcium every day. Dairy products (milk, yogurt, and cheese) are the easiest way to get this amount via diet (three servings every day of a dairy product). If one does not eat a lot of dairy products, calcium-fortified orange juice is a good substitute and calcium supplements are also acceptable. Once postmenopausal, all women should increase their calcium intake to 1200 mg per day, and those who are not using hormones should try to increase their intake to 1500 mg. The Calcium Information Center (1-800-321-2681) can suggest ways to maximize your calcium intake via diet and vitamin use.

Recently, women with MS were found to be at higher risk for vitamin D deficiency. This, too, can contribute to the development of osteoporosis. Although this deficiency may simply be due to inadequate intake of the vitamin, it may also result from insufficient exposure to the sun. People with MS who stay out of the sun in order to avoid becoming overheated, may also be depriving themselves of the 10 minutes or so of sun exposure per day that provides adequate amounts of vitamin D. In order to ensure that you are getting an adequate amount of this important vitamin, you can take it in pill form (400–600 IU per day). Unfortunately, vitamin D is not found in many foods other than fortified milk.

Alendronate (Fosamax®) is a nonhormonal medication, available since 1995 for postmenopausal women, that prevents bone resorption, decreases fractures of the spine, hip, and wrist by up to 50 percent, and treats existing osteoporosis. If osteoporosis is a significant problem for a postmenopausal woman, this drug can be beneficial; it will not, however, address the full range of symptoms typically managed with HRT.

Raloxifene (Evista®), an osteoporosis prevention drug, was approved for postmenopausal women in 1997. This drug increases bone mass (although not as significantly as estrogen), reduces the risk of spinal fractures (but not hip fractures), and lowers LDL ("bad" cholesterol) levels. Unlike estrogen, raloxifene does not stimulate the uterine lining, so there is no need for progesterone, the second hormone that is often combined with estrogen in HRT. In addition, raloxifene does not increase breast cancer risk, and may even reduce it. Raloxifene does, however, slightly increase a woman's risk for blood clots and may cause hot flashes to recur during the first few months of use.

I have read a lot about natural alternatives to HRT. Could a healthy diet, in combination with natural supplements, be as beneficial for me as taking hormones?

The answer depends on what you are trying to accomplish. A healthy lifestyle (including 30 minutes per day of exercise, 5 days a week; not smoking; a low-fat, high-fiber diet; adequate calcium intake; and regular medical checkups) will be more effective than herbs in promoting your wellness as you join the 50 million women in America over 50. This kind of healthy lifestyle will help to prevent the cardiovascular disease that kills more women than the next 16 causes of death combined.

For symptom relief at menopause, meditation, massage and acupuncture may be helpful. For hot flashes, vitamin E, up to 400 IU a day, and soy (drink, powder, or tofu) may be helpful. The herbs typically recommended to address menopausal symptoms (evening primrose oil, black cohosh and dong quai), have not been found to yield consistently positive results. If you do opt to try these, be sure to inform your physician and start with low doses.

Recommended Readings

Birk, K. & Kalb, R. Fertility, pregnancy, and childbirth. In R. Kalb (ed.) *Multiple Sclerosis: A Guide for Families.* New York: Demos Medical Publishing, 1998, pp. 61–71.

Birk, K. General health and well-being. In R. Kalb (ed.) *Multiple Sclerosis: A Guide for Families.* New York: Demos Medical Publishing, 1998, pp. 151–162.

Doress-Worters P, Laskin Siegal D. *(The New) Ourselves Growing Older.* New York: Peter Smith, 1996.

Dorman, CD. *Living Well with MS.* New York: HarperCollins, 1993.

Haseltine, FP, Cole, SS, & Gray, DB. *Reproductive Issues for Persons with Physical Disabilities.* Baltimore, MD: Paul H. Brookes Publishing, 1993.

Krotoski, D, Nosek, MA, & Turk, MA. *Women with Physical Disabilities: Achieving and Maintaining Health and Well-Being.* Baltimore, MD: Paul H. Brookes Publishing, 1996.

North American Menopause Society. *Menopause Guidebook.* (North American Menopause Society, P.O. Box 94527, Cleveland, OH. 44101-4527; tel: 800-774-5342).

A comprehensive 50-page booklet published by the leading organization devoted to improving women's health through menopause and beyond. The booklet, along with the Society's "Menopak," are free with a $5.00 shipping and handling charge.

Resources for Rehabilitation

A Woman's Guide to Coping with Disability. Lexington, MA: Resources for Rehabilitation, 1994.

Rogers J, Matsumura, M. *Mother to Be: A Guide to Pregnancy and Birth for Women with Disabilities.* New York: Demos Medical Publishing, 1991.

Selected publications available from your local chapter of the National Multiple Sclerosis Society (800-Fight-MS):

◇ *Genes and Susceptibility* (EG 750)
◇ *On: Pregnancy* (EG 749)
◇ *Hormones in Multiple Sclerosis* (EG 765)
◇ *Facts and Issues* (reprints of articles that originally appeared in the National MS Society magazine, *Inside MS*, covering such topics as pregnancy, fatigue, energy management, sexuality, genes and MS susceptibility)

14

Employment

Phillip D. Rumrill, Jr., Ph.D., CRC*

The working role is one of the most valued in American society. A person's work not only determines what he or she does on a day-to-day basis, but also helps to define who that person is. The work that provides a person's income and economic stability also defines his or her role in the community, and a significant part of that person's self-esteem is tied to occupational status within the community.

Most adults spend at least half their waking hours on work-related activities, making work the single most time-consuming task in their lives. People spend much more time working than in any other life role, including that of spouse, parent, or friend. So, when a disease like multiple sclerosis (MS) affects people's ability to do their job, it threatens not only their economic and social status, but also their sense of who they are.

People with MS are a qualified, experienced, and capable group of workers. In fact, more than 90 percent of people with MS have worked at some time in their lives, and approximately two-thirds are still employed at the time of diagnosis. As the illness progresses, however, there is a sharp drop in labor-force

*With grateful acknowledgment of materials from the first edition written by Donna Kulha.

participation. At the present time, only 25 percent to 40 percent of Americans with MS are employed. A number of research studies have been conducted over the years concerning employment and MS, but we still do not have a clear understanding as to why one person with MS keeps his or her job while another, with a similar degree of disability, leaves the work force. Factors that have been identified as predictors of employment difficulty and/or job loss for people with MS include:

◇ mobility impairments
◇ working in a job that requires significant physical exertion
◇ cognitive impairments
◇ a poor relationship with one's employer
◇ negative attitudes on the part of co-workers
◇ a progressive course of the illness

Given the negative impact that job loss can have on a family's economic circumstances and overall sense of well-being, it is important to identify ways to help people with MS continue working as long as they wish to do so. The first step is to remind people who are working while coping with MS that the decision to leave the work force is theirs and theirs alone. *There is no reason for a physician to prescribe unemployment as part of a person's treatment regimen; there is no evidence that removing oneself from the work force has a positive impact on health status.* If and when a person is considering disability-related retirement, the choice should be made in consultation with significant others. Before making the important decision to work or not to work, people with MS will want to be fully informed about the laws, services, and resources that can assist them in maintaining their employment.

Comprehensive psychosocial services, the state Vocational Rehabilitation program, occupational therapy, job retention programs, and consumer advocacy strategies have been developed to support people's efforts to continue on the job while coping with MS. Education for people with MS and their employers and co-workers, proactive approaches to legal rights, and legislative initiatives are also vital means of keeping people with MS in the work force.

For example, the *Americans with Disabilities Act* (ADA) of 1990 was the first comprehensive legislation passed by any country in the world to prohibit discrimination on the basis of disability. The ADA guarantees full participation in society for people with disabilities in much the same way as the Civil Rights Act of 1964 guaranteed the rights of all people regardless of race, sex, national origin, and religion. The four areas of social activity covered by the ADA are employment, public services, public accommodations, and communications (telephone systems).

As it pertains to employment, the ADA requires employers with 15 or more employees to provide reasonable accommodations for qualified employees with disabilities. For people with MS, reasonable accommodations may include:

◇ modifications to the work schedule as a means of combating fatigue (e.g., an abbreviated work week or an extended lunch break during which to rest)
◇ flexibility in the manner or location in which work is performed (e.g., home-based employment)
◇ provision of equipment (e.g., a closed-circuit magnification machine for a person with a visual impairment)
◇ renovations of the work environment (e.g., modification of rest rooms to accommodate a motorized scooter)

It should be noted that reasonable accommodations are determined on a case-by-case basis, and that employers are NOT required to do any of the following:

◇ eliminate a primary job responsibility from a person's job description
◇ lower production standards that are applied to all employees
◇ provide personal use items (e.g., a cane, wheelchair, eyeglasses)
◇ excuse a violation of conduct rules
◇ provide accommodations that constitute an undue hardship, i.e., changes or modifications that would prove too costly or disruptive to the operation of the business

Before becoming eligible for a reasonable accommodation, the worker or applicant must disclose his or her disability status to the employer and make a request for the accommodation in question.

This does not mean, however, that the person must disclose his or her underlying diagnosis or disabling condition. **An employer *never* has the right to know that you have MS**, only that you are a person with a disability who needs an accommodation to perform an essential function of the job you hold or wish to hold.

Although reasonable accommodations are an important part of the ADA, the employment protections available to people with disabilities go far beyond on-the-job accommodations. Under Title I of the ADA (the employment section), people with disabilities have the civil right to enjoy the same benefits and privileges of employment as their non-disabled co-workers. This means that personnel decisions (e.g., hiring, promotion, layoff, termination) must be made without respect to the person's disability status. Workers may not be harassed on the basis of their disabilities, and the compensation they receive must be commensurate with their qualifications and productivity irrespective of disability. Provided below are key terms and definitions related to the ADA.

Individuals with disabilities. Individuals (1) with a mental or physical impairment that substantially limits one or more life activities, or (2) have a history of such an impairment, or (3) are perceived (even erroneously) as having such an impairment.

Qualified individuals with disabilities. Under Title I of the ADA, the term "qualified" applies to an individual with a disability who meets the skill, experience, education, and other job-related requirements of a position held or desired and who, with or without reasonable accommodations, can perform the essential functions of the job.

Essential job function. Essential job functions are narrowly defined to include fundamental job duties, as opposed to marginal ones. A job function is more likely to be "essential" if it requires special expertise, if a large amount of time is spent on that function, and/or if that function was listed in the written job description prepared before the employer advertised for or interviewed job applicants.

Reasonable accommodations. These refer to an employment-related modification that an employer must make in order to ensure equal opportunity for an individual with a disability to (1) apply for or test for a job; (2) perform essential job functions; and/or (3) receive the same benefits and privileges as other employees. The employer is required to provide a reasonable accommodation for known disabilities (e.g. where the disability is obvious or the applicant/employee informs the employer of the disability). Although each case must be evaluated individually, some common examples of on-the-job accommodations include:

◇ restructuring of existing facilities
◇ restructuring of the job
◇ modification of work schedules
◇ reassignment to another position
◇ modification of equipment
◇ installation of new equipment
◇ provision of qualified readers and interpreters
◇ modification of application and examination procedures and/or training materials
◇ and flexible personal leave policies

Undue hardship. An accommodation might prove to be an undue hardship for the employer if its implementation resulted in a significant difficulty or expense. Factors to be considered in making this determination include (1) the nature and net cost of the accommodation; (2) the impact of the accommodation on the operation of the facility involved, taking into account the facility's overall resources and the number of its employees; and (3) the manner in which the employer's business operates, taking into account its size and financial resources. In asserting that an accommodation is an undue hardship, an employer must rely on actual, not hypothetical, costs and burdens.

The *Family and Medical Leave Act* (FMLA) of 1993 is another federal law with important implications for employed people with MS and other disabling conditions. The FMLA has enabled thousands of American employees to retain their jobs while taking unpaid leaves of absence to attend to important family health concerns. The law requires employers in the public and private sectors to hold workers' jobs open and continue paying health insurance premiums while employees take time off to treat and/or recover from illnesses or injuries. *It also provides leave for employees who must attend to the health care needs of their family members.* For example, a person whose elderly parent needs transportation to medical appointments, or extra care following an acute illness, could request unpaid leave to attend to the parent's needs.

Any employer who has 50 or more employees residing within a 75-mile radius of the work location is covered by the FMLA. Employees are eligible for protection under this law if they have worked at the job for at least one year (no fewer than 1,250 hours within the 12 months preceding the requested leave date) and have (or have a family member who has) a serious health condition. Under this law, a *serious health condition* is defined as any illness, injury, impairment, or course of treatment that renders a person unable to perform essential job functions. The term is broader and more inclusive than the ADA's definition of *disability*, which means that someone with MS could be considered to have a serious health condition under the FMLA but not meet the ADA's standard for *disability*. Unlike the term *disability*, *serious health conditions* pertain to both temporary and permanent conditions (e.g., pregnancy, or birth or adoption, and surgery, as well as chronic illness).

Under the FMLA, employers are required to provide up to 12 weeks of unpaid leave per calendar year for an eligible employee who is coping with a serious health condition. The 12 weeks need not be taken consecutively, and the employer must allow the worker to return to the same or a similar, equivalent position. The right to return to work following unpaid leave can be denied only to key employees—those earning the highest 10 percent of salaries—and only when holding open the jobs of these employees would create substantial and grievous long-term economic injury to the employer's operations. The employer's burden of proof for this exception is more stringent than for the ADA's defense of undue hardship.

The following questions illustrate some of the important employment issues faced by people with MS. Although the chapter discusses the relevance of the ADA and FMLA to various employment-related problems and concerns, the information in the chapter should not be used as personal legal advice. These questions and answers are intended to provide a background for your own personal planning and problem solving. If and when you have questions about your particular employment situation, your best strategies will be to:

◇ consult the literature and other resources listed at the end of the chapter

◇ consult with your local chapter of the National Multiple Sclerosis Society

◇ seek any additional help or advice from an attorney who specializes in labor law

Americans with Disabilities Act

I'm interviewing for a new job. Do I need to tell a potential employer about my diagnosis? If I do need to disclose, what am I required to say?

The issue of disclosure is one of the most important, and potentially complicated, employment concerns for people with MS. As a matter of law, you have no obligation to disclose anything about your disability status or underlying diagnosis during a job interview. Your employer <u>never</u> has the right to know your diagnosis, and people with MS and other disabilities are generally encouraged to leave medical information out of any discussion with a prospective employer. The only time you need to disclose the fact that you are a person with a disability is when you believe that you will need a reasonable accommodation to perform one or more of the job's essential functions. If your disability is obvious, and if you are certain that you would need on-the-job accommodations, you may wish to mention your accommodation needs during an interview. If you opt for that strategy, it is important to focus on the skills and strategies you use to overcome disability-related work limitations—not on how difficult it would be for you to perform a particular function. People are also encouraged to accompany disclosure of their disability status with a specific plan for the accommodations that would be most beneficial in performing the job. That way, you take all of the uncertainty out of the accommodation process; employers are much more likely to approve a strategy that you have identified than they are to engage in the process of identifying what your needs are, especially during a job interview.

If your disability is not obvious to the employer, and you do not foresee any need for reasonable accommodations in your current health situation, there is generally no reason to mention disability at all. If your disability does not affect your job performance, think of it as you would any other circumstance in your life. If the fact that you are having marital problems does not affect your job performance, is it any of your employer's business? How about your credit history? What church you go to? These issues have no bearing on your ability to do your job, so you probably would not bring them up in an interview. Think of your disability in the same manner, and always err on the side of maintaining your right to privacy. You can always add more information about your disability status if the situation calls for it, but you can never recapture your privacy if you make a full disclosure during a job interview.

When checking my references, can a potential employer ask how MS has affected my work in the past?

Absolutely not. Again, the prospective employer never has the right to know that you are a person with MS. Even if you disclose your diagnosis of MS, he or she cannot inquire about it with your references. The employer may ask for an assessment of your ability to perform the job for which you have applied, or an explanation of the kind of worker you were for the referencing employer. If you do not wish to disclose your MS or disability status to a prospective employer, it is important to ask your references who might be aware of your diagnosis not to mention any medical or disability-related information. Ask them to focus on your characteristics as a worker, not on personal issues that have no bearing on your employability.

After being offered a job, I was told that I need to pass a physical examination. What should I do?

Take the physical, and be honest with the physician. He or she may not disclose any diagnostic information to the employer. Also know that the ADA requires physical examinations to be job-specific. In other words, if you have applied for a job as an administrative assistant, the employer may not test you to determine whether you can lift 50 pounds over your head. In fact, medical examinations can include only the physical tasks required for the particular job in question. Physical examinations also must be conducted post-offer; in other words, the employer must first make a determination that he or she wants to hire you before requiring the physical examination. Although the job-specific and post-offer nature of physical examinations enhances your protection as a person with a disability, the employer may withdraw the job offer if the examining physician determines that you are physically unable to perform the job. Of course, the employer would be legally required to consider reasonable accommodations to overcome your physical limitations, but the accommodations must enable you to do the job or else you would not be deemed qualified for that particular position.

I use a cane on bad days and I may need one on the day of my job interview. Should I tell the interviewer that I have MS?

In general, the answer is no. You may wish to disclose your disability status at that time, but this is only necessary if you believe that your mobility impairment would interfere with your ability to do the job. On the other hand, some people prefer to get everything out in the open. A woman with MS once asked, "How can I expect my employer to be honest and open with me if I won't be honest with him? MS is nothing to be ashamed of, so why can't I just let him know? That might make him even more understanding of my needs." It is important to note here that there is certainly nothing wrong with disclosing your MS diagnosis if you choose to do so. Whether and how much you disclose to a prospective employer is entirely up to you, as long as you remember that getting everything out in the open vis-à-vis MS is a courtesy to your employer, not a legal obligation.

One possible risk associated with being open about your diagnosis is that your employer may have inaccurate conceptions of what MS is and how it affects individuals. Even if your only symptoms are fatigue and mild tremors, your employer might view you as a safety risk because a former employee with MS lost her balance periodically. *Given the highly individualized nature of MS, telling an employer you have MS tells him or her absolutely nothing about your ability to do the job.* Therefore, given the potential for misconceptions based upon most employers' limited experience with people who have MS, your best strategy is usually to restrict discussions of your disabilities to non-medical, functional terms.

For the employer's part of the job interview, he or she may inquire about your needs for reasonable accommodations if you have an obvious disability and he or she believes that you would need accommodations to perform the job's essential functions. It is perfectly acceptable for an interviewing employer to say, "I see that you use that cane to help you walk, and this job requires the worker to push a cart filled with supplies to different parts of the building. Would you need any accommodations to do that?" At this point, it is important to think about accommodations that you might need to perform that function, and to discuss those strategies openly with the employer. Here again, the main purpose of this dialogue is to identify ways to help you be a productive worker, not necessarily to share medical information that may be of limited utility in arriving upon an accommodation plan. The employer may also ask you to demonstrate how you would perform any or all essential functions of the job, even if he or she does not routinely ask other job applicants to do so.

I have been offered a job, and the question of medical benefits arises. Can I be denied coverage under my employer's health insurance plan because of a diagnosis of MS?

Title I of the ADA prohibits employers from entering into contracts that discriminate against people with disabilities. This includes contracts related to health insurance. Employees with disabilities must be given the same coverage that is available to all other employees. Additionally, an employer cannot refuse to hire you because his or her insurance company will not cover you, or if covering you increases the employer's health care premiums. However, an employer may offer health insurance coverage that contains preexisting condition exclusions or limits certain procedures, provided that those exclusions or limitations pertain to ALL employees.

The Health Insurance Portability and Accountability Act of 1996 (see Ch. 15) provides some protections for employees with disabilities who change jobs. The Act enables a person with a preexisting medical condition to join his or her new employer's health insurance plan and be exempt from preexisting condition exclusions, *as long as the employee does* not interrupt his or her insurance coverage. The best advice for people with MS who leave a job is to continue their health insurance benefits as long as is allowable and then transfer their coverage to the new employer's plan.

Given the complexity of health care coverage in the United States, it might be tempting to conceal your MS from an insurance company during your enrollment process. This is not advisable, because any insurance company can discontinue your coverage if it learns that you have lied about your medical history on application forms. Remember also that your employer has no right to read any medical information that you submit to insurance companies.

My wife has had MS for many years. Am I required to disclose this information if I am offered a job at a company that will be providing my family's health insurance coverage? Will my wife's medical costs be covered by this new coverage?

If your employer has a grace period during which you can enroll family members in health insurance plans without disclosing medical information, that is always your best option. If the grace period passes, you should report to the insurance company (not to the employer) whatever medical information is requested. Your wife may be subject to preexisting condition exclusions, but many employers offer multiple insurance plans from which to choose. Whenever possible, you should select the plan (usually a managed care plan) which does not contain preexisting condition exclusions. As managed care companies continue to move toward flat-fee (capitation) contracts with health care providers (paying providers a certain amount of money per insuree to serve whatever medical needs are presented), the likelihood of having MS excluded from coverage as a preexisting condition stands to decrease. Also, you cannot be denied an employment opportunity because your wife has MS; the ADA prohibits discrimination against people whose family members or associates have disabilities.

I have just been told that I have a definite diagnosis of MS. Should I quit my job?

There is no reason to quit your job just because you have been diagnosed with MS. There is no evidence that unemployment will have a positive effect on your health status; in fact, many experts believe that people who work are psychologically and physically healthier than those who do not. With advancements in assistive technology, medical treatment, and societal attitudes toward people with disabilities, people with MS and other potentially disabling conditions are able to maintain their jobs longer than ever before. Keep in mind, as well, your legal rights under the ADA and FMLA—those laws were put into place to enable you to keep working as long as you wish to do so. If and when you decide to stop working, it is important that you weigh all important factors (e.g., family circumstance, financial needs, health status) with input from significant others, health care professionals, and your employer. The fact that you have been diagnosed with MS should not be the determining factor in this exceedingly important decision, and you will know better than anyone else when and if it is time to stop working.

I have been with the same company for three years and have recently been diagnosed with MS. How do I decide whether or not I need to disclose this information?

In general, the best reason for disclosing your disability status is that you foresee a need for a reasonable accommodation on your job. If symptoms of your illness are obvious to others, if they have begun to interfere with your job performance, and/or if you have been receiving feedback from your employer that there are problems with your performance, you may want to approach your employer about possible accommodations. Although you do not have to disclose the underlying cause of your disability (i.e., your MS), it is important to frame your disability status in functional terms: I am a person with a disability, and I have been having difficulty performing X and Y on my job. I would like to discuss some ways to accommodate these difficulties—some strategies that will enable me to continue being a productive employee.

It is also important to note that you need not reference the ADA specifically in your discussions with your employer. In fact, the National Multiple Sclerosis Society advocates a win-win approach to on-the-job accommodations, in which the employee with MS keeps his or her legal protections out of the dialogue with the employer to every extent possible. The best rationale for reasonable accommodations is that they will help you to maintain or enhance your productivity on the job. This benefits both you and the employer, and it demonstrates your willingness to engage in a cooperative, non-adversarial process of identifying and implementing cost-effective accommodations. This approach is almost always more effective than invoking your civil rights in a formal way, or threatening to sue your employer if he or she does not meet your needs. The best advice about disclosure and the accommodation request process is to:

◇ be direct but friendly
◇ frame your disability-related work limitations in functional terms
◇ focus on your accommodation needs rather than your medical diagnosis
◇ emphasize the mutual benefits of providing you with on-the-job accommodations
◇ use your legal rights and recourses under the ADA if and only if your employer refuses to provide an appropriate accommodation to meet your stated needs

If I decide to disclose at work, who should be the first to know, and how much information should I be prepared to offer?

Your immediate supervisor is usually the person to whom you should first disclose. The supervisor may wish to involve other representatives of the employer, particularly a human resources specialist or a department manager. Your co-workers have no legal right to know anything about your disability status, but you may wish to let them know what is going on as a courtesy. Communications to co-workers about your disability should come from you, not your employer, and should include only the information needed to help them understand your circumstance. In any disclosure, it is important to focus on the symptoms or effects of your disability which specifically affect your job performance. It is usually best to refrain from providing clinical, medical descriptions of any kind. Even if you choose to disclose your MS, avoid using such terms as exacerbation, attack, progressive, and disease. You may wish to write out your disclosure statement and rehearse how you will say it with a friend or advisor. Your local National Multiple Sclerosis Society staff can also help you in determining whether, how, and to whom you should disclose.

All my MS symptoms are invisible. Do I have to tell my employer that I have been diagnosed with MS?

No. The only time it is necessary to disclose the fact that you have a disability is when you feel that you might need an on-the-job accommodation. If your symptoms are invisible, and if they

do not pose any problems for you in doing your job, there is neither a need nor any advantage for you to mention anything about
this personal aspect of your life.

**The people in my office know about my MS. My symptoms are
not very visible and my colleagues and supervisor have trouble
understanding about my good days and bad days. I'm happy to
work long hours when I am feeling good but sometimes I'm just
not able to. How much am I required to explain to them about
my condition?**

You are not required by law to discuss the nature or course of your
illness. However, you may want to share the fact that your symptoms are more noticeable on some days than on others as a means
of helping your employer and co-workers better understand your
needs. For people whose MS is characterized by exacerbations and
remissions, the best strategy is often to develop a contingency plan
for dealing with bad days or an unexpected relapse. In developing
this kind of contingency plan, you may not be discussing a particular accommodation strategy, but rather a general strategy for covering your shift on days when you cannot work your full schedule.
Although the employer is only required to accommodate *current*
limitations under the ADA, setting up a contingency plan for
potential limitations can be an effective way of establishing a cooperative, non-adversarial arrangement that meets your need for time
off and your employer's need for personnel coverage.

**Most of my symptoms are not visible to others. Fatigue and
memory problems pose the greatest problems at work for me.
Are these invisible impairments covered by the ADA?**

Yes. Physical or mental impairment need not be visible or obvious to substantially limit functioning in one or more major life
activities, as per the ADA's definition of disability which was
cited in the beginning of this chapter. The important standard
regarding your symptoms is whether they pose problems for you
in doing your job. Remember, a qualified person under the ADA
is one who possesses the minimum credentials required for the
job and who can perform essential functions of that job—with
reasonable accommodations if required. Fatigue and cognitive
impairments are among the most common symptoms of MS, and
there are a number of proven strategies to help people overcome
those effects while doing their jobs. Contact your local chapter of

the National Multiple Sclerosis Society for additional information on easy-to-implement job accommodations.

Is every employee covered under the ADA?

Only those employees who have disabilities, have records of disabilities, or are perceived as having disabilities, are protected by the ADA. Having a diagnosis of MS does not automatically qualify one as a person with a disability under the ADA. The prevailing standard involves the functional aspects of the diagnosis—that is, whether the impairment substantially limits functioning in one or more major life activities.

More specifically, only those employees with disabilities who work for a covered employer are protected under the ADA. Title I of the ADA covers employers with 15 or more employees in both the public and private sectors. Native American tribes, the federal government, and tax-exempt private membership clubs are not required to comply with the ADA's employment provisions. The Rehabilitation Act of 1973 prohibits the federal government and employers receiving federal funds from discriminating against workers on the basis of disability, but the ADA's protections are farther-reaching and more stringent.

Who is responsible for deciding what accommodations I need: my doctor, my employer, my union, my lawyer or myself?

Ideally, you and your employer make a joint and mutually-acceptable decision regarding which accommodations to implement. Title I of the ADA requires that employee and employer engage in a cooperative dialogue to assess the worker's needs, identify accommodation options, and implement a reasonable accommodation that is agreeable to both parties. In that process, input can be sought from medical professionals, unions, and (if the collaborative process has broken down) attorneys. In general, the accommodation process works best when most of the decision making is done by the employee and employer, with a minimum of assistance from partisan advocates. Other resources that might be enlisted in identifying cost-effective accommodations include rehabilitation counselors, assistive technology specialists, rehabilitation engineers, ergonomists (specialists in the study of workplace design and safety), and physical or occupational therapists.

Who decides if a requested accommodation is reasonable?

When a qualified individual with a disability requests an accommodation, the employer must make a reasonable effort to provide an accommodation that is effective for that individual. An accommodation does not have to be made if it presents an undue hardship to the employer. Undue hardship refers to accommodations that would be too expensive or disruptive for a particular business to handle. The employer's determination of undue hardship can be challenged in court or before the Equal Employment Opportunity Commission (EEOC).

Who pays for the accommodations that are made (e.g., adaptive equipment, building renovations, schedule changes)?

In most cases, the employer will be required to pay the costs of the accommmodation unless it presents an undue hardship. In determining whether an accommodation represents an undue hardship, the cost that will be considered is the actual cost to the employer. Specific federal tax credits and deductions are available to employers who make accommodations required by the ADA, and research indicates that the majority of on-the-job accommodations used by people with MS cost nothing or very little to implement. A vocational rehabilitation counselor in your area can tell you about local funding sources that might help pay for some accommodations.

My boss says that the accommodations I have requested are too expensive. What should I do now?

Before developing a plan for appeal, it is important to understand that the courts in ADA lawsuits have given the employer considerable discretion in determining what constitutes an undue hardship. Your best bet is to meet again with your employer. In that meeting, discuss possible alternatives to your desired accommodation that might be less expensive; *the ADA entitles you to a reasonable accommodation, not necessarily your first choice.* If you simply cannot reach an agreement, your next step is to file a complaint with the EEOC, which oversees ADA Title I enforcement. Not only does the EEOC investigate complaints and make a determination about the legal merits of the complaint, it attempts to resolve employee-employer conflicts in a non-litigious manner. Should you proceed with a formal complaint to the EEOC, it is advisable to retain an attorney who specializes in disability and/or employment law. If the EEOC complaint does not result in a satisfactory resolution to your concern, you may wish to file a lawsuit against your employer in civil court. Remedies available to people with disabilities under Title I of the ADA include hiring, reinstatement, punitive damages, compensatory damages, and court orders to stop discriminatory conduct.

I have requested several accommodations that have been denied on the basis that these changes would substantially alter my job description. What recourse do I have?

Your employer is not required to provide accommodations that would substantially alter your job description. Restructuring of the job, one of the types of reasonable accommodations listed in ADA regulations, applies only to minor, or marginal duties of the job. Essential functions of the job, which are delineated on a written job description, are not subject to restructuring.

I feel that I need further advice at this point, from a lawyer, a union representative, or the National Multiple Sclerosis Society. Can I be fired from my job for seeking outside advice or support?

Absolutely not. Title I of the ADA protects people with disabilities from harassment, intimidation, or retaliation on the part of employers. You have every right to avail yourself of legal or other kinds of advice, and you cannot be penalized or punished for it. Just to be on the safe side, though, there is probably no good reason to tell your employer that you have sought outside counsel.

My co-workers resent the accommodations that have been made for my disability. How can I improve the situation?

Many experts would recommend that you educate your co-workers about MS and how it affects you. That is certainly an option, but remember that you have absolute rights to privacy under the ADA. You have no legal obligation to let your co-workers know what is going on, but informing them about your condition may, in some cases, help them understand that you are not receiving preferential treatment. As with any form of disclosure, the standard you should apply in deciding whether to inform your co-workers about your MS is how much information do they need in order to understand your situation.

I have requested a promotion at work, but I was told that they are hesitant to put me in a more responsible position because I could have an exacerbation. Is a company allowed to take that position with me?

An employer cannot limit, segregate, or classify a person with a disability in any way that negatively affects him or her in terms of job opportunity and advancement. Promotion and other personnel decisions must be based on factual evidence about the person's ability to do the job, not on any assumption, speculation, or stereotype about the worker's disability status. Given that your employer already knows you have MS, your best strategy in this situation may be to try to alleviate your supervisor's concerns about your job performance. The supervisor has a responsibility to the company to ensure that any position is filled by a person who is capable of handling the work. If your supervisor is concerned that you might miss work because of exacerbations, review with him or her your prior work history and attendance record. If your MS is of the exacerbating/remitting type, discuss with your supervisor how you would plan to handle the work load during a period of disease flare-up. If you have not experienced frequent exacerbations in the past, your supervisor may be basing his or her judgement about you on inaccurate information regarding MS. As a courtesy to the supervisor (although you have no legal obligation to do so), you might want to ask your physician to write a letter on your behalf explaining that exacerbations are not necessarily part of the MS picture. Additionally, the National Multiple Sclerosis Society has literature designed to answer employers' questions about the disease. If the company continues to deny you a promotion, and you believe that you are qualified to do the job in spite of your symptoms, you might want to contact the EEOC or consult an attorney.

My employer has accommodated all my requests, but I am still having difficulty doing my job. I have been offered a position in another department, but it would mean a demotion and a cut in pay. Do I have to take this position? If I don't, can my employer fire me from my present position?

According to the law, an employee with a disability can be reassigned to a different position that is equivalent in terms of pay and job status, assuming that he or she is qualified for the position and that such a position is vacant or will be vacant within a reasonable amount of time. If no such equivalent position is available, and if no accommodations would enable you to remain in the current position, your employer can reassign you to a lower-grade position. In such a situation, your employer does not have to maintain your salary at the level of your former position unless the same is done for other employees who are reassigned to lower-grade positions. Finally, your employment can be terminated if all requested accommodations have been provided, no equivalent position is available, and you cannot perform the essential functions of your current job.

Under what circumstances can I be fired from a job because of my MS?

You can be terminated from your job if you can no longer perform the essential functions of the position even with the help of reasonable accommodations. You can also be terminated if the accommodations you need to perform essential job functions are too expensive or would pose an undue hardship for the employer. However, the employer is required to make an effort to find more suitable, alternative positions for you within the company. In other words, you cannot be terminated because of your inability to perform essential job functions until every reasonable effort has been made to accommodate your limitations.

I feel that I can no longer do my job the way I used to do it. How will I know if and when it's time for me to retire?

It is time for you to look into other options if you have researched and requested all possible accommodations to assist you in doing your job, yet still find you cannot adequately perform the essential job functions. Be sure to investigate other positions that may be available within your company. Other options include job retraining that would enable you to continue working in some other field, volunteer work, Social Security Disability Insurance, and long-term disability.

How do I figure out if I am eligible for Social Security Disability Insurance (SSDI) or Supplemental Security Income (SSI)?

Both SSDI and SSI are programs run by the Social Security Administration. The medical requirements for disability payments are the same under both programs, and disability is determined by the same process. For a person with MS, the recognized areas of impairment may include gait, vision, cognition, and fatigue. Eligibility for SSDI is based on prior work history, whereas SSI disability benefits are made solely on the basis of financial need. Applications for SSDI require a five-month waiting period from the determination of disability to the start of benefits. Twenty-four months after the initial waiting period, the person becomes eligible for Medicare insurance coverage (see Chapter 15). There is no similar waiting period for SSI benefits; individuals eligible for SSI based on financial need are covered by Medicaid (see Chapter 15). To be eligible for SSDI, a person must: (1) have worked and paid Social Security taxes (FICA) for enough years to be covered under Social Security and to have paid at least some of these taxes in recent years; (2) be considered medically disabled (i.e., too disabled to work); and (3) not be working or working but earning less than the Substantial Gainful Activity (SGA) level of $700 per month ($1,110 for beneficiaries who are blind). In determining a person's gross earnings, certain employment-related expenses will be deducted from the calculation if the person is paying expenses out of pocket and not otherwise being reimbursed for them. These deducted expenses include some types of attendant care services, transportation-related costs, medical and non-medical equipment costs, medication costs, and some types of residential modifications.

The SSDI payment amount is based on a worker's lifetime average earnings covered by Social Security. The payment amount will be reduced by worker's compensation payments and/or public disability payments. Those individuals who are receiving payments from private disability insurance companies may find that these payments are reduced by whatever amount they subsequently receive from SSDI. The SSDI payment amount is not affected by other (non-work) income or resources.

To be eligible for SSI based on a medical condition, a person must (1) have little or no income or resources; (2) be considered medically disabled (i.e., too disabled to work); and (3) initially not be working or be working but earning less than the SGA level of $700 per month (this restriction does not apply to beneficiaries who are blind). As with SSDI, certain out-of-pocket employment-related expenses will be deducted from the calculation of the person's gross earnings.

Once you begin to receive SSI benefits, work activity will not bring an end to SSI eligibility as long as you remain medically disabled. Even if you cannot receive SSI income maintenance checks because the amount of money you earn exceeds the SGA, eligibility for Medicaid may continue indefinitely. The SSI payment amount is based on the amount of other income, your living arrangements, and the state in which you reside. The basic payment is known as the federal benefit rate; this rate is adjusted each year to compensate for inflation and cost of living increases. Most states pay an additional amount known as a state supplement. The amount and qualifications for these supplements vary from state to state.

What happens if I retire on disability and then find in six months or a year that I feel able to go back to work? Would that jeopardize my chances of getting disability in the future?

There are many work incentives available if you decide to return to work while receiving SSDI benefits. These incentives provide support over a period of years to allow any disability beneficiary to test his or her ability to work and gradually become self-supporting and independent. You have at least four years to test your ability to work. During the first 12 months (trial work period) you will receive full SSDI payments. Following the initial nine of these twelve months, you begin a three-year extended period of eligibility. If you stop working any time during this period, you can restart your cash benefits without a new application, demonstration of your disability, or waiting period. Your Medicare benefits will also continue during this three-year period. Once Medicare stops due to renewed work activity, you can elect to buy coverage as long as you remain disabled. If you become disabled again within five years after the prior period of disability ended, you do not have to go through another five-month waiting period to get benefits, nor do you have to wait to become reeligible for Medicare.

I can no longer work full-time and am receiving SSDI. What would happen to my SSDI if I returned to work on a part-time basis?

As long as you earn under $700 per month (the establish cutoff for Substantial Gainful Activity), you will continue to receive SSDI. However, if your earnings are greater than SGA, you will be considered gainfully employed and your SSDI payments will be stopped following your trial work period. Keep in mind that in calculating your gross income, the Social Security Administration will deduct certain types of employment-related expenses that directly affect your ability to get to and perform your job and that you have personally paid for without other reimbursement.

What is vocational rehabilitation and how do I find out if I am eligible for this type of program?

The Rehabilitation Act of 1973 provides for services designed to enable people with disabilities to become or remain employed. Although this is a program mandated by federal law, it is carried out by individually-created state agencies. Each state agency has its own name and slightly different program. Vocational rehabilitation services are defined as an eligibility program rather than an entitlement program. This means that you must demonstrate eligibility by having a physical or mental disability that results in a substantial handicap to employment. There must also be a reasonable expectation that vocational rehabilitation services might help you to become more employable. As can be seen in the wording of these criteria, there will obviously be some variation from agency to agency in determining any one person's eligibility. Many vocational rehabilitation agencies operate under an Order of Selection mandate, whereby services are prioritized for those applicants who have the most severe disabilities. Your first step is to contact the vocational rehabilitation program in your state to ask for information about eligibility and application procedures.

An important work incentive provided by the Social Security Administration is called Continued Payment Under a Vocational Rehabilitation Program. This incentive provides that people receiving SSI or SSDI who improve medically to the point that they are able to return to work can continue to receive their benefits if they are participating in any approved vocational rehabilitation program whose services are likely to enable them to resume working.

What types of services might be provided by my state's vocational rehabilitation program?

The state's vocational rehabilitation services might include:

◇ a thorough rehabilitation evaluation to determine extent of disability and need for treatment to correct or reduce the disability

◇ vocational guidance and counseling

◇ medical appliances and prosthetic devices if needed to increase your ability to work
◇ vocational training to prepare you for gainful employment
◇ provision of occupational equipment and tools
◇ job placement and follow-up
◇ post-employment services

Keep in mind that although these programs are mandated by federal law, they tend to vary considerably from state to state.

What is a PASS Plan?

The Plan for Achieving Self Support is a work incentive available for people who are receiving SSI. It allows them to design individualized plans to achieve specified work goals. Under the plan, a disabled person is allowed to set aside income and/or resources for a specified period of time in order to obtain education or training, purchase work-related equipment, set up a business, or for any other reasonable expense related to becoming financially self-supporting. During this period, the income and resources set aside for the plan are excluded from the SSI income and resource restrictions.

Family and Medical Leave Act

How do I determine if my employer is covered by the Family and Medical Leave Act (FMLA) or if am eligible to request unpaid leave under that law?

To be considered a covered employer under the FMLA, your employer must have at least 50 employees residing within a 75-mile radius of the work facility. Companies or agencies with fewer than 50 employees are not covered. You are eligible to request unpaid leave if you have at least one year (1,250 hours worked within the last 12 months) and have (or have a family member who has) a serious health condition. A serious health condition is defined under the FMLA as any illness, injury, impairment, or regimen of treatment that renders one unable to perform any essential function of his or her job. The term *serious health condition* is broader and more inclusive than the ADA's definition of *disability*. This means that a person with MS could be a person with a serious health condition under the FMLA but not meet the ADA's standard as a person with a disability. Unlike the term *disability*, *serious health conditions* pertain to both temporary and permanent conditions. Examples of commonly invoked *serious health conditions* under the FMLA include pregnancy, birth or adoption of a child, surgery, chemotherapy, and chronic illnesses.

How do I go about requesting FMLA leave?

The first step is to notify your employer, preferably in writing, that you need the leave time. You must state that you have a serious health condition, but you do not need to tell your employer that you have MS. Be specific about the dates of your leave, keeping in mind that you can take as many as 12 weeks off during each calendar year. If the need for your leave is foreseeable (e.g., elective surgery, birth of a child), the law requires you to give 30 days advance notice. If the need for the leave is unforeseeable (e.g., an unexpected exacerbation of your MS), the FMLA requires that you provide "reasonable notice," but leaves that term undefined in the regulations.

Once you have issued your request for leave, the employer has two business days to respond to your request. If your employer does not respond within two days, you are automatically considered eligible for the leave you have requested. Your employer may ask for documentation of your serious health condition from a health care provider. In submitting this verification, the provider should adhere to the following conditions as a means of safeguarding your privacy:

1. The statement should verify the need for a medical leave without disclosing the underlying medical condition.
2. The information reported should be job-related (e.g., need for, length of, and timing of the medical leave).
3. The statement of verification should avoid any discussion of the possible future effects of the serious health condition.

To further protect your privacy, the following conditions apply within the workplace:

1. Leave requests are supposed to be processed by a designated, knowledgeable person so that discussion with the employee's supervisors and co-workers is limited.

2. Supervisors should be notified of facts related to the circumstances of the leave, not about specific aspects of the employee's (or a relative's) serious health condition.
3. Records related to medical leave must be maintained in a separate file from the employee's personnel records.

My wife has MS and needs to see her neurologist once every three months. The doctor is some distance from us, so the visits take pretty much the whole day. I am the only person who can drive her to these appointments. Can I request time off for this purpose under the FMLA?

You can request time off for this purpose, provided that your employer is covered by the FMLA and you meet the criteria of an eligible employee as defined above. The FMLA allows eligible employees to take time off to help family members with their serious health conditions. Family members under the FMLA include spouses, parents, and dependent children. You must follow the same request procedures as would be required if you were taking time off to attend to your own health, and the employer may request documentation of your wife's serious health condition.

Recommended Readings

Bowe F. *Reasonable Accommodation Handbook.* Parsippany, NJ: American Telephone and Telegraph Corp., 1983.

Dejong GB. The Americans with Disabilities Act and the current state of U.S. disability policy. *Journal of Disability Policy Studies* 1990;1:3.

LaRocca NG. *Employment and Multiple Sclerosis.* National Multiple Sclerosis Society, 1995.

Mancuso LL. The ADA and employment accommodations: What now? *American Rehabilitation,* Winter 1990–1991.

National Multiple Sclerosis Society. *Employment Initiatives for People with Multiple Sclerosis,* 1992.

Ostberg K. *Using a Lawyer . . . What to Do If Things Go Wrong: A Step-by-Step Guide.* New York: Random House, 1990.

President's Committee on Employment of People with Disabilities. Arkansas Research and Training Center in Vocational

Rehabilitation. *Applying for Technology in the Work Environment,* 1990.

Rao S. Cognitive function in MS. II: Impact on employment and social functioning. *Neurology* 1991;41: 692-96.

Rumrill P. *Employment Issues and Multiple Sclerosis.* New York: Demos Medical Publishing, 1996.

Sumner, G. *Project Alliance: A job retention program for employees with chronic illnesses and their employers.* National Multiple Sclerosis Society, 1995.

Szymanski E. & Parker R. *Work and disability: Issues and strategies in Career Development and Job Placement.* Austin, TX: Pro-Ed, 1996.

Selected publications available from your local chapter of the National Multiple Sclerosis Society (800-FIGHT-MS):

◇ *ADA and People with Multiple Sclerosis* (ECS 6021)
◇ *The Win-Win Approach to Reasonable Accommodations: Enhancing Productivity on Your Job* (ES 6025)
◇ *Living with Multiple Sclerosis* (ES 0087)
◇ *Information for Employers* (ER 6002)
◇ *Should I Work: Information for Employees*—(ER 6001)
◇ *Working with MS*—Mary Elizabeth McNary, M.A., CRC. One in a series of workbooks entitled *Living Well with MS,* written for, and by, individuals who have been living with MS for some time.

Recommended Resources

President's Committee on Employment of People with Disabilities
1331 F Street NW
Washington, DC 20004-1107
1-202-376-6200 (voice)
http://www.50.pcepd.gov/pcepd

◇ *Americans with Disabilities Act, A Summary*
◇ *Employer Incentives When Hiring People with Disabilities*
◇ *Ready, Willing and Available*

Equal Employment Opportunity Commission
1801 L Street NW
Washington, DC 20507
1-202-663-4264 (Voice)
http://www.eeoc.gov

◇ *The Americans with Disabilities Act: Your Employment Rights as an Individual with a Disability*
◇ *The Americans with Disabilities Act: Your Responsibilities as an Employer*
◇ *ADA: Questions and Answers*
◇ *Facts About the American Disability Act*
◇ *Facts About the Disability-Related Tax Provisions*

Multiple Sclerosis Society of Canada
250 Bloor Street East, Suite 1000
Toronto, Ontario M4W 3P9
1-416-922-6065 (1-800-268-7582 Division Offices)
http://www.mssoc.ca

National Multiple Sclerosis Society
733 Third Ave.
New York, NY 10017
1-800-344-4867
http://www.nmss.org

Canadian Council on Rehabilitation and Work
500 University Ave, Suite 302
Toronto, ON
M5G IU7
1-416-260-3060
http://www.ccrw.org

The Job Accommodation Network
West Virginia University
P.O. Box 6080
Morgantown, WV 26506-6080
1-800-526-7284
http://janweb.icdi.wvu.edu

JANCANA-The Job Accommodation Network of Canada
45 Sheppard Avenue East, Suite 801
Toronto, Ontario M2N 5W9
1-416-250-7490 (Voice and TDD)

National Organization on Disability
910 Sixteenth St. NW
Suite 600
Washington, DC 20006
1-202-293-5960 (voice)
http://www.nod.org

Disabled American Veterans
807 Maine Ave., SW
Washington, DC 20024
1-202-554-3501
www.dav.org

The Foundation on Employment and Disability
3820 Del Amo Blvd
Suite 201
Torrance, CA 90503

Operation Job Match
2021 K St NW
Suite 100
Washington, DC 20006

National Business and Disability Council
201 I.V. Willets Road
Albertson, NY 11507-1595
1-516-465-1515
http://www.business-disability.com

15

Insurance Issues

Robert Enteen, Ph.D.

Obtaining insurance can be a complex and stressful process, particularly for people who are dealing with the added uncertainties of multiple sclerosis. But the effort you make to examine your insurance needs and explore the available options is well worth your while, because insurance can provide vitally important financial protection for you and your family. The aim of this chapter is to simplify the process for you.

While there are many types of insurance, the four that are usually most important to people affected by MS or other disabling conditions are *health* (including hospitalization and major medical coverage), *disability*, *long-term care*, and *life* insurance. Although this chapter addresses all of these, particular emphasis is given to health insurance. This should not be surprising in view of the lifelong, unpredictable, and varying medical and allied health needs that confront many people with MS. Disability insurance—whether government or private—is also extremely important since it provides income to replace the wages lost when one must leave the workforce because of a disability. Long-term care insurance, which covers an array of home, community, and nursing home services, is important for selected segments of the MS population. Life insurance is less frequently and urgently sought by most people with MS, because it generally has less relevance for one's day-to-day needs.

The following commonly asked questions and answers provide a simple, useful overview of insurance. Because insurance is complex, and because insurance planning is such a central component of financial and "life" planning, you are urged to use the chapter as a starting point, rather than as a complete and sufficient guide to making insurance decisions. At the end of the chapter, several sources are listed to which you can later turn for additional, comprehensive information and advice.

What are the different types of health insurance I need to know about?

There are more than a dozen different types or "categories" of health insurance plans and a tremendous number of variations among plans within each category. Fortunately, three very simple distinctions take us a long way toward understanding health insurance options. They are "government" vs. "private" options; "fee-for-service" plans vs. "managed care" plans; and "group" vs. "individual" coverage. Virtually any plan you select will reflect some combination of these; for example, it may be a government-provided, group, managed care plan; or a private, fee-for-service plan, purchased on an individual basis.

◇ *Government options.* Millions of Americans are eligible for government insurance programs based on: their current or past employment in a government agency or program; because they meet legally mandated benefit "entitlement" requirements; or because they are the family members of living or deceased people who are or were eligible for these insurance programs. The chief types of government health insurance are Medicare, Medicaid, VA (veterans) benefits, CHAMPUS, CHAMPVA, the Federal Employee Health Benefits Program (FEHB), and state or local government employee insurance programs.

◇ *Private options.* The chief types of private health insurance include group coverage provided by an employer or membership organization, individual (or individual and family) plans, risk pools, Blue Cross and Blue Shield "Open Enrollment" Plans, and Medicare Supplement (or "Medigap") insurance.

◊ *"Fee-for-service" plans.* In general, if you are covered under a fee-for-service plan, you may use the services of any appropriately credentialed physician or allied health provider you wish. To the extent that you use "covered" services—that is, services that are eligible for coverage under your particular contract—and so long as you meet all of the policy and procedural requirements for using such a service, your plan will either pay a specific sum (a part or the total cost of your care) to your provider or reimburse some or all of your costs directly to you if you pay the provider.

◊ *"Managed care" plans.* In contrast, a managed care plan generally combines the financing and delivery of appropriate care for covered individuals by prior arrangements with *selected* providers. Currently, the chief forms of managed care are HMOs (health maintenance organizations), PPOs (preferred provider organizations), and POS (point-of-service) plans.

How do I know which types of health insurance I'm eligible for?

Every health insurance plan has its own eligibility requirements. Because they can be complicated, some basics of eligibility for each type are presented here.

◊ *Medicare.* Medicare is the largest federal health insurance program. It is the chief source of coverage for the elderly and for certain people with disabilities, including at least 40,000 people with multiple sclerosis. Medicare's coverage is fairly comprehensive, providing both hospital ("Part A") and medical ("Part B") protection. Regrettably, its coverage is quite limited for long-term care services such as nursing home stays, and does not include prescriptions.

Many people are surprised to learn that Medicare is not limited to people aged 65 or above. A person who has MS (or any other disabling condition) and is under age 65 may qualify for Medicare benefits if he or she meets the eligibility requirements for Social Security Disability Insurance (SSDI) benefits (see Chapter 14 for a discussion of SSDI eligibility). Applications for SSDI generally require a five-month waiting period from the date of the disability determination to the start of SSDI benefits. Twenty-four months after this initial waiting period, the individual becomes eligible for Medicare coverage.

◇ *Medicaid.* Medicaid is a medical assistance program for certain individuals and families with low incomes and assets. In addition to offering comprehensive hospital and medical protection (including prescriptions), Medicaid also provides coverage for an array of long-term care services, including nursing home stays. Far fewer people with MS are eligible for Medicaid than for Medicare because their family income and assets are usually too high to meet the Medicaid requirements.

Medicaid is a joint program of the federal government and each state government. Although the federal government contributes money to the Medicaid program, each state administers its own Medicaid program. Medicaid differs from Medicare in another key respect: Medicaid coverage varies from state to state save for certain core (Medicaid "mandated") benefits available in every state's program. Thus, it is important to learn the specifics of Medicaid coverage in your own state.

◇ *Veterans' benefits.* The U.S. Department of Veterans Affairs offers comprehensive "VA" health care to veterans with "service-connected" disabilities and to disabled veterans whose disabilities are not service-connected who meet certain eligibility criteria. Of particular relevance to readers of this book, onset of multiple sclerosis in a veteran may be considered to be service-connected under specified conditions (referred to as the "7-Year Rule").

◇ "CHAMPUS"—the Civilian Health and Medical Program of the Uniformed Services—is a health benefit program for all seven uniformed services: the Air Force, Army, Navy, Marine Corps, Coast Guard, Public Health Service, and the National Oceanic and Atmospheric Administration. CHAMPUS does *not* cover active duty service members (the "sponsors"), but only their families, as well as retired service members and their families.

◇ "CHAMPVA"—the Civilian Health and Medical Program, Department of Veterans Affairs—is a federal program providing medical care to certain eligible survivors and dependents of veterans. These include the following, provided they are *not* eligible for Medicare Part A or CHAMPUS: the spouse or children of a veteran if the veteran has been judged by the VA to have a permanent and total service-connected disability; the surviving spouse or children of a veteran who died as a result of a service-connected condition, or who, at the time of death, was judged permanently and totally disabled from a service-connected condition; the surviving spouse or children of a person who died while on active duty.

◇ *Federal Employee Health Benefits Program (FEHB).* The Federal Employee Health Benefits program provides a choice of health plans for federal civilian employees. There is a federal government contribution toward the cost of premiums. FEHB coverage is available immediately, from the date of enrollment, without a medical examination or restrictions due to the subscriber's age or physical condition. If certain conditions are met, the FEHB offers continued protection for the subscriber and eligible family members after the subscriber's retirement from federal service, and for eligible family members after the enrollee's death.

◇ *State and local government employee programs.* In general, state and municipal governments offer health benefit plans to their employees and eligible family members. Although the choice of options is typically not as broad as the FEHB program offerings, it is not uncommon for employees and their families to have a choice of two or more options.

◇ *Employer, membership, or other group health plans.* An employer typically offers group coverage to its employees, and often to the employees' families as well. Group coverage is also offered by many membership organizations, including labor unions, trade associations, professional societies, and fraternal organizations. Additionally, group coverage can be obtained on the basis of a shared characteristic other than "membership" as, for example, through a church group, college alumni association, or credit card holder group. Ordinarily these "sponsors" contract with an insurance company or managed care organization to provide a specific combination of benefits for all enrollees. In recent years, sponsoring organizations have increasingly begun to offer a choice of plans, each with special features, so that a prospective enrollee can choose the plan best suited to his or her own and family members' needs.

In general, group health insurance is less costly than individual or individual and family coverage. This is because the insurer can "share" or "spread" the risk of paying out money for services across a number of enrollees. While some enrollees will prove to be relatively heavy users of care, and therefore will be costly to the insurer (costing more than the premiums paid by them or on their behalf), others will use little or no care, and therefore will be less costly enrollees (the premiums paid for their enrollment will be greater than the amount the insurer has to pay out for their care). In contrast, there is less opportunity for the insurer to spread risk and offset or limit its potential payout in individual or individual and family plans (see following); thus, higher premiums are usually charged.

◇ *Individual and family plans.* Individual and family plans, as the names suggest, are purchased by individuals to cover themselves or themselves and their family members. In general, purchase is made either through an insurance agent or broker, or directly from the insurance company or managed care organization. As the individual owns and pays directly for the coverage, it is "portable." Therefore, in contrast to most employer group coverage, the individual can retain the plan even if he or she changes employment or becomes disabled and has to leave the place of employment. While the cost of premiums for this type of insurance may be higher than employment-based coverage, it may be less expensive in the long run because continuity of coverage is assured.

◇ *Blue Cross and Blue Shield "open enrollment" plans.* Blue Cross and Blue Shield is not a single company. Rather, it is a nationwide federation of local, independent community health services corporations. In most cases, these operate under state laws as not-for-profit service organizations. The plans contract with physicians, hospitals, and other health care facilities and providers to offer health care to "subscribers" (insureds).

In return for their not-for-profit status (they are allowed to operate under special state laws and regulations, and with a special tax exemption), the "Blues" accept special responsibility for addressing needs of the public. Traditionally, they have acted as the "insurers of last resort" for people who could not obtain or afford insurance through commercial plans. Most importantly for readers with MS or other disabilities, some Blues organizations offer "open enrollment" hospital coverage, or hospital and medical coverage, to anyone in their territory, even if an applicant has a preexisting condition. (Typically, open enrollment plans include waiting periods before benefits are paid for services needed by subscribers for their preexisting conditions.)

Policies available under open enrollment vary among the Blues. They range greatly in price, coverage, and other features. There is also variation in *when* open enrollments are available and in how well they are advertised. For example, some Blues have continuous open enrollment throughout the year. Others only open their doors to all applicants during specified times of the year (often only in June and December). Thus, readers who want to investigate this option need to call their local Blue Cross and Blue Shield organization and learn whether and when open enrollment is possible, along with the details of the plan(s) offered.

◇ *Medicare supplement (or "Medigap") plans.* Medicare pays a large part of the health care costs of its insureds, but the insured individual remains responsible for Medicare deductibles and co-insurance, and for services and excess provider charges not covered under Medicare. These additional costs can be substantial. In response to these unpaid costs, many private insurers offer Medicare Supplement (also called "Medigap") plans to supplement Medicare services and to cover Medicare beneficiary costs.

Initially, there was a bewildering array of Medigap plans on the market and many questionable marketing practices, such as companies selling several overlapping plans to the same individual. To address these problems, the National Association of Insurance Commissioners developed ten standardized Medigap plans, called "A," "B," "C," and so on through plan "J." While each plan differs in the specific coverage offered, a given plan is always the same wher-

ever it is sold in the United States (thus, if you purchase
plan B in New York, it will be identical to a plan B purchased in California, Nebraska, or elsewhere). It is important to note, however, that individual companies charge
different amounts for the same plan. Thus, insurance company X may charge substantially more for plan B than the
insurance company Y does for an identical plan B. So it
pays to shop around.

◇ *"Risk pools."* Over the past twenty years, a number of states
have created "risk pools" to provide protection for state
residents who are otherwise uninsurable. The pools offer
guaranteed availability of health insurance to individuals
regardless of their health status. A common eligibility
requirement is that an applicant must prove that he or she
has been denied coverage by at least two commercial insurers. Among people in need of risk pools are those who have
been denied coverage by private (for-profit) insurers
because of a preexisting condition such as multiple sclerosis.

The costs and coverage within pools vary greatly among
states that have them, but there is a fairly standard design.
In general, the state legislature enacts a law requiring that
all commercial insurers doing business in the state join
together to create an insurance association or pool to offer
insurance to individuals who meet eligibility requirements. One member insurer serves as the administrator of
the pool, managing the plan under guidelines for benefits,
premiums, deductibles, and other matters established in
the state's law.

◇ *COBRA.* Health benefit provisions in the Consolidated
Omnibus Budget Reconciliation Act of 1985 are designed
in part to ensure that people who lose employment-related
group health insurance benefits because of job termination
or reduction in job hours can buy group coverage for themselves and their families for limited periods of time. The
law generally covers group health plans maintained by
employers with twenty or more employees. It applies to
plans in the private sector as well as those sponsored by
state and local governments. COBRA does not apply to
plans sponsored by the federal government and certain
church-related organizations.

If the employee has worked for a company subject to the federal COBRA law, and must leave work for almost any reason, that individual (and covered family members) will be able to maintain the same coverage for eighteen months, at only 2 percent above the group premium. If an employed person leaves work, and in the first eighteen months establishes eligibility for Social Security Disability Insurance, then the group coverage can be extended to a total of twenty-nine months, although there may be an increase in premiums from months nineteen to twenty-nine.

For companies that are not subject to COBRA, a standard conversion to another health plan may be offered. This coverage will generally be less comprehensive than in the employer group plan and will likely cost more than the premium charged within the group.

To find out if you and your family members are eligible for COBRA, ask the employee benefits manager at your company and read the plan booklet. As there are deadlines for gaining COBRA coverage, it is up to you to learn what they are and apply in a timely manner if a relevant life event occurs to you or others in your family.

What is a "preexisting condition" and what implications does such a condition have for access to insurance?

Within the insurance industry, a preexisting condition, whether due to illness (such as MS) or injury, is defined as "a physical or mental condition of an individual which (1) first manifested itself prior to the application for, or issuance of, his or her insurance policy; or (2) existed prior to application or issuance and for which treatment was received." In other words, a preexisting condition is one that began before the insurance was applied for and continues to exist; or began and was treated before the time that the application for insurance is made. While the wording may differ from one insurer or policy to another, the effects are generally the same: your application will either be denied or you will receive coverage, but it will contain various limitations and exclusions that temporarily or permanently reduce the protection your policy provides.

The basis of the restrictions concerning preexisting conditions lies in the concept of "risk." In the world of insurance, risk means chance of loss. Insurance companies base their approval of an application, the coverage they offer, and the premiums they charge, on a calculation of the financial risk they take on by covering a particular individual or group. Risk is a measure of the likelihood that the insurer will have to pay out some of the money it collects in premiums, in the form of direct payments to providers, reimbursement of insured individuals who themselves pay the providers, or direct provision of care (as in the case of some HMOs).

The main insurance difficulty confronting people with preexisting conditions such as multiple sclerosis is that they are typically viewed by insurers as presenting a higher than standard risk. This explains why individuals with MS encounter difficulty obtaining affordable coverage that is adequate for their current or expected medical needs, particularly relating to their preexisting condition. Some conditions are viewed by insurers as presenting a higher risk than others. While the understanding and medical management of MS have improved in recent years, most insurers continue to view all people with MS as "high risk." The National Multiple Sclerosis Society and other MS advocates work continuously to improve insurer understanding of MS and to improve insurance options for people affected by this disease.

Which type of health insurance is best for me?

Your health insurance should cover (1) standard risks of illness and injury for yourself and your family; and (2) special needs if any member of your family has a condition such as multiple sclerosis that may require special, major, costly, and/or continuing or long-term medical attention. It is up to you to identify and become familiar with your health insurance options. In the end, you must make the decision based on your own and your family's estimated present and future needs (and associated future financial risk) and the adequacy and cost of various coverage plans.

Most people try to identify one health insurance plan that will meet all of their needs now and in the future. An alternative (and perhaps more realistic) approach is to identify your present and potential health insurance needs and then find a combination of plans or policies to address them. A person with MS should probably think in terms of the following personal and family health insurance needs:

1. hospitalization for MS and other preexisting conditions;
2. hospitalization for all other conditions;

3. major medical for MS and other preexisting conditions;
4. major medical for all other conditions;
5. long-term care.

How do I begin to identify my present and future needs?

Start by considering the key components of standard coverage. A "typical" adequate plan will include both (1) hospitalization (hospital, surgical, and medical) coverage, and (2) major medical insurance. Hospitalization insurance is the most essential and common type of health insurance because it offers protection against the enormous costs that can be incurred by even a brief hospital stay and related in-hospital medical services. Hospitalization coverage is available to individuals, families, and group members. Typically, it involves either a small deductible or no deductible at all.

In view of the rapid increase in costs of health care in recent years and the wide and increasing range of out-of-hospital services available, "major medical" insurance is an important complement to hospitalization coverage. Major medical typically involves a deductible that the insured person must pay without any reimbursement. After the deductible is met, the insurer generally pays a percentage (e.g., 80 percent) of covered expenses; the insured pays the remaining portion of the expense (e.g., 20 percent), called "co-insurance." Many major medical policies include an annual individual and family out-of-pocket maximum—a dollar limit on how much the insured(s) must pay in combined deductibles and co-insurance before the insurer assumes responsibility for 100 percent of any additional covered expenses.

Once these essential insurance protections have been determined, consideration should be given to:

◇ any significant medical condition that you or your family members have (or are at significant risk for in the future);
◇ your/their past health care utilization due to the condition(s);
◇ the prognosis—that is, the likely future course of the condition and consequent likely future use of services.

In regard to future service need and use, your best source of advice is your (or your family member's) primary care physician.

When there is a major preexisting condition, a specialist often fills the role of primary physician. For example, neurologists often serve as the primary physicians for people with multiple sclerosis. In such cases, it is the specialist who should be consulted about likely future medical care needs.

If you determine that certain types of services will likely be especially important to you or your family member (e.g., physical therapy, psychotherapy, inpatient rehabilitation, nursing care), you should seek out plans that provide appropriate levels of coverage for these needs, without imposing problematic limitations on use of relevant services.

How do I identify my options?

Once you have determined your own needs and those of your family members, you must begin to identify the relevant options available to you. Because many insurance plans exclude people with MS and other preexisting conditions, this process can be difficult, time-consuming, and frustrating. Following is a checklist of avenues you should explore:

√ Are you employed? If so, are you eligible for coverage under your employer's plan? If you are a fairly new employee, is there a grace period during which you (or your family) can enroll automatically, without being questioned and chosen based on your (and their) health status? If your employer does not have a plan, or if you cannot be covered under it due to MS, will your employer pick up some or all of the cost of insurance you purchase elsewhere?

√ Are you taking a new job or considering a change in employers? If so, does your prospective employer offer a health insurance plan in which you can enroll?

√ Are you married? If so, does your spouse have an employer group plan under which you might be insured? If your spouse is a new or recent employee, is there a grace period during which you can enroll automatically with no reference to the fact that you have MS? If you are rejected on first try, can you reapply at some future date? What new documentation should you submit at that time (e.g., medical support indicating that you have had few or no MS symptoms and related services during the interim)?

√ If you have left employment due to disability or some other reason, are you eligible for COBRA or another "continuation or conversion" option?

√ Does your state insurance law include provision for a COBRA-like policy? Contact your state insurance department to find out.

√ If you are close to exhausting your COBRA coverage, will you now have an opportunity for a "standard conversion," even if it means less coverage at higher cost?

√ If you have established eligibility for Social Security Disability Insurance (SSDI) (see Chapter 14), are you aware that after twenty-four months on SSDI you become automatically eligible for Medicare?

√ If you are leaving SSDI and returning to work, are you aware that you may be able to continue or repurchase your Medicare coverage? Will your new employer offer a group plan in which you can enroll despite your MS?

√ Are your family's combined income and assets low enough that you might qualify for your state's Medicaid program? The formula excludes such items as the value of your house or your first car.

√ Are you on active duty or a veteran? Are you the family member of an active duty, retired, or deceased veteran? If so, have you checked with the U.S. Department of Veterans Affairs? CHAMPUS? CHAMPVA?

√ Does the Blue Cross and Blue Shield organization serving the community in which you live offer an "open enrollment," either year-round or at certain times of the year?

√ Have you contacted your state insurance department to learn whether your state has a "risk pool" for otherwise uninsurable state residents?

√ Are you (or is your spouse) a member of any professional societies or fraternal organizations? Have you checked with them to see if they offer health insurance options to members (and perhaps to their families)? Have you looked into health insurance programs through your credit cards, church, alumni association, or any other group that is offering such a program?

√ Have you contacted your state insurance department to learn whether there are any other, or "special," or "recently enacted" programs for state residents that increase the number of health insurance options, including those for people with multiple sclerosis or other disabling conditions?

√ Have you contacted the insurance committees of your state legislature to learn whether there are any bills pending that might increase your options if enacted?

√ If you are in crisis and lack health insurance, have you contacted your local or state health department to learn about free or low-cost services for which you might be eligible?

√ If you are a student, have you checked to see whether you are eligible for coverage under your parents' insurance? If you are a college student, does your college or university offer a plan you can afford and for which you are eligible?

√ If you are a recent graduate, looking forward to employment in the near future, or a working person temporarily between jobs, have you contacted insurance companies to learn whether they offer short-term plans for which you would be eligible?

√ If you are frequently hospitalized, or hospitalized for a substantial number of days each year, have you received mail offers of "hospital indemnity" insurance for which you would be eligible without reference to your multiple sclerosis? Does your professional or fraternal organization offer such coverage?

√ Have you contacted insurers to learn whether you would be eligible for a catastrophic excess plan through your professional or fraternal organizations?

√ If any sources tell you they would not cover you because of your MS (and you deem it in your interest to buy partial coverage, even if it is not optimal for needs related to your MS), have you asked whether they will sell you a plan that excludes or limits coverage for your MS while providing protection for the range of standard health needs?

√ Have you contacted local HMOs and physician networks in your area to see whether they will enroll you despite your multiple sclerosis?

Once I've identified one or more options, on what basis should I make my choice?

Insurance plans are complex. The complexity of your decision increases dramatically when you identify two or more plan options and try to compare them. Following is a fairly simple grid (see Figure 15.1) that you can use to analyze a single plan or to compare plans. Listed down the left are factors you should consider when choosing health insurance. If you are comparing plans, list each one across the top of the page. In this way, you can "break the plans down" into their components and judge or compare them on those factors of greatest interest to you.

Remember as you review your options that not all of your coverage has to come from a single source—you can distribute your insurance needs over several plans. For example, one plan that will not cover preexisting conditions may provide excellent and

Figure 15-1.   Plan Comparison Grid

Factor	Plan		
	1	*2*	*3*
Plan Coverage in Relation to Your/Your Family's General Medical Needs (list specific services here, and rate)			
Plan Coverage in Relation to Your/Your Family's Special (e.g., MS-related) Medical Needs (list specific services here, and rate)			
Coverage Limitations and Exclusions			
Preexisting Condition Waiting Period			
Choice of Providers			
Access to Neurologist Expert in MS Care			
Cost —premiums —individual and family deductibles —% coinsurance for key services —out-of-pocket maximum —(for managed care plans) cost to you if you use non-plan providers			
Premium Rate Guaranteed?			
Policy Renewal Guaranteed?			
Yearly and Lifetime Maximums on $ of Coverage			
Company Reputation/Financial Rating			

inexpensive coverage for other hospitalizations. Another may cover preexisting conditions but charge a higher premium.

Do I need to tell an insurance company that I have MS when I apply to join their plan?

You should respond honestly and fully to any questions asked of you by a broker, by an insurer through its agent, or on an application form. Both you and the insurer have legal rights, responsibilities, and duties in contracting for health insurance. Your duties and responsibilities include communicating facts (for example, about your health history and current health) that are relevant to the insurer's decision whether to accept you for coverage, and on what terms. The insurer is entitled to cancel your contract if you either intentionally or unintentionally fail to provide information that would have influenced the insurer's decision when it considered whether to cover you. The same is true if you falsely present relevant information, including facts about your health history or current status. In health insurance applications, all facts relating to your current or past health are considered relevant. In short, you should avoid any false representations of facts, and any omissions, on relevant matters.

In general, insurers will ask about your past and current health, often including a checklist of conditions; if you check any conditions, the insurer may ask for explanations of these. Moreover, insurers will typically ask a "blanket" additional question such as "Have you had/do you have any other health conditions not indicated above?"

The key exception to the foregoing is where the insurer simply does not ask directly *or by implication* for such information. For example, when you join a new company and are offered entry into their plan, the card you fill out may have no health-related questions; this is because employees in that company are automatically permitted entry into the plan, regardless of their health. Similarly, there is often a grace period during which your spouse can enroll without providing medical information; after the grace period, if he or she wishes to join, medical information may be required.

Are new treatments for MS, such as Betaseron®, Avonex®, or Copaxone®, covered by health insurance?

Here, as in other insurance matters, plans vary greatly in their coverage. In the end, you must investigate coverage under any plan you have or are considering. Many private insurance companies cover the new disease-modifying agents that have been approved by the FDA for treatment of relasping-remitting MS as part of their prescription drug coverage provisions. Many others do not. Among those that do cover the drug, coverage varies. Many impose *deductibles* (generally modest ones), *co-insurance* (ranging from nominal, e.g., $5.00, to substantial, e.g., 30 percent of the total yearly cost), and/or *yearly caps* on the total amount they will pay (for example, $2,000). They may require submission of some documentation of "medical necessity" from your neurologist and then undertake a prior authorization review. Some companies may require that you purchase the medications at designated pharmacies.

Virtually all state Medicaid programs cover Betaseron®, Avonex®, and Copaxone®, but you must contact the agency in your state to confirm this and to learn the specifics of the coverage they offer (how much, with what co-pays or dispensing fees, and so on).

In line with its current prescription policy, Medicare does not cover any of the disease-modifying agents. However, many states have special drug assistance programs that will help to cover the cost for state residents who are Medicare beneficiaries. Call your state insurance department and ask whether such a program exists in your state. Additionally, some Medicare managed care plans will cover these medications. If you are enrolled in a Medicare managed care plan, call the appropriate plan administrator to learn about your eligibility for coverage.

If you have problems or questions regarding coverage for Betaseron®, Avonex®, or Copaxone®, call the manufacturers' customer service numbers to ask about financial assistance (see Appendix B). Explain the situation and ask if you qualify for a subsidy from them to cover the costs of the drug. They will explain their policies and give you instructions on how to apply for assistance.

Regarding coverage of other new MS treatments, nearly all insurers require that a treatment has been approved for prescription use by the U.S. **Food and Drug Administration** (FDA) before they will even consider paying for it. A drug that has not been FDA-approved will likely not be covered. Even if a drug is FDA-approved, it may only be approved for particular uses or patients. For example, currently Betaseron®, Avonex®, and

Copaxone® have only been approved for use by people with exacerbating-remitting MS. If you do not meet this criterion, you may not be able to obtain coverage for any of these drugs, even if your insurer covers the drug for other plan enrollees (who do meet the FDA approval criterion).

People participating in clinical trials of an experimental treatment may receive coverage through the research administrators or clinicians conducting the trials. If you are considering entering a trial, ask if they will have to pay some or all of the cost of the experimental agents you will receive.

Our 21-year-old daughter has recently been diagnosed with MS. She is about to graduate from college and become ineligible for coverage under our family health insurance policy. Will she be able to get health insurance of her own?

While there is no assurance that she can get coverage, there are many options for her to explore. In most parts of the country, her surest route to coverage may be to take a job with a large company that offers a group health insurance plan to its employees. Large companies often pay some or all of their employees' insurance premiums. If she lives in or moves to one of the several states that have enacted "open enrollment" legislation in recent years, she will also be assured of the opportunity to buy individual coverage, as long as she can pay the relatively high premiums. She should call the insurance departments in those states in which she has an interest to learn whether they have enacted open enrollment legislation. For additional ideas, refer to the list of possible avenues for obtaining insurance on pages 346–348.

What is managed care and how does it work for someone with MS?

Managed care is a system of organizing health care that integrates the financing and delivery of health care to covered individuals through arrangements with selected providers. The providers are available to furnish a relatively comprehensive array of health services (although many plans lack coverage for durable medical equipment such as wheelchairs or for care in the home). Explicit standards are used by the managed care organization to select health providers for participation in the plan. Formal policies and procedures exist for ongoing quality assurance and utilization review in the provision of care to enrolled individuals. There are generally significant financial incentives for enrollees to use providers and procedures associated with the plan, rather than using "out-of-plan" providers.

The most common and best known form of managed care is the "health maintenance organization" (or HMO). In return for a fixed, periodic payment, the HMO providers offer a wide range of health care services, including preventive care. The HMO may have a single central facility, several branch sites, or may exist as an array of individual providers and facility locations that have contracted to provide service for the HMO. Two common forms of HMO are the "staff model," in which physicians and other providers are employees of the HMO; and the "individual practice association" (or IPA), in which physicians and other providers maintain their personal practices but agree to serve as HMO providers, under the terms of the HMO, when caring for an HMO enrollee. In the traditional HMO, an enrollee who goes "out-of-plan" does not receive coverage for those outside services (save in special cases such as emergencies).

The second most common managed care arrangement is the "preferred provider organization" (or PPO). In this arrangement, physicians and other providers contract with the PPO sponsor to reduce their fees when a member of the PPO comes to them for service. Plan members choosing to use out-of-plan providers receive *some* coverage, but less than if they had used one of the "preferred providers."

A new and increasingly popular hybrid, aimed at controlling costs while retaining consumer choice of providers, is the "point-of-service" HMO. Combining aspects of HMOs and PPOs, the point-of-service plan functions as an HMO, but provides some (limited) coverage for out-of-plan providers. Thus, a person who chooses to consult an out-of plan provider will generally receive coverage, but less than if he or she had stayed within the HMO for that care.

Managed care organizations work the same way for people with MS as they do for other enrollees. However, some studies and individual anecdotes raise some concerns. These concerns relate primarily to the inadequacy of access to MS experts. For example, the managed care organization may have very few (or no) providers (neurologists or others) who are expert in caring for people with multiple sclerosis. Or they may have such specialists, but the enrollee can only receive a referral to one if his primary care provider ("PCP"—generally a family physician or internist) chooses to make the referral. Because the managed care organization places great emphasis on saving money, the PCP may have major financial or other incentives to limit referrals to specialists. Informal surveys suggest that MS enrollees who have adequate access to MS specialists are generally pleased with their managed care experience. When they have inadequate access, they are usually dissatisfied with the managed care organization. PPOs try to address this problem by offering some coverage for out-of-plan consultations or treatment, but they are often more costly than HMOs. Point-of-service HMOs attempt to address this problem by combining the key features of HMOs (comprehensive care and low cost) with that of PPOs (covered access to out-of-plan providers, although typically at higher cost than staying in-plan).

In short, people with MS may fare well in managed care organizations—especially point-of-service HMOs—*if* the plan they choose is a comprehensive one and, most importantly, provides ready access to MS specialists. When considering a managed care plan, one should make sure to ask about access to providers with expertise in MS care and about coverage for the kinds of equipment or home care that are sometimes needed by a person with MS.

If my company switches over to one of the new managed care plans, will I be denied coverage because of my MS?

You should have the same rights to enrollment under the managed care plan as you had when the employer group coverage was a fee-for-service plan. If you do not, ask your employer (generally the benefits manager) about this and appeal the decision. If unsuccessful, contact your state insurance department to determine whether the employer has acted legally in excluding you from transferring to the new plan, while allowing other employees to make the transfer. This problem is more likely to arise in very small companies than among large ones.

What is long-term care insurance (LTCI) and will I be eligible for it now that I have MS?

Long-term care includes a wide range of medical, social, and support services. These services are designed for elderly people and chronically ill or disabled individuals who live in the community or in extended care facilities, and need ongoing or periodic assistance throughout their lives. Long-term care services are generally categorized as in-home assistance, community care, or institutional care.

In evaluating a person's dependence on others for assistance with everyday activities, insurance companies usually divide personal functioning into two categories: *activities of daily living* (ADLs) such as feeding, bathing, dressing, toileting, bowel and bladder continence, and getting into and out of a chair; and "instrumental activities of daily living" (IADLs), including household and community activities such as meal preparation, doing laundry, grocery shopping, managing money, making telephone calls, doing light work, getting around outside, and going places that are beyond walking distance.

Most standard health insurance plans of the sort described previously in this chapter provide only very limited long-term care coverage or none. However, many private insurance companies market long-term care insurance policies that cover some, many, or all of these services. Moreover, government programs such as Medicaid (and Medicare for certain situations) cover some or many such services.

Private long-term care insurance is not appropriate for everyone. Its main purpose is to protect against catastrophic costs associated with expensive services over a long period. In view of the risk to insurers, these policies are often costly. Thus, you may be well-advised not to use the coverage unless you have more than modest family assets to protect, as well as a sufficient income that you can readily afford the high premiums for good long-term care insurance. Of course, if you do have sufficient income and assets, this insurance may be extremely valuable to you and your family. To determine if it is right for you, contact any of the following and ask for their booklets advising consumers about long-term care insurance:

◇ your state insurance department (generally located in the state's capital city);

◇ National Association of Insurance Commissioners (NAIC) at 816-842-3600;

◇ Health Insurance Association of America (HIAA) at 800-277-4486 or 202-223-7780;

◇ American Association of Retired Persons (AARP) at 202-434-2230.

Experience suggests that relatively few insurers offering LTCI will sell to people with MS. The few in each state that do offer it tend not to advertise this fact. Moreover, they will generally decide only on a case-by-case basis. Some preliminary research suggests that they will consider people (1) whose initial MS diagnosis was made at least five but preferably ten years ago or more; (2) who currently exhibit no significant disabling MS symptoms—who have no ADL deficiencies and function independently; (3) whose "recent" medical records are free from evidence of recurrent need to treat MS-generated symptoms; and (4) who are in good general health.

To find coverage, three approaches appear to be most useful:

◇ a comprehensive survey of companies listed by the National Association of Insurance Commissioners and your state insurance department;

◇ a focused search concentrating on companies that have publicly announced that they are willing to consider applications from people with MS (good sources are your friends and acquaintances with MS who have themselves purchased this coverage from certain companies); and

◇ consultation with specialized brokers who handle the policies of several companies selling LTCI.

What is disability insurance and am I eligible for it now that I have MS?

Disability insurance is more aptly called "disability income insurance." It is a form of health insurance that provides periodic payments to replace your regular income when you cannot work as a result of illness, injury, or disease. Generally, a minimum number of days when you are unable to work are required before your "sick pay" ends and your disability insurance begins. "Short-term disability insurance" typically provides partial coverage (e.g., 60 percent) of your lost earnings for a period of about six months. If your inability to work extends beyond that period and you continue to be eligible, you begin to receive "long-term disability benefits."

There are both private (including employer-provided) and government forms of disability insurance. The most common and important form of government disability insurance for people with multiple sclerosis is Social Security Disability Insurance (SSDI), as described in Chapter 14. A person may be found eligible for SSDI who has worked and paid social security taxes (FICA) for at least ten years (five of which must be in the ten years prior to leaving the workforce), and meets the criteria for medical and vocational disability.

If you are employed by a company that has a group disability insurance plan for its employees, you should be eligible for this coverage. If you have the opportunity to purchase disability insurance through your employer or any professional or fraternal organization to which you belong (or would be willing to join), you should try to do so. By virtue of your membership in one of these groups, you may automatically be entitled to the basic amount of disability insurance that is offered to the entire group, regardless of your MS diagnosis or other medical history. This basic coverage is called "guaranteed-issue coverage." Your MS diagnosis would prevent you from buying coverage over and above this basic amount, but you would still be assured of some basic coverage. Since organizations may offer this type of group coverage only as a one-time incentive for membership, one strategy is to join as many organizations as you can that offer this type of group disability coverage. These multiple group memberships would thus enable you to piece together adequate coverage. It is certainly in your best interest to obtain disability coverage while you are actively working; it is virtually impossible to obtain disability coverage once a person leaves work due to disability.

How will the fact that I have MS affect my ability to obtain life insurance?

Life insurance is typically a less urgent matter for people with MS than is health insurance. The reason seems clear: life insurance is protection against a future (perhaps very distant) eventuality. In contrast, health insurance may be vitally important any or every day in protecting you against the substantial costs that you may incur, unpredictably, due to multiple sclerosis or any other medical problem.

For those who want to obtain life insurance, there are companies that will sell it to you. You must shop around to find them since many will refuse coverage for a person with MS. Often the amounts of life coverage they will sell to you are less than standard, and you may be charged higher premiums than non-disabled applicants.

How does the Americans with Disabilities Act (ADA) deal with the insurance questions of someone with chronic illness and/or disability?

In June 1993, the U.S. Equal Employment Opportunity Commission (EEOC) ruled that under the Americans with Disabilities Act (ADA): (1) employers cannot refuse to hire people with disabilities due to concern over the effects on the employer's health insurance costs; and (2) employees with disabilities must generally be given "equal access" to any employer health insurance. That is, the ADA prohibits employers from limiting benefits that single out a particular disability, a discrete group of disabilities such as cancers, or disability in general. Additionally, the ADA requires that these rules apply both to employers that buy commercial insurance *and* to self-insured employers (even though this group is free from certain other insurance laws and regulations). Moreover, the burden is on the challenged employer, rather than the employee, to prove that differential treatment of an employee with a disability was not "subterfuge."

Much remains to be done to test the full implications of the ADA in protecting the insurance rights of individuals with MS and other disabilities. While many lawsuits have been launched, at this writing the number of case law rulings remains fairly limited.

What is the Health Insurance Portability and Accountability Act (HIPAA), how does it affect people with MS?

The Health Insurance Portability and Accountability Act (also known as the Kassebaum-Kennedy Bill), passed by Congress in 1996, contains important provisions—both positive and negative—for persons with MS.

The *positive* aspects of the bill:

◇ **Preexisting condition exclusions**: Insurance companies are now prevented from denying coverage *for more than one year* for pre-existing health conditions, including MS.
◇ **Portability of coverage**: Because the bill limits exclusions on preexisting conditions, and requires guaranteed avail-

ability of health insurance to anyone who has employment-based coverage, workers will not be "locked" into jobs or prevented from starting their own businesses for fear of losing their health insurance coverage.

◇ **Individual coverage:** The bill guarantees the availability of individual coverage to those who have had employment-based insurance *for at least 12 months*, and who are ineligible for, or have exhausted coverage under, COBRA. [COBRA allows employees of large companies to extend their health coverage for up to 18 months after they leave a job.] *All protection is linked to continued coverage. Do not let your group health coverage lapse for more than 62 days even if it means that you need to purchase expensive COBRA protection to maintain your coverage.*

◇ **Guaranteed renewal:** Under this bill, insurers are required to renew coverage for individuals and groups as long as premiums are paid.

The *negative* aspects of the bill:

◇ The bill does not provide any protection for individuals who are covered by individual policies. The limits on exclusions for preexisting conditions apply only to those individuals who have been enrolled in group plans for at least 12 months.

◇ The legislation provides no assistance to the millions of Americans who are uninsured. Nor does it do anything to address the very high cost of health insurance for those who are struggling to maintain their coverage.

◇ Loopholes in the law have enabled insurance companies to circumvent the intent of the legislation. The U.S. General Accounting Office has reported that many health insurers have begun charging higher premiums to people who attempt to exercise their rights under Kassebaum-Kennedy. This has had the effect of excluding them from purchasing coverage. In addition, some insurers are reported to have created financial disincentives for their agents by refusing to pay them commissions for policy sales to applicants with preexisting conditions. These are only two of the loopholes that have been identified in the law and accompanying regulations. As the impact of these loopholes becomes increasingly clear, it is hoped that efforts will soon be made to address them.

Is any progress being made toward improving health insurance coverage for people with MS?

The past two to three years have been disappointing in terms of progress in assuring health insurance protections for uninsured and underinsured Americans, including many people with MS. While there has been, and continues to be, much legislative "sound and fury," there have been regrettably few if any improvements. Indeed, in some respects, our health insurance "system" in 2000 protects far fewer people than it did a few years ago.

Consider the following:

◇ Perhaps most telling, the number of people without health insurance has risen continuously, from approximately 37 million in the early 1990s to over 43 million today.

◇ Five years ago, the health insurance industry used scare-tactic commercials to lead the campaign that defeated the Clinton initiative to assure health insurance for all Americans. Ironically, in May 1999, the industry proposed enormous new federal subsidies to address the alarming increase in uninsured people. In announcing the proposal, the head of the industry's chief trade association made it clear that most of the money would be passed on to health care providers rather than to the public.

◇ In 1997, Congress created the Children's Health Insurance Program, providing $39 billion over ten years to enable states to improve health insurance for children in low-income families. Yet, by the end of 1999, only a small portion of the available money had been spent, and far fewer children had gained protection than was intended. By some estimates, the number of uninsured children has actually increased since 1997, and now stands at about 10.7 million. One partial explanation is that in many states, more children have been dropped from Medicaid coverage than have acquired coverage under the new program.

◇ Similarly dramatic has been the failure to date of the Mental Health Parity Act of 1996. This law was designed to equalize group plan mental health benefits in comparison with coverage for physical conditions. Here, too, insurers have circumvented the law by using loopholes that enable them to set differing limits on the number of covered out-patient visits and hospital days, and by charging differing co-payments and deductibles for mental and physical health services.

◇ As of this writing (August, 1999), congressional efforts to enact a "Patients Bill of Rights" have been stalled by parti-san politics.

On a more positive note, Congress passed the Work Incentives Improvement Act of 1999 (WIIA). WIIA will make it easier for individuals with disabilities to continue working or return to work *while still being able to gain access to or retain government-sponsored health care coverage (Medicare and Medicaid).* In addi-tion, the bill will expand vocational rehabilitation options for peo-ple with disabilities and improve the dissemination of informa-tion regarding these new work incentives. Specifically, WIIA will:

◇ Expand access to Medicare by 54 months, for a total of 102 months, for SSDI beneficiaries earning *more than* $700 per month. The additional 54 months will help individuals earn the 30 work credits necessary to purchase Medicare at a lower premium when they complete their 102-month period of extended eligibility.

◇ Give states the option to allow working individuals with disabilities who have annual incomes up to $75,000 to buy into Medicaid on a sliding fee scale.

◇ Give states that participate in the above program the option to allow individuals who become ineligible for Medicaid because their condition improves (but who still have a severe medical impairment) to buy into the program.

◇ Give states the option to participate in a Medicaid demon-stration program for workers with a *potentially* disabling condition who would be expected to meet the SSI defini-tion of disability if they did not receive medical services. The expanded program will offer an opportunity for health care coverage for individuals who would otherwise have difficulty obtaining insurance.

◇ Allow expedited re-entry into SSI or SSDI for those who have returned to work but again become unable to work and file a request within 60 months of the last date of benefit coverage.

◇ Provide a ticket to SSDI and SSI beneficiaries to obtain employment services, vocational rehabilitation services, and other support services such as assistive technology from an employment network of their choice to help them enter the workforce.

This new piece of legislation has the potential to make it easier for many individuals to enter or re-enter the workforce without jeopardizing their access to government-sponsored health care coverage. The ultimate impact of the legislation, however, will depend on the willingness of individual states to take advantage of the legislation's provisions. The individual states will need to be willing to assume their share of the costs of the specific provisions.

In addition, a federal judge in New York struck down a provision in HIPAA that originally threatened to reduce the availability of long-term care for people with MS and other severe disabilities. With the exception of the very wealthy, most Americans with severe disabilities have looked to Medicaid to finance long-term care services. Medicaid is the program that provides the health benefit component of state public assistance benefits. In order to be eligible for Medicaid assistance, an individual must meet strict financial requirements, including a limit of $2000 in savings (not counting the value of the family home if the spouse is still in residence). Over the past several years, attorneys and financial planners had developed a variety of legal and proper strategies for ensuring a person's eligibility for Medicaid. The provision in HIPAA, recently stuck down by the federal judge, had made it illegal for attorneys and tax planners to advise people seeking Medicaid eligibility on ways to shield their assets. Describing the provision as unconstitutional, Attorney General Janet Reno has stated that it will not be enforced by the Justice Department.

Perhaps the fundamental health insurance improvements we need will come only when uninsured and underinsured Americans become numerous enough, and angry enough, that legislators and corporations can no longer ignore their demands—or can no longer appease the public by passing high-sounding legislation that is then skirted in reality.

Until then, the greatest protection for people with MS and others concerned about their health insurance protection is to remain informed, and active. Obtain booklets from your state insurance department. Study them to learn your legal rights and obligations in your state. Read your insurance policy carefully, if you have one, and learn to use your benefits to your greatest advantage. Keep abreast of federal and state bills aimed at improving coverage. And make your voice and your vote heard by your elected representatives. What sounds good on paper, and in the halls of Congress and state legislatures, will mean nothing if it doesn't create genuine improvements.

Recommended Readings

Enteen R. *Health Insurance: How to Get It, Keep It, or Improve What You've Got (2nd edition)*. New York: Demos, 1996.

This book is the most comprehensive introduction available on health insurance. It includes health insurance basics, techniques for determining your health insurance needs, descriptions of nearly two dozen options, what to do when something goes wrong, and many state-by-state listings of where to turn for advice or assistance.

Isaacs SL, Swartz AC. *The Consumer's Legal Guide to Today's Health Care: Your Medical Rights and How to Assert Them*. Boston: Houghton Mifflin, 1992.

Government Agencies and Private Organizations

There are a variety of organizations and government agencies that can provide you with useful information and advice, generally at no cost. Your state's insurance department, listed in the blue pages of your phone book, offers information and assistance about virtually any insurance matter. Other useful government agencies include your state office on aging, the agency on developmental disabilities, health department, social services department (Medicaid), Medicare office, workers' compensation agencies, and veterans' affairs agencies. Although the names of these departments and agencies may differ somewhat from state to state, they can generally be located by calling telephone information in your state's capital city. The Appendixes in Robert Enteen's book, *Health Insurance* (cited previously) provide numerous listings with addresses and phone numbers.

American Association of Health Plans (1129 20th St., N.W., Suite 600, Washington, DC 20038; Tel: 202-778-3200). Provides information about health maintenance organizations.

American Association of Retired Persons (AARP) (Tel: 202-434-2277). Disseminates valuable information on all types of insurance.

Association of Managed Healthcare Organizations (601 13th St., N.W., Suite 370 South, Washington, D.C. 20005; Tel: 202-434-4565). Provides information about Preferred Provider Organizations.

Center for the Study of Services (Write to The Consumer Guide to Health Plans, 733 15th Street, N.W., Suite 820, Washington, D.C. 20005; Tel: 800-475-7283). Ranks managed care plans and publishes its findings.

Consumer Federation of America (CFA) (1424 16th Street, N.W., Washington, D.C. 20036; Tel: 202-387-6121 or 212-387-0087). This insurance consumer advocacy group publishes a useful life insurance guide called Taking a Bite Out of Insurance.

Health Insurance Association of America (Tel: 202-223-7780). The chief private source of information about health, disability, and long-term care insurance.

16

Long-Term Care

Debra Frankel, MS, OTR

It is not possible to predict what the future holds for any one individual with multiple sclerosis. While for many the disease remains mild, others will experience more severe problems and disability. While remaining optimistic about the future is important, it is also helpful to think ahead about the different possibilities that may be in store.

This chapter answers questions about long-term care options. Long-term care encompasses all the services available to those people with an illness or disability who need help in performing activities of daily life, such as dressing, showering, preparing meals, managing their home, and so forth. Long-term care refers to a wide range of services, including housekeeping, personal care assistance, adult day health care, respite care, support for caregivers, housing options, and nursing home care. This chapter addresses questions about these services and programs, describing what they are, how much they cost, and how to determine when you might need them. The chapter also identifies ways you can cope with the complex feelings that may accompany the decision to use these services and programs.

It is unlikely that you will need to use many of the programs described here. However, planning and preparing for an unpredictable future is generally a better strategy than waiting to make difficult decisions until you are in the midst of a crisis. This will give you the comfort and security of knowing that you have this information in the event you ever need to use it.

My husband's MS is getting much worse and we're having a hard time managing without help. We need to decide what to do next. How can we talk about this together? I feel guilty about not being able to do it all and my husband feels like he's a burden to the family. Every time I bring it up, it turns into an argument. What can we do?

Facing up to difficult realities and planning for an unknown future are a stressful part of living with MS for every member of the family. Family members may feel overwhelmed with added responsibilities, scared about an unpredictable future, guilty about not being able to manage it all, and angry about the changes MS has forced upon them. The person with MS may feel discouraged about needing to ask for help, ashamed of becoming more dependent, and guilty or angry about the changes MS has imposed on the family. Sometimes these strong feelings interfere with a family's ability to talk calmly about these matters. At a time when family members may need to make important decisions about the future, their feelings can become barriers to honest and effective communication.

Sometimes, just giving family members a chance to air their feelings and voice their points of view in a planned family meeting is the best way to address these issues. It often works best to lay some ground rules, such as no interrupting, taking turns speaking, agreeing to disagree on some topics, and recognizing that this is a hard conversation for everyone to have.

Some families enlist the services of a care manager or case coordinator to help them focus on the decisions at hand and identify available resources. In addition, talking to a family counselor may promote mutual understanding and help to separate the emotions from the objective realities that need to be confronted.

Acknowledging to one another that talking about these harsh realities is usually unpleasant and often frightening, but deciding that you are in it together, can be the beginning of more open communication.

What is a care manager?

Care managers (also called care coordinators or case managers) are health professionals who specialize in providing information, referral, advocacy, and coordination of health and social services to individuals who need assistance with personal care and health care. They usually have a background in social work, nursing, counseling, gerontology or another healthcare field. A care manager can provide a range of personalized services to the individual and his or her family, including:

◇ helping to identify needs;
◇ arranging for home care or other long term services (e.g. adult day health care, nursing home care);
◇ providing crisis intervention;
◇ offering counseling and support;
◇ reviewing financial and insurance questions;
◇ acting as a liaison to family members who are far away.

The manager may charge a flat fee or hourly rate. When hiring, ask for the person's credentials, references, and a written agreement or contract regarding fees and work to be performed. Be sure to clarify whether expenses (e.g., phone charges, mileage) are included in the fee or will be charged separately. The services of a care coordinator or case manager are generally not covered by insurance, although it is always best to check with your specific insurance carrier. The benefit of hiring someone to help you and your family navigate through the complex system of long term services may be well worth the cost.

Contact the National Association of Professional Geriatric Care Managers at 520-881-8008 or *www.caremanager.org* for more information or to locate a care manager in your area.

Home Care

My wife needs more help now and I have to be at work all day. What kinds of in-home services are available to her?

Home care services include:

◇ housekeeping—basic homemaking tasks, light cleaning, errands, laundry, and cooking;
◇ personal care—assistance with dressing, bathing, grooming, transfers, exercise, and toileting;

◇ nursing care—assistance with medications, catheter-care, and other medical procedures;

◇ rehabilitation services—occupational therapy, physical therapy, speech therapy and social work;

◇ companionship—conversation, supervision, company and entertainment.

Depending on your insurance coverage, any or all of these may be available in your home.

Who provides home care services?

The two primary options available when hiring help at home are: 1) using a home care agency or 2) finding and hiring someone on your own. There are benefits and drawbacks to both options.

Professional home health care agencies select, train, and supervise their staff of homemakers, home health aides, nurses, therapists and social workers. The agency manages record keeping, scheduling, coordinating and insurance billing—all of which can lift a burden from an already overwhelmed family. Agency rates vary, however, and home care through an agency can be costly. Also, the agency's scheduling practices may not offer you flexibility in terms of the helpers' available hours.

Hiring privately offers you greater control. You can decide who comes to your home and negotiate their schedules, salaries, and responsibilities. In most cases, this option is less costly because the arrangements are made without the involvement of a third party. While it is unlikely that an insurance company will pay for someone you hire on your own, Medicaid (in certain states) will pay for personal care assistants hired independently through Independent Living or Personal Assistance Programs.

When hiring someone privately, it is useful to explore local colleges and churches, or put a notice in the local paper. Word of mouth is often the best method of identifying potential helpers. You might even be able to recruit a volunteer through a high school community service program, a retired senior volunteer program, or through your church or synagogue. However you decide to recruit candidates, it is critical to screen each person carefully and obtain personal references.

Who pays for home health care?

Medicare, Medicaid, and private insurance cover some home care services. However, there are usually strict eligibility criteria and limitations on coverage.

◇ Medicare will only pay for personal care or homemaker services if there is also a need for skilled care (nursing or rehabilitation services). Medicare does not generally cover ongoing care.

◇ Medicaid will cover personal care services on an ongoing basis for eligible persons in some states. Other states may offer personal care assistance programs that allow you to hire on your own and receive public funding to pay your helpers. Check with your local chapter of the National MS Society or public health department to find out what types of personal care assistance programs are offered in your area.

◇ Private insurance and HMOs may cover some home care services through an agency—usually for a limited period of time. They, like Medicare, may require that you need a skilled service along with personal care or homemaker services.

◇ If you are a veteran, you might also want to check with the Veteran's Administration to see if you are covered for home health care.

◇ Some long-term care insurance policies also provide coverage of home health services. Each policy is different, so check your policy document or call your insurance agent for details.

◇ Some people over the age of 60 might find that their local Council on Aging offers assistance with home care.

If you are paying privately for agency assistance, some home health agencies offer a sliding fee scale, allowing individuals to pay according to their ability to do so. Generally, the cost of hiring a helper privately will come out of your own pocket. You are well advised to comply with Social Security regulations in hiring household help. The Social Security Administration can explain your responsibilities when paying assistants in your home.

The cost of not asking for help can also be very high for you and your partner, individually and for your relationship. The stress of too much responsibility and the consequences of unattended needs can be overwhelming. Don't wait for a crisis to begin using helpers at home.

I feel uncomfortable having strangers come into my house. What can I do to feel more secure about that?

A home health agency usually conducts a careful screening and interview process with its potential employees. The agency provides training and supervision of its employees, so you can generally feel confident about the helpers you have hired from a home health agency. If you feel uncomfortable about the behavior of anyone coming to your home from an agency, alert the agency immediately.

When hiring on your own, remember that you are in charge. Prepare a *written* job description that clearly outlines your needs and expectations. It is recommended that you conduct a lengthy interview and require three references whom you can contact personally. In some states, you can conduct a criminal background check on a potential employee. Check with your state government as to whether they have a Criminal History Systems Board that enables you to conduct a Criminal Offender Record Information (CORI) check. Also, have a family member or friend present during the interview to get another person's reaction. It is important to trust your instincts when hiring. If something makes you uncomfortable, do not hire that individual, even if he or she "looks good on paper."

Once you have decided to hire a particular individual, establish a trial period during which you and the employee will have an opportunity to evaluate how things are going. At the end of the trial period, you have the option to terminate the person's employment if you are dissatisfied with his or her behavior, manner of speaking to you, job performance, or if something just doesn't feel right.

Other ways to protect yourself include: keeping track of how much cash you have in the house; keeping checkbooks, credit cards and other valuables safely out of view; keeping track of your medication supply; discussing finances only with family and trusted friends; requiring receipts for any shopping done on your behalf; and asking friends or relatives to stop by periodically when your helper is on duty.

I've been depending on my children to help me get up and dressed in the mornings. Sometimes I think it's good for them to learn how to handle this kind of responsibility, but at other times I wonder if it will be harmful for them. Is it all right for kids to help out at home?

Children of parents with MS may have extra responsibilities around the house. Such tasks as doing laundry, taking out the trash, cleaning up and preparing meals can help youngsters learn valuable life skills. As long as youngsters have time to enjoy their own age-appropriate activities, these extra responsibilities are not harmful to them (even though they may complain from time to time!). However, children should not be involved in the personal care of a parent. It is inappropriate to ask a child to assist a parent with toileting, showering, dressing, and other personal activities. Wherever possible, arrange for assistance from adult family members, friends, and home health agencies for this type of care. You can contact your local chapter of the National MS Society for help in finding personal care assistance.

My mother comes to my house every day to cook and clean and help me out. I need her help and I appreciate it, but I would like to give her a much-needed break. Do you have any ideas?

Respite care is a service that provides family caregivers a break from their caregiving responsibilities. Respite care might involve hiring a personal care assistant or home health aide to fill in at home and provide caregiving and/or companionship for a set number of hours each week, or weeks each year. Resources and/or funding for respite care may be available from your local National MS Society chapter.

Some families are able to make arrangements with friends to stay with the person with MS for an evening, afternoon or weekend, so that the family caregiver can have a break and the individual with MS a change of routine. Respite can also be provided by having the person with MS admitted to a nursing facility for a few days or weeks so that round-the-clock care is available while family caregivers are away or taking a break. A planned respite provides a refreshing break from routine for everyone. Caregivers need time to attend to their own needs.

Adult Day Care

Since leaving work because of my disability, I seem to be spending all my time at home alone. Getting out has just become too tiring and difficult for me to manage. My doctor is encouraging me to get out of the house more regularly. She suggested I try an adult day care program. What is adult day care?

Adult day centers provide a planned, daytime program that includes a variety of health, social, and support services in a supervised setting. This is a community-based service designed to meet the needs of people who, due to a disability or illness, may need personal assistance, health monitoring, socialization, and/or supervision. Specific services might include: social activities, meals, rehabilitation therapies, nursing care, personal care, and counseling.

How will I know what kind of adult day health program is right for me, and who is going to pay for it?

There are several types of adult day care: *Social day care* offers minimal personal care assistance and emphasizes social activities and mental stimulation. *Adult day health care* offers moderate personal care assistance, health monitoring, and rehabilitation therapies. There are also programs that are specifically geared to those with cognitive impairments.

A high quality, adult day health center will do a thorough assessment to determine your needs and interests, and offer you the opportunity to ask questions and observe the program. They should also work with you to develop an individualized plan (to be re-evaluated periodically) that meets your social, recreational, and health needs. In general, you are looking for a program that:

◇ provides a full range of services in a safe and secure environment;
◇ offers a flexible schedule of full- or part-time care;
◇ has well-trained staff and volunteers and a low staff to participant ratio;
◇ adheres to state and national standards and guidelines.

Most adult day programs are targeted to seniors, although some may offer special activities for younger participants. You can often determine whether a program is right for you by asking about the types of activities offered and the age and disability range of the participants. It is also important to check a program's references and talk to two or three participants about their experience. The National Adult Day Services Association (*www.nadsa.org;* 202/479-6682) can provide information about choosing a program.

Fees for adult day care vary, depending on the region of the country and the range of available services provided by the center. Daily fees may range from $10 to $150/day. Medicaid provides funding for adult day care, including transportation to and from the program, for eligible individuals. Some private insurance or HMOs may partially cover adult day care or specific services provided as part of a program (e.g. occupational or speech therapy). Medicare may also cover some components of the program (e.g., rehabilitation therapies), but does not cover the cost of the program in full. Some private long-term care insurance policies cover adult day care. Check with your agent or refer to your policy documents. If you do not have coverage and are paying privately, ask the center if they offer a sliding fee scale.

Housing Options

My husband and I have heard that there are some apartments where housekeeping and meals, and even some personal care services, are included in the rent. Is that a good choice for someone with MS?

You are referring to a new housing/health care option called assisted living. Assisted living residences combine housing, personalized supportive services, and health care designed to meet the needs (both scheduled and unscheduled) of those who require help with activities of daily living. These programs foster independence and resident choice while providing a safe and supportive environment.

The types of services offered at these programs usually include: three meals a day served in a common dining area (apartments also have their own kitchens or kitchenettes), housekeeping services, transportation, personal care assistance, emergency call systems, medication management, health promotion programs, social activities, and laundry services. Assisted living programs may offer single rooms, studio apartments, or one-two bedroom apartments. They may be free standing or housed with other residential options such as nursing homes or independent living units.

Today, most residents of assisted living facilities are elderly. However, more and more younger, disabled individuals and couples are finding that these programs meet their needs.

How much does assisted living cost, and how can we tell if a facility is adequate for our needs?

Costs vary with the program and the types of services needed by the residents. Monthly fees (including rent and services) range from $1,000-$4,000 per month. Some programs offer a basic fee with additional charges for special services. Most residences offer month-to-month arrangements although some may require a long-term commitment. Make sure you understand fully the costs and services available.

Regulations and licensing requirements for assisted living programs vary from state to state. Residences must comply with local building codes and fire safety regulations and some states require that staff be certified and receive special training. When considering a particular program, you will want to look into: state licensure and certification requirements, staff credentials and ratios of staff to residents, services and activities offered, costs, contracts, accessibility, availability of common areas, security, quality and size of living space, menus and special dietary requirements. It is very important to read informational materials and contracts very carefully and be a cautious consumer. Marketing brochures can be misleading or unclear as to costs and availability of services. Contact the Assisted Living Facilities Association (ALFA) at *www.alfa.org* or 703/691-8100 for a directory of facilities in your area.

I'm living alone and feel less secure now because I need more help than I used to. Do I have any options that would allow me to feel more secure and independent?

An emergency response system (ERS) can offer a sense of safety and security to many people who live by themselves. An ERS usually consists of a call button (worn as a necklace or bracelet) that can be pushed if you fall or need emergency help. Once activated, the system alerts an attendant at the system headquarters who will try to contact you to determine your needs. The attendant will then contact pre-determined family members, neighbors, or local fire/emergency services to respond to your call. The call device can be worn in the shower and to bed, and the system is in operation 24 hours a day.

Another option is to find a roommate who, in exchange for rent, can offer some personal care assistance and/or companionship. Other personal care and home care assistance options are described in the answers to previous questions.

Home modifications might also help you feel safer and more independent. Widening doorways, creating an accessible bathroom, building a ramped entrance, or purchasing adaptive equipment, can often enable someone to stay at home safely and more independently. A consultation with an occupational therapist or home modification specialist will help you identify your options.

Other housing opportunities or innovative programs may exist in your community. Such options might include:

◇ congregate housing, in which several people with disabilities share common space and personal care services while each has a private room and/or bath;

◇ cooperatives, in which people who have similar needs share personal care assistants;

◇ adult foster care, which places a disabled adult with a "foster family" that provides companionship, supervision, and, perhaps, personal care.

Check with your local chapter of the National MS Society for information about housing and independent living options that may be available in your area.

Caregiver Issues

I feel fully consumed by my responsibilities as a caregiver. I love my wife and don't want to become resentful of the demands MS has placed on me. What can I do?

The responsibilities of caregiving may cause family members to neglect their own health and personal needs. It is important for your wellbeing to be attentive to your personal needs for leisure time, exercise, and the pursuit of personal interests. You deserve to have your own needs met, and a person who is feeling less overwhelmed and frustrated will be more effective and patient as a caregiver.

Try to arrange respite care—that is, time when you are relieved from caregiving responsibilities. You can hire help through a home health agency or see if other family members or friends will agree to stay with your wife while you have time for yourself. Your wife might enjoy the change of company as well! Your local chapter of the National MS Society can refer you to community agencies and facilities that provide respite care. Some chapters are also able to provide funding for respite care.

You might also want to consider joining a caregivers' support group. The sharing of experiences and mutual support provided by these groups can be invaluable. Talking to others in a similar situation (as well as to your health care providers) can also help you learn how to distinguish between real, or immediate, needs and unduly demanding behaviors. This may help you set limits and clarify with your partner the best ways you can provide help and still take care of yourself. Contact the National MS Society chapter near you, as well as the Well Spouse Foundation (*www.wellspouse.org*; 800/838-0879) and the National Family Caregiver's Association (www.nfcacares.org; 800/896-3650). These organizations also offer excellent newsletters and resource information.

I recently felt so tired and worn out that I shouted at my husband and pushed him into his wheelchair when I was helping with a transfer. My loss of control frightened him (and me) and I felt terrible afterwards. How we prevent this from happening again?

When people are frustrated, overwhelmed, and stretched beyond their emotional and physical capabilities, they may lash out verbally and physically. While carepartners can control such impulses most of the time, *there are situations in which even the most thoughtful, loving person can lose control.* People with MS, who must depend on others, are very vulnerable to abusive treatment or neglect. They too, however, can lose control, lashing out physically or verbally at the people who care for them. When tensions mount and family members are troubled by their own behavior or the way they are being treated, it is time to seek professional help. If you would be embarrassed or ashamed for someone to see your behavior or overhear the way you speak to your partner, you know it is time to seek help. No one in a family should have to accept abusive treatment. When this situation occurs, it means that the family is in need of additional resources to address relationship issues and conflicts, improve communication, and ease the stresses on the care partnership. Your local chapter of the National MS Society can direct you to a counselor who is sensitive to the stresses experienced by those living with chronic illness.

Nursing Home Care

We just aren't able to manage any more at home; my wife needs someone with her almost all the time now. How do you know when you've reached the limit of what you can do at home?

The answer to this question will differ for each family, but is usually a function of many factors:

◇ number of family members and friends available to help;
◇ financial resources of the family;
◇ level of disability of the person with MS;
◇ the needs and wishes of the person with MS;
◇ health status of the caregiver;
◇ types of support available in the community.

While it is never an easy conclusion to draw, nursing home placement may be the best option if the resources available to you in your home are insufficient to meet the family's needs.

Is a nursing home the right choice for someone with severe MS?

When care needs exceed the resources available at home, nursing home placement is a reasonable and viable choice. A nursing home can provide the full range of necessary services and may well enhance the quality of life of someone who is unsafe or socially isolated at home.

There are many misconceptions about nursing home care, and most people find that their fears about nursing home life are never realized. In fact, life in a nursing home can offer many benefits, including more opportunities for socialization and recreational activities, peace of mind, safety, security, and 24-hour professional care and supervision. While many people perceive a nursing home as "the end of the road," it can provide those who need it a positive, comfortable, and healthy alternative. Furthermore, the person living in a nursing home can return home for holidays and special visits, or on a more permanent basis if there is a significant change in his or her condition.

While most nursing homes are geared to the elderly, some facilities have special programs for young and middle aged residents. Some nursing facilities actually specialize in MS care. Be sure to ask each facility for the age range of its residents.

What is the cost of nursing home care and how do people pay for them?

Nursing home care can range from $100-$400/day, and Medicaid is the most common source of payment. To qualify for *Medicaid*, an individual is required to have very limited assets. Your state Division of Medical Assistance can give you information about Medicaid eligibility. To qualify for Long Term Care Medicaid, you may have to demonstrate the need for skilled nursing care and for help with specific activities of daily living. These requirements tend to vary from state to state.

Medicare will cover up to 100 days of skilled nursing or rehabilitation under certain circumstances. You can call the Social Security Administration at 800/772-1213 or visit *www.medicare. gov* for specific information.

Private long-term health insurance often covers a portion of the daily nursing home rate and may cover other services you receive there as well. Be sure to read your policy carefully as there are often caps and limitations on coverage.

Private health insurance and *HMOs* generally do not cover the cost of nursing home care. However, there may be some services that are covered, e.g., physical therapy or durable medical equipment. Again, it is important to check your policy carefully.

Finances are often the most confusing and misunderstood part of the whole process of finding and entering a nursing home. Be sure to ask questions. You may also want to consult a lawyer or care manager who can help you understand the complexities of financing long-term care.

My husband and I are beginning to look for a nursing home for him. What should we be looking for in making our choice?

Ask for referrals from your physician and other healthcare providers, friends, local chapter of the National MS Society, and other families with MS. Try to plan ahead and visit as many facilities as possible. You might also want to check the results of government surveys and report cards conducted by your state. It is important to be an informed (but skeptical) consumer, accepting that even the best facility will not be perfect or ideal. If possible, the person with MS should be involved in visiting and selecting a facility. This involvement can make a critical difference in his or her future adjustment in the new situation. When choosing a nursing home, look for the following:

◇ a current operating license from the state
◇ an administrator who has a current state license
◇ certification for Medicaid and Medicare
◇ a location that suits the resident and makes it convenient for family and friends to visit
◇ clean, accessible, bright and roomy bedrooms and living areas
◇ common space for activities and entertaining
◇ an inviting dining area
◇ appetizing food
◇ a physician who is available for emergencies
◇ residents who are well groomed and dressed appropriately
◇ a friendly, skilled, caring, and accommodating staff
◇ adequate staffing [Staffing will vary depending on the shift, and the level of care required by residents on a particular floor or unit. The ratio can range from 4-10 residents for each nursing assistant. Talk to the staff at the facility, and to other residents and their families about their feelings regarding staffing patterns.]
◇ an active resident council, or other ways in which residents can participate in the life of the home
◇ a Residents' Bill of Rights
◇ privacy
◇ an appropriate range of activities, trips and social events

◇ availability of rehabilitation activities
◇ ability to bring personal belongings
◇ a volunteer program
◇ a generous visiting policy
◇ security and safety

Once your husband has moved into the nursing home, it is recommended that you visit during different shifts, make unannounced visits, and ask him about the quality of care he is receiving. Even after your husband has moved into a facility, it is possible to make a change or transfer if either or both of you are dissatisfied with the care. A nursing home checklist is available from the Health Care Financing Administration and can be obtained by calling 800-638-6833 or visiting their web site at *www.hcfa.gov/medicare/*medicare.htm.

My mother-in-law cannot understand how we have could have come to the decision to have my wife live in a nursing home. She is making me feel so guilty! How do we handle it when family members disagree about such important decisions?

Decisions like these are often complicated by intense feelings, and harsh realities are obscured by our wishes that things were different. Try to sit down together as a family and talk honestly about the situation. Talk about the resources you have used, the solutions you have tried, and the thought processes that went into making this decision. Do your best to give a clear picture of the situation—the personal care that is needed, your safety concerns, the impact of caregiving on other family members, the financial factors, and medical issues. This will help distinguish the objective reality from the sadness, frustration, and anger that family members may be feeling. If communication breaks down, consider seeing a family counselor who can facilitate a reasoned, calm discussion. While family members may not ultimately agree, they might become more sensitive to your point of view and understand the decision you have reached.

My wife will soon be moving into a nursing home. Are there any strategies we can use to make the transition a smooth one?

For the person entering a nursing home, as well as family members, the days before and after the move can be filled with anxiety. As with every transition, there will be fears and doubts. With care and understanding, planning and help, the uncertainties of adjusting to nursing home life can be minimized.

If possible, arrange for several visits to the facility prior to moving day. On the day of the move, you and other family members can help your wife set up her room. It helps to bring along personal possessions to create a welcoming space. You can also begin to help your wife begin to learn her way around. You and other family members and friends might plan on staying for the first meal or activity, and meeting other residents and staff.

Anger and depression are not uncommon reactions to moving into a nursing home. Your wife may withdraw initially, or seem angry or bitter. You may find yourself the target of these angry feelings even if you and she made this decision together. It will be important to share your feelings with one another, tap into social and mental health services that are available to you both, and enlist religious or spiritual supports to help ease the transition.

Your wife's adjustment can also be helped along by frequent visits from you and other family members and friends, invitations to join family gatherings outside the nursing home, and reassurances that family relationships will remain caring and strong in spite of the change in living arrangements. Your own adjustment is important as well. Do not hesitate to seek the support of family, friends, your clergyman, or a counselor.

It is important to keep in mind that caring and caregiving do not end because your loved one is no longer living with you. You may find yourself more relaxed and more emotionally available to your wife once you feel less overwhelmed and frustrated with providing the physical care yourself. Be prepared to get involved in the life of the nursing home. Your involvement and visibility in the home will keep you aware of the quality of ongoing care, help you identify and solve problems before they grow, and help you create a new kind of relationship with your spouse.

My wife and I have done a lot of talking about this decision, but now that it's decided, I feel guilty and unsure. I even feel embarrassed to tell our friends. Is this really the right thing?

You and your family may have second thoughts as the move gets closer. Remind yourself that you have carefully thought about this decision, reviewed the options, and debated the pros and cons before arriving at your decision. Review the benefits of the move—the increased security, professional care, and companionship of others. As with all major life transitions, you can expect this decision to be accompanied by anxieties and doubts. With the support of nursing home staff, family, and friends, however, these problems can be minimized.

You may feel that some family members or friends are being judgmental, but this may just be a reflection of your ambivalence and guilt, rather than reality. You need not feel compelled to defend your decision to anyone outside your family, as they have not walked in your shoes. Try to focus on the benefits of the move and avoid the people in your life who cannot be supportive and helpful to you during this difficult transition.

Recommended Readings

Miller, D. & Crawford, P. (1998) The Caregiving Relationship. In R. Kalb (ed.) *Multiple Sclerosis: A Guide for Families.* New York: Demos Medical Publishing.

Selected publications available from your local chapter of the National Multiple Sclerosis Society (800-FIGHT-MS):

◇ *A Guide for Caregivers*—(ES 6010)
◇ *On: Hiring Help at Home*—(EG 752)
◇ *Facts and Issues*—(reprints of articles that originally appeared in the National MS Society magazine, *Inside MS,* covering a variety of topics, including hiring home help)

Recommended Resources

Assisted Living Facilities Association (ALFA) (Tel: 703-691-8100; Internet: *www.alfa.org*)
Health Care Financing Administration (Tel: 800-638-6833; Internet: *www.hcfa.gov/medicare/medicare.htm*)
National Association for Home Care (Tel: 202-547-7424; Internet: *www.nahc.org*)
National Association of Professional Geriatric Care Managers (Tel: 520-881-8008; Internet: *www.caremanager.org*)

National Council on Aging (Tel: 800-424-9046; Internet: *www.ncoa.org*)

National Family Caregivers Association (Tel: 800-896-3650; Internet: *www.nfcacares.org*)

Social Security Administration (800-772-1213; Internet: *www.medicare.gov*)

Well Spouse Foundation (Tel: 800-838-0879; Internet: *www.well-spouse.org*)

17

Life Planning

Laura Cooper, Esq.

The purpose of this chapter is to highlight some of the ways in which individuals with multiple sclerosis and their family members can take action and problem-solve *now* in an effort to safeguard the family's well-being *in the future*. Of all the topics in the book, this may be the one that people are most reluctant to explore. The questions touch on topics relating to severe or incapacitating disability, long-term care, financial security, and self-determination in regard to medical decisions and treatment. Although most people with MS will never have to deal with many of the questions that are raised here, there is no way to predict exactly who will be confronted with severe disability and who will not. Therefore, the chapter is designed to help you think about ways to safeguard the future for yourself and your family in the event that the MS becomes severely disabling. Having engaged in this type of long-range thinking and planning, you can feel more secure no matter what the future brings.

The legal and financial questions raised here are meant to provide you with some basic information about these complicated issues. Complete, in-depth answers would necessarily be more complex than could be dealt with in a single chapter. Not only are each family's circumstances unique, but also the laws governing many of these issues differ somewhat from state to state, and from country to country. Therefore, the chapter is designed to help you identify questions you might want to raise with an attorney and/or certified financial planner who is familiar with the laws of the state (or province) in which you live. The type of attorney to consult about this type of disability-related planning is one who specializes in "elder law" or in disability planning (see Recommended Resources). Your local chapter of the National Multiple Sclerosis Society can help you locate a qualified professional in your area to help you with life planning.

What is the difference between a living will and a health care proxy and why do I need to have one or both of them?

Every competent person has the right to accept or refuse medical care. Unfortunately, illness or injury can intrude on the decision-making process, limiting a person's ability to communicate or carry out his or her wishes when the time for a decision arrives. What actually happens is that although the person retains the *right* to make a decision, the *legal ability* to exercise the right may be lost due to the incapacity to make such decisions. When an individual is judged legally incompetent (through unconsciousness or severe cognitive impairment, for example), health care providers do not need to abide by the person's choices if those choices conflict with medical judgments. If, however, personal choices about medical treatment have been made in advance and incorporated into a legally enforceable **advance directive**, the legal ability to make decisions is protected even after the person becomes incapacitated. Health care providers can then be directed by the wishes that the person made clear in advance, even if those wishes conflict with medical judgments.

Advance medical directives take the form of written documents in which competent persons state their medical decisions for the future. This can be accomplished in two ways: (1) via a **living will**, in which you outline specific instructions for your health care providers; or (2) by a **health care proxy** (also known as a power of attorney for health-care decision-making), in which you designate another person, who knows and would be sympathetic to your desires, to make medical decisions for you in the event that you become too incapacitated to make them for yourself.

Although the living will and health care proxy are both known as advance directives, they differ in the type of directive that is involved. A living will establishes certain treatment guidelines that are to be followed in the future (e.g., an instruction that no "extraordinary measures" are to be used to prolong life in the event of permanent unconsciousness). A health care proxy does not establish treatment guidelines directly. Instead, it appoints a trusted individual to act as your agent and make any necessary decisions in the event that you cannot act for yourself. A health care proxy can incorporate provisions of a living will by requiring that the health care proxy follow any directives that you have included in your living will. Because it is almost impossible to predict all the circumstances that might arise during an illness, it would be difficult for you to include an exhaustive list of advance directives in a living will. Hence, a health care proxy is necessary, in addition to a living will, if you wish to preserve completely the right to self-determination; any decision that is not determined by the directives in your living will would then be made by the person you have entrusted to speak for you. Consequently, a good set of advance directives will include both a living will and a health care proxy, or a single document incorporating both items.

Advance medical directives are recommended for all adults, with or without chronic illness or disability. In fact, many hospitals now routinely ask any person being admitted whether he or she has made an advance directive. Once you have written your directives, be sure to give copies to your health care providers and close family members so that they can be informed of your wishes.

If my husband does not execute an advance directive, how will medical decisions be made for him if he becomes unable to make those decisions for himself?

Once it has been determined that an incapacitated person cannot make decisions and has not left specific directives, family members are usually considered to be the appropriate decision-makers. In theory, most courts agree that even in the absence of a proxy, family members are the appropriate decision-makers. In practice, however, health care providers are not required to follow the family's decisions (to withhold or remove life support, for example) if the providers question the good faith or the medical advisability of those decisions. Therefore, appointing a proxy would provide a safeguard in the event that health care providers hesitate to follow the requests of the incapacitated person as understood or interpreted by family members. Since proxies are considered to directly exercise the wishes of the incapacitated person, health care providers cannot disregard any proxy decisions that conform to the terms of the advance directive.

It is precisely because of this issue that an important legal distinction must be made between a "proxy" and a "surrogate." A proxy is named in the advance directive and is therefore chosen directly by the incapacitated individual. A surrogate is someone who is legally appointed by the court and is *not*, therefore, considered to be directly exercising the wishes of the incapacitated person. For example, if no valid health care proxy exists, a surrogate may be appointed to make the incapacitated person's decisions. This surrogate may be empowered to make these decision in one of two ways: (1) by virtue of a legal relationship (e.g., spouse, parent, or adult child) that automatically gives the person the authority to make surrogate decisions; or (2) by court-appointment as a guardian.

The extent to which you can enforce decisions concerning your husband's future care will depend on whether you are acting as his proxy or as his surrogate. If your husband named you as his proxy, you are acting for him and have the same authority as if he were making his own decisions. If you were named his surrogate decision-maker by some other process of law, your decisions will only be honored if you are thought to be acting in good faith, and if his health care providers think your decisions are medically advisable.

My wife has experienced significant cognitive changes as a result of her MS. Her memory, judgment, and decision-making abilities are severely impaired. How can we make sure that she will get proper care if I die before she does?

Assuming that your wife executed a health care proxy naming you as her proxy prior to her severe cognitive impairment, and also designated your successor, this successor could take over if you were to die or become legally incapacitated and unable to make decisions for her. However, if your wife executed a proxy without designating your successor, your death would leave her in the same position as if she had not designated a proxy at all.

If your wife did not execute a health care proxy, the court will generally appoint surrogate (substitute) decision-makers according to a hierarchy established by state law, with close relatives being given priority over more distant relatives. Thus, if no valid proxy exists, you would probably be appointed her surrogate decision-maker and then replaced by another surrogate if you became incapacitated or died.

A surrogate chosen by the court does not have the power to delegate his or her surrogate decision-making authority to other persons. Therefore, if you acquired your ability to make medical decisions for your wife as a court-appointed surrogate rather than as her designated proxy, the court will simply appoint another surrogate in the event that you die or become incapacitated. As a surrogate, you cannot control in any legal or formal way who this successor will be. However, there are steps that you can take to try to assist the court to make an appropriate decision in such a matter. The best strategy is to define her wishes, as you understand them, in a "values history" form. The purpose of such a form is to assist you in describing your wife's feelings and preferences concerning her health as you understand them. Values history forms are usually available from elder law attorneys.

In addition to making decisions about your wife's medical care, you will also want to try to ensure that sufficient resources will be available after your death (or during your life if you are also incapacitated and are using substantial resources for your own care) to provide for that care. The best way to do this is to develop plans to increase, protect, and preserve your assets.

The medical expenses related to my husband's MS are already pretty high. If he should need nursing care in the future, we would be unable to afford it. We earn salaries, but nowhere near enough to cover nursing care in addition to our living expenses. Are there any ways to handle this problem?

The first step in assessing what money is available for long-term care is to identify all of your joint income and assets. Once you have a complete picture of income and assets, you need to take steps to protect as many of those assets as possible against the expense of long-term care or other extraordinary costs. For example, you want to make sure that you have adequate insurance to protect against catastrophic losses, that you make careful investments, and that you protect your credit rating. If regular in-home or outside care does become necessary, try to determine which of the necessary services might be at least partially covered by government programs or private insurance, and which are available at low cost. Finally, extended family members should begin to think about their financial contributions. While there may be no immediate need for money from relatives, planning for possible long-term care expenses will allow you to determine when financial assistance from relatives might be required. The earlier the possibility is discussed, the easier it will be for people to plan and provide for it.

If you do not have enough resources to pay for long-term services, you will need to try to create a source of money to cover the costs. People with a significant amount of "whole life" insurance, or a home with a significant amount of equity in it, have two possible avenues for raising the necessary cash. The whole life insurance policy may have a high enough cash value to provide you with a lump sum of cash via a policy loan that does not have to be repaid until the death of the insured person. You would probably, however, be required to make annual interest-only payments on the loan. You might also be able to convert home equity into cash while continuing to live in the home. The mechanism for doing this is called a "reverse mortgage," which is basically a loan against the value of a home that does not require repayment until the borrower sells or otherwise (permanently) leaves the home. For information about reverse mortgages, contact the National Center for Home Equity Conversion (see Recommended Resources).

If you find that you still cannot obtain the resources necessary to pay for your husband's long-term care, your only realistic, available option is for your husband to become eligible for Medicaid, the state health care program for low-income individuals (see Chapter 15). The amount of your joint income and assets, in conjunction with the requirements of your state Medicaid program, will determine whether Medicaid would provide care at-home or would only cover your husband's care in a residential nursing facility. Since at-home care is more expensive than residential nursing care in many states, Medicaid will refuse to pay for a person to receive nursing care at home if the family's assets or income are above a certain level.

I need to apply for Medicaid if my wife and I are going to be able to pay for my nursing home care. How do I go about becoming eligible for Medicaid coverage?[1]

You need to be very careful when trying to make your income and assets low enough to qualify for Medicaid coverage (see Chapter 15). Medicaid rules severely restrict protective transfers of income and assets. In other words, the rules prohibit you from reducing your assets simply by taking them out of your own name and "giving" them to children or other relatives. To understand how complex these issues are, it helps to understand the basic rules. Any assets transferred out of a person's name during the thirty-month period prior to entering a nursing facility or applying for Medicaid is generally considered a non-valid transfer and will delay eligibility for Medicaid.

There are, however, certain exceptions to this thirty-month rule. Medicaid rules allow a couple to change the title on their home when one partner enters a nursing facility and permit the at-home spouse to keep some assets and income. The family may also keep a low-value car and some personal belongings. Additionally, there are certain individuals to whom a person is permitted to transfer anything at any time, including a minor child who is blind or disabled. The person applying for Medicaid may transfer any assets to his or her at-home spouse as long as the spouse does not transfer it to anyone else within thirty months

[1]Some policy-makers think that planning for Medicaid qualification is unethical. Until the recent advent of long-term care insurance, however, no reasonable, social alternative was provided for middle-class Americans to provide for payment of their own long-term care. Even recently, if a young person was diagnosed before such time as he or she could reasonably be held responsible for obtaining and paying for long-term care insurance, that person would still be considered uninsurable and therefore still be unable to provide direct payment for necessary care. Thus, because our social and financial market and political structures essentially preclude uninsurable middle- or lower-class people with MS from providing for their own needs, the use of Medicaid planning to *qualify* for Medicaid cannot be considered unethical for these people. They are simply using financial planning to quality for Medicaid because they do not have sufficient funds to obtain needed long-term care. This is distinctly different from the practice of trying to preserve significant assets for inheritance by obtaining Medicaid funding for long-term care.

for less than its true value. A couple is also permitted to invest liquid assets in their home by paying off an outstanding mortgage, making home improvements, or buying a new home for more money than the present home is worth. Of course, an additional benefit of paying off the mortgage or increasing the value of the home is to make more equity available in case a reverse mortgage might be useful at a later time. Whatever you do, however, must result in a home in which the at-home spouse actually resides.

In addition to reducing your assets in order to qualify for Medicaid, it will be necessary to deal with your various income sources. If your wife, as the well spouse, has enough independent income (from her own employment, for example) to support herself, and if you receive your care in a skilled nursing facility, you may be able to set up an income-cap trust (also known as a "Miller" trust) for any personal income you personally receive over the Medicaid qualifying amount. The essential problem here is that all of one spouse's income and assets are deemed to be available to the other spouse if they are living together (but not if they are divorced).

However, if you move into a nursing facility for more than a month, most states have income eligibility limits that use a "name-on-the-check" rule. (Since individual states may have their own versions of this rule that place other restrictions or limits on exempt income, you should check with your state Medicaid agency for more specific information.) Essentially, after the first month in the nursing facility, any income that is received in your wife's name is generally not counted toward the state's maximum income limit for your own Medicaid eligibility. Therefore, the only income that remains at issue after your first month in the facility is income received in your name. If that income is still too high for you to be eligible for Medicaid, a trust can be set up to divert that income so that you can still become Medicaid-eligible.

The main function of an income-cap trust is to change the way that Medicaid measures your available income. In this type of trust, any income over the Medicaid limit is sheltered for special needs. The money in trust cannot be used for basic support or for services that are covered by Medicaid. The trust will have a "trustee" who administers any income of yours that goes into the trust, and the trustee can use the funds only to pay for items or services, not covered by Medicaid, that would provide you with some benefit. Money in the trust cannot be used for your wife, and the state will be entitled to the proceeds of the trust after your death (up to the total amount already spent by Medicaid on your care). It is important to keep in mind that each state's Medicaid agency may impose different requirements on the trust. If you are considering an income-cap trust, you should contact your state Medicaid agency for information about the specific requirements for this type of trust, and consult with an attorney familiar with your state's laws.

If, after examining your income and assets, you and your wife determine that Medicaid would be your only option to pay for nursing care, you should start as quickly as possible to arrange the "ownership" of your funds so that you will be immediately eligible for Medicaid when the time comes. This not only includes transferring assets in acceptable ways (taking into account the ineligibility period or transfer restrictions), but also arranging your income sources, to the extent possible, so that income is in your wife's name. While it is not usually possible to put your own pension or Social Security checks in your wife's name, it may be possible to put other sources of income such as investments in her name.

If you desire to have your nursing care at home rather than in a nursing facility, and you are not able to make yourself eligible under your state's income limitations, a last resort may be to obtain a divorce that divides your income and assets in such a way that you are left with transferable assets and no disqualifying income sources. While this may be a distressing option to consider, it might make it possible for you to live together and yet redistribute your assets in order to make yourself eligible for Medicaid. Since some state Medicaid programs do not recognize divorce settlements for Medicaid-qualification purposes, be sure to consult your state Medicaid agency about its restrictions.

Our 46-year-old daughter has progressive MS. She is fairly well at the present time, but we would like to make financial provision for her in our estate planning. What is the best way for us to do this?

You need to develop a cohesive estate plan in which you accomplish the following: (1) decide who will get your property when you die; (2) set up procedures to make sure that your property passes to others free from probate or with the lowest possible probate fees; (3) set up ways to pass your property to others while reducing or avoiding taxes; and (4) set up a mechanism to manage property you are leaving to others who might be unable to manage it themselves, including your disabled daughter.

In general, the method you choose to distribute your assets will involve either a will, a trust, or both. In using estate planning tools to protect your daughter, it would be advisable to consult an experienced attorney; the law is quite complex and mistakes in planning could have unfortunate consequences. For example, a problem that is commonly overlooked in estate planning is the effect that inheritances or gifts can have on a person's eligibility for public benefits such as Medicaid. Under certain circumstances, it might be preferable to limit or eliminate the transfer of assets to your daughter so that she is not put in the position of missing out on valuable (government) social services (see Recommended Readings).

A written will probably will serve as the cornerstone of your financial estate plan. A will is a binding legal document that determines how your estate should be distributed after you die. In addition to distributing property, wills may be used to handle certain personal affairs such as ensuring that your disabled daughter is cared for properly in the event that she becomes legally incompetent. Parents and guardians may use wills to name their successors. Such designations, depending on the state in which they are made, may be legally binding or of invaluable assistance to a court in any necessary guardianship proceedings. These designees are known either as "successor" or "testamentary" guardians.

A trust is a binding legal arrangement in which a person transfers assets to another person, known as a trustee, who manages it for the named beneficiary. This arrangement may be made as part of a will, in which case it is called a "testamentary" trust, or it may become effective during your lifetime, in which case it is called a "living" trust. Additionally, a living trust may be changeable during your lifetime ("revocable") or it may be fixed ("irrevocable"). A trust can be used to select a trustee who will look out for the financial and personal interests of your daughter without the need for a guardian, and it may result in substantial tax savings. The disadvantages of a trust may include complexity, cost, and the possibility that changing circumstances will leave the trustee without the most appropriate options. Although trusts may come in many forms, the most important for this purpose include:

◇ *Contingent testamentary trusts*—proceeds of an estate go first to the surviving spouse and then are held in trust for your daughter after the spouse's death;

◇ *Living trust with a pour-over provision*—allows property to be added to the trust for your daughter after your death;

◇ *Discretionary trust*—carefully defines the amount and kind of discretion that the trustee will have in distributing or withholding benefits;

◇ *Sprinkling trust*—allows you to instruct the trustee, in the event that the trust has more than one beneficiary, to distribute the benefits unequally according to the unique needs of each of those beneficiaries;

◇ *Life insurance trust*—ensures that the benefits of a life insurance policy will be managed properly.

It is advisable to consult with an estate planning attorney in order to make sure, given your financial and social circumstances, that the best strategies are used to ensure that your daughter will be protected both financially and socially once you pass away. In many states there are experts in estate planning for families with children who have disabilities. You can obtain current information about such experts by contacting the National Information Center for Children and Youth with Disabilities as well as the September 1996 issue of *Exceptional Parent* (see Recommended Resources).

My husband has recently been diagnosed with MS. He is the primary breadwinner right now while I am home with our young children. Should we be doing any kind of special planning, financial or otherwise, now that he has MS?

Most definitely. You and your husband should create a financial plan that includes insurance and other protection planning, as well as a comprehensive estate plan that also includes the advance directives discussed previously. Financial planning is the methodical process of assessing your total assets and liabilities, as well as future income potential and anticipated expenses, and then using that information to determine your best options for meeting future needs and wants. Planning should be done as soon as possible and then revised periodically or as new circumstances dictate.

The planning process may include the assessment of a myriad of financial options, including insurance plans, annuities, pensions, home equity, and availability of government benefits. Certified financial planners and lawyers may be valuable in sorting though the options and identifying the possible legal and tax consequences of various choices and choice combinations. Because your husband is the primary breadwinner, you will need to pay special attention to disability, life, health insurance, and long-term care issues so that your income stream will be protected if his disease progresses and he becomes unable to work. You might also want to be thinking about the type of employment you would seek in the event that you need to provide additional income for the family. If you would need further training in a particular area in order to become employed, you might want to think about taking some courses now. Then, in the event that your husband becomes unable to continue working, you would feel less financially vulnerable and more prepared to take on the breadwinner role.

Saving for the future was hard enough before I got MS. How can my wife and I plan for our financial future now that I have such an unpredictable illness?

Your first priority should be to increase the rate of retirement savings as much as you possibly can, since MS may shorten the time you have before retirement. You should also make sure that your financial plan includes consideration of the potential future need for government benefits, as described previously.

Next, it is important for you to safeguard yourself and your family from the potential extraordinary costs of the unpredictable illness. When you are planning for such risk, the sensible approach is to assume that the worst will happen, and assess what your needs would be if the worst were to occur. You should never plan for the best; such a strategy is doomed to fail in all but the most ideal and infrequent circumstances. By planning for the worst, even though the best is what you hope for, you will feel pleasantly surprised and adequately prepared if less than the worst comes your way.

Consider, for example, the following grim scenario. If you, as your family's primary breadwinner, become disabled, the continuation of your family's entire health insurance package might be jeopardized if it is based on your employment. Additionally, you would need to provide income replacement for any time that you were not working, including finding income supplements for added expenses attributable to any disability you might incur. You might find it difficult or impossible to increase your life insurance to provide financial security for your family members in the event of your death. And, even upon returning to work (assuming that you were able to do so, and that you could obtain adequate health insurance coverage from your employer following a period of disability), you might find that you were no longer as productive as you were before your disability occurred, and therefore could not earn as much money. You might even lose your job altogether. All of these possibilities are frightening, to say the least. If you planned for all of them, you might be able to preserve whatever lifestyle you had before your disability occurred. If you adequately planned for none or only part of them, and you were handed a significant disability for a substantial period of time, your family's quality of life would no doubt be negatively affected.

The ultimate question in this circumstance is how can a person deal with the financial risks attributable to ill health but still maintain adequate income and savings? The answer to this question lies mostly in devising a strategy of protection planning for the risk of ill health. The object of this kind of protection planning is to find ways to lessen the risks—e.g., to make yourself and your loved ones as "bullet-proof" as possible, given whatever unpleasant surprises your MS or other health conditions might bring your way. As described in Chapter 15, your best strategy is to devise an insurance package that covers your family's five separate elements of health risk: (1) major medical coverage for any preexisting conditions such as the MS that may be excluded from your primary policy; (2) major medical coverage for all other conditions; (3) hospitalization for the excluded health condition(s); (4) hospitalization for all other conditions; and (5) some provisions for long-term services. You should also make special efforts to obtain adequate life and disability insurance that is not contingent upon your or someone else's employment (see Chapter 15 for a discussion of ways to obtain these types of insurance after you have been diagnosed with MS). Once your savings rate is on target, and your assets are protected from depletion with sufficient insurance, you are well on your way to financial security despite the potential intrusion of disability.

I have progressive MS and seem to be slowly getting more disabled. My husband and I want to protect the money we have saved toward our children's educations and our own retirement but we both know that my medical expenses may grow considerably if my MS gets much worse. Are there any strategies to deal with this?

The most important strategy is to maintain a "stop-loss" in insurance coverage. This refers to the maximum out-of-pocket expense you will have to absorb before you are completely insured for the medical costs. There are two basic elements to this strategy. The first is to obtain adequate basic major medical and hospitalization coverage that has a built-in "stop-loss" provision that limits your maximum out-of-pocket expenses in any calendar year. The second element is to obtain a good "catastrophic" or "excess" major medical policy. These policies are usually available to members of large organizational groups, and your diagnosis will not necessarily exclude you from eligibility for these group policies. Although you will be excluded from some, others will only impose a waiting period (perhaps a year or two) before you can claim benefits for your preexisting condition. The benefit of such a policy is that it provides an additional measure of protection by increasing the maximum lifetime benefits available, as well as enlarging the scope of expenses that may be covered for your illness. For example, many of these policies expressly provide for custodial (as opposed to skilled nursing) long-term care, a benefit that is specifically excluded in most major medical policies. Additionally, these policies are relatively inexpensive, so their expense is usually manageable in addition to your usual major medical coverage.

Another strategy you might consider if you find that you are spending a significant amount of time in the hospital is to collect multiple hospital indemnity insurance policies. These policies will pay you a specific indemnity—or dollar amount—for every day that you are in the hospital. These can be real money-makers if you are hospitalized with any frequency due to your MS or related conditions. Additionally, many of these policies can be obtained without preexisting condition exclusions (usually only with waiting periods). These policies can be obtained from many organizational groups and are fairly inexpensive. Unless you find yourself having more than sporadic, brief hospitalizations, you might only want to carry a single good policy of this type to help pay for the deductibles and co-payments you may have when you are hospitalized. Keep information on other available indemnity policies for which you qualify in a file. Then, if your amount of hospitalization increases to a point that justifies the cost of multiple premiums, you can sign up for additional policies.

A good certified financial planner who is well-versed in disability issues should be able to assist you in putting together an adequate insurance portfolio for your needs.

Although this chapter comes at the end of the book, its more suitable placement might well be at the very beginning. Effective planning means looking ahead in an effort to make the future as workable and predictable as it can possibly be in the face of life's uncertainties. MS only adds to those uncertainties. Every chapter in this book is designed to help you familiarize yourself and your family members with the possibilities inherent in living with this type of unpredictable chronic illness. While many people will never experience much of what is described in these pages, being educated about the disease and the resources that are available to help you will enable you to feel more prepared to deal with whatever the future brings.

Recommended Readings

Cooper L., *Insurance Solutions: Plan Well, Live Better. A Workbook for People with Chronic Illness or Disability*. New York: Demos, 2000.

Garner RJ, Coplan RB, Raasch BJ, Ratner CL. *Ernst & Young's Personal Financial Planning Guide*. New York: John Wiley & Sons, 1995.

Isaacs SL, Swartz AC. *The Consumer's Guide to Today's Health Care*. New York: Houghton Mifflin, 1992.

Matthews J. *Beat the Nursing Home Trap: A Consumer's Guide to Choosing & Financing Long-Term Care (2nd edition)*. Berkeley, CA: Nolo Press, 1993.

Mendelsohn S. *Tax Options and Strategies for People with Disabilities (2nd edition)*. New York: Demos Medical Publishing, 1996.

Pond JD. *The New Century Family Money Book*. New York: Dell Publishing, 1993.

Roberts R. *The Veteran's Guide to Benefits*. New York: Signet, 1989.

Russell LM, Grant AE, Joseph SM, Fee RW. *Planning for the Future: Providing a Meaningful Life for a Child with a Disability After Your Death (2nd edition)*. Evanston, IL: American Publishing, 1993.

Recommended Resources

American Association of Retired Persons (AARP) (Tel: 202-434-2277). Disseminates valuable information on all types of insurance.

Center for Medicare Advocacy (Tel: 860-456-7790; Internet: *www.medicareadvocacy.org*). Provides assistance to people with disabilities (and their advocates) in areas of Medicare, educational materials, home care, and referrals.

Center for the Study of Services (Tel: 800-475-7283; Write to *The Consumer Guide to Health Plans*, 733 15th Street, N.W., Suite 820, Washington, D.C. 20005). Ranks managed care plans and publishes its findings.

Consumer Federation of American (CFA) (Tel: 202-387-6121 or 212-387-0087; Write to CFA, 1424 16th Street, N.W., Washington, D.C. 20036). This insurance consumer advocacy group publishes a useful life insurance guide called *Taking a Bite Out of Insurance*.

Health Insurance Association of America (Tel: 202-824-1600). Has useful booklets for consumers, such as *A consumer's Guide to Medicare Supplemental Insurance*.

National Academy of Elder Law Attorneys, Inc. (1604 N. Country Club Road, Tucson, AZ 85716; tel: 602-881-4005). If you send them a stamped, self-addressed, legal-sized envelope, they will send you a brochure entitled "Questions and Answers When Looking for an Elder Law Attorney."

National Association of Personal Financial Advisors (800-366-2732). They will send you names of association members in your area.

National Center for Home Equity Conversion (Reverse Mortgage Locator, National Center for Home Equity Conversion, 7373 147th Street, Suite 115, Apple Valley, MN 66124; tel: 612-953-4474).

National Committee for Quality Assurance (NCQA) (Tel: 800-839-6487; Internet: *www.ncqa.org*). Collects information on managed care plans, including HMOs and rates them on factors such as physician credentials and subscriber turnover, publishes its findings, and accredits the plans. The accreditation report is provided free-of-charge upon request, or can be accessed via the NCQA website.

National Information Center for Children and Youth with Disabilities (P.O. Box 1492, Washington, D.C. 20013; tel: 800-695-0285; 202-884-8200).

People's Medical Society (Tel: 610-770-1670). Publishes useful information about health insurance. Resource directory in the September 1996 issue of *Exceptional Parent*.

Glossary

Abductor muscle   A muscle used to pull a body part away from the midline of the body (e.g., the abductor leg muscles are used to spread the legs).

ACTH (adrenocorticotropic hormone)   ACTH is extracted from the pituitary glands of animals or made synthetically. ACTH stimulates the adrenal glands to release glucocorticoid hormones. These hormones are anti-inflammatory in nature, reducing edema and other aspects of inflammation. Data from the early 1970s indicate that ACTH may reduce the duration of MS exacerbations. In recent years it has been determined that synthetically produced glucocorticoid hormones (e.g., cortisone, prednisone, prednisolone, methylprednisolone, betamethasone, dexamethasone), which can be directly administered without the use of ACTH, are more potent, cause less sodium retention and less potassium loss, and are longer-acting than ACTH.

Activities of daily living (ADLs)   Activities of daily living include any daily activity a person performs for self-care (feeding, grooming, bathing, dressing), work, homemaking, and leisure. The ability to perform ADLs is often used as a measure of ability/disability in MS.

Acute Having rapid onset, usually with recovery; not chronic or long-lasting.

Adductor muscle A muscle that pulls inward toward the midline of the body (e.g., the adductor leg muscles are used to pull the legs together).

ADLs *See* Activities of daily living.

Adrenocorticotropic hormone (ACTH) *See* ACTH.

Advance (medical) directive Advance directives preserve the person's right to accept or reject a course of medical treatment even after the person becomes mentally or physically incapacitated to the point of being unable to communicate those wishes. Advance directives come in two basic forms: (1) a living will, in which the person outlines specific treatment guidelines that are to be followed by health care providers; (2) a health care proxy (also called a power of attorney for health care decision-making), in which the person designates a trusted individual to make medical decisions in the event that he or she becomes too incapacitated to make such decisions. Advance directive requirements vary greatly from one state to another and should therefore be drawn up in consultation with an attorney who is familiar with the laws of the particular state.

Affective release Also called pseudo-bulbar affect; a condition in which episodes of laughing and/or crying occur with no apparent precipitating event. The person's actual mood may be unrelated to the emotion being expressed. This condition is thought to be caused by lesions in the limbic system, a group of brain structures involved in emotional feeling and expression.

Afferent pupillary defect An abnormal reflex response to light that is a sign of nerve fiber damage due to optic neuritis. A pupil normally gets smaller when a light is shined either into that eye (direct response) or the other eye (indirect response). In an afferent pupillary defect (also called Marcus Gunn pupil), there is a relative decrease in the direct response. This is most clearly demonstrated by the "swinging flashlight test." When the flashlight is shined first in the abnormal eye, then in the healthy eye, and then again in the eye with the pupillary defect, the affected pupil becomes larger rather than smaller.

AFO   *See* Ankle-foot orthosis.

Ankle-foot orthosis (AFO)   An ankle-foot orthosis is a brace, usually plastic, that is worn on the lower leg and foot to support the ankle and correct foot drop. By holding the foot and ankle in the correct position, the AFO promotes correct heel-toe walking. *See* Foot drop.

Antibodies   Proteins of the immune system that are soluble (dissolved) in blood serum or other body fluids and which are produced in response to bacteria, viruses, and other types of foreign antigens. *See* Antigen.

Anticholinergic   Refers to the action of certain medications commonly used in the management of neurogenic bladder dysfunction. These medications inhibit the transmission of parasympathetic nerve impulses and thereby reduce spasms of smooth muscle in the bladder.

Antigen   Any substance that triggers the immune system to produce an antibody; generally refers to infectious or toxic substances. *See* Antibody.

Aspiration   Inhalation of food particles or fluids into lungs.

Aspiration pneumonia   Inflammation of the lungs due to aspiration.

Assistive devices   Any tools that are designed, fabricated, and/or adapted to assist a person in performing a particular task, e.g., cane, walker, shower chair.

Assistive technology   A term used to describe all of the tools, products, and devices, from the simplest to the most complex, that can make a particular function easier or possible to perform.

Ataxia   The incoordination and unsteadiness that result from the brain's failure to regulate the body's posture and the strength and direction of limb movements. Ataxia is most often caused by disease activity in the cerebellum.

Atrophy   A wasting away or decrease in size of a cell, tissue, or organ of the body because of disease or lack of use.

Autoimmune disease   A process in which the body's immune system causes illness by mistakenly attacking healthy cells, organs, or tissues in the body that are essential for good health. Multiple sclerosis is believed to be an autoimmune disease, along with systemic lupus erythematosus, rheumatoid arthritis, scleroderma, and many others. The precise origin and pathophysiologic processes of these diseases are unknown.

Autonomic nervous system The part of the nervous system that regulates involuntary vital functions, including the activity of the cardiac (heart) muscle, smooth muscles (e.g., of the gut), and glands. The autonomic nervous system has two divisions: the sympathetic nervous system accelerates heart rate, constricts blood vessels, and raises blood pressure; the parasympathetic nervous system slows heart rate, increases intestinal and gland activity, and relaxes sphincter muscles.

Axon The extension or prolongation of a nerve cell (neuron) that conducts impulses to other nerve cells or muscles. Axons are generally smaller than 1 micron (1 micron = 1/1,000,000 of a meter) in diameter, but can be as much as a half meter in length.

Axonal Pertaining to the axon.

Axonal damage Injury to the axon in the nervous sytem, generally as a consequence of trauma or disease. This damage may involve temporary, reversible effects or permanent severing of the axon. Axonal damage usually results in short-term changes in nervous system activity, or permanent inability of nerve fibers to send their signals from one part of the nervous system to another or from nerve fibers to muscles. The damage can thus result in a variety of symptoms relating to sensory or motor function.

B-cell A type of lymphocyte (white blood cell) manufactured in the bone marrow that makes antibodies.

Babinski reflex A neurologic sign in MS in which stroking the outside sole of the foot with a pointed object causes an upward (extensor) movement of the big toe rather than the normal (flexor) bunching and downward movement of the toes. *See* Sign.

Bell's palsy A paralysis of the facial nerve (usually on one side of the face), which can occur as a consequence of MS, viral infection, or other infections. It has acute onset and can be transient or permanent.

Blood-brain barrier A semipermeable cell layer around blood vessels in the brain and spinal cord that prevents large molecules, immune cells, and potentially damaging substances and disease-causing organisms (e.g., viruses) from passing out of the blood stream into the central nervous system (brain and spinal cord). A break in the blood-brain barrier may underlie the disease process in MS.

Brain   That part of the central nervous system that is contained within the cranium (skull).

Brainstem   The part of the central nervous system that houses the nerve centers of the head as well as the centers for respiration and heart control. It extends from the base of the brain to the spinal cord.

Brainstem auditory evoked potential (BAEP)   A test in which the brain's electrical activity in response to auditory stimuli (e.g., clicking sounds) is recorded by an electroencephalograph and analyzed by computer. Demyelination results in a slowing of response time. This test is sometimes useful in the diagnosis of MS because it can confirm the presence of a suspected lesion or identify the presence of an unsuspected lesion that has produced no symptoms. BAEPs have been shown to be less useful in the diagnosis of MS than either visual or somatosensory evoked potentials. *See* Visual evoked potential; Somatosensory evoked potential.

CAT scan   *See* Computerized axial tomography.

Catheter   A hollow, flexible tube, made of plastic or rubber, which can be inserted through the urinary opening into the bladder to drain excess urine that cannot be excreted normally.

Central nervous system   The part of the nervous system that includes the brain, optic nerves, and spinal cord.

Cerebellum   A part of the brain situated above the brainstem that controls balance and coordination of movement.

Cerebrospinal fluid (CSF)   A watery, colorless, clear fluid that bathes and protects the brain and spinal cord. The composition of this fluid can be altered by a variety of diseases. Certain changes in CSF that are characteristic of MS can be detected with a lumbar puncture (spinal tap), a test sometimes used to help make the MS diagnosis. *See* Lumbar puncture.

Cerebrum   The large, upper part of the brain that acts as a master control system and is responsible for initiating thought and motor activity.   Its two hemispheres, united by the corpus callosum, form the largest part of the central nervous system.

Cerebral   Pertaining to the cerebrum.

Chronic   Of long duration, not acute; a term often used to describe a disease that shows gradual worsening.

Clinical finding   An observation made during a medical examination indicating change or impairment in a physical or mental function.

Clinical trial   Rigorously controlled studies designed to provide extensive data that will allow for statistically valid evaluation of the safety and efficacy of a particular treatment. *See also* Double-blind clinical study; Placebo.

Clonus   A sign of spasticity in which involuntary shaking or jerking of the leg occurs when the toe is placed on the floor with the knee slightly bent. The shaking is caused by repeated, rhythmic, reflex muscle contractions.

Cognition   High level functions carried out by the human brain, including comprehension and use of speech, visual perception and construction, calculation ability, attention (information processing), memory, and executive functions such as planning, problem-solving, and self-monitoring.

Cognitive impairment   Changes in cognitive function caused by trauma or disease process. Some degree of cognitive impairment occurs in approximately 50–60 percent of people with MS, with memory, information processing, and executive functions being the most commonly affected functions. *See* Cognition.

Cognitive rehabilitation   Techniques designed to improve the functioning of individuals whose cognition is impaired because of physical trauma or disease. Rehabilitation strategies are designed to improve the impaired function via repetitive drills or practice, or to compensate for impaired functions that are not likely to improve. Cognitive rehabilitation is provided by psychologists and neuropsychologists, speech/language pathologists, and occupational therapists. While these three types of specialists use different assessment tools and treatment strategies, they share the common goal of improving the individual's ability to function as independently and safely as possible in the home and work environment.

Combined (bladder) dysfunction   A type of neurogenic bladder dysfunction is MS (also called detrusor-external sphincter dyssynergia—DESD). Simultaneous contractions of the bladder's detrusor muscle and external sphincter cause urine to be trapped in the bladder, resulting in symptoms of urinary urgency, hesitancy, dribbling, and incontinence.

Computerized axial tomography (CAT scan)   A non-invasive diagnostic radiology technique for examining soft tissues of the body. A computer integrates X-ray scanned "slices" of the organ being examined into a cross-sectional picture.

Condom catheter   A tube connected to a thin, flexible sheath that is worn over the penis to allow drainage of urine into a collection system; can be used to manage male urinary incontinence.

Constipation   A condition in which bowel movements happen less frequently than is normal for the particular individual, or the stool is small, hard, and difficult or painful to pass.

Contraction   A shortening of muscle fibers that results in the movement of a joint.

Contracture   A permanent shortening of the muscles and tendons adjacent to a joint, which can result from severe, untreated spasticity and interferes with normal movement around the affected joint. If left untreated, the affected joint can become frozen in a flexed (bent) position.

Coordination   An organized working together of muscles and groups of muscles aimed at bringing about a purposeful movement such as walking or standing.

Corpus callosum   The broad band of nerve fiber tissue that connects the two cerebral hemispheres of the brain.

Cortex   The outer layer of brain tissue.

Corticosteroid   Any of the natural or synthetic hormones associated with the adrenal cortex (which influences or controls many body processes). Corticosteroids include glucocorticoids, which have an anti-inflammatory and immunosuppressive role in the treatment of MS exacerbations. *See also* Glucocorticoids; Immunosuppression; Exacerbation.

Cortisone   A glucocorticoid steroid hormone, produced by the adrenal glands or synthetically, that has anti-inflammatory and immune-system suppressing properties. Prednisone and prednisolone also belong to this group of substances.

Cranial nerves   Nerves that carry sensory, motor, or parasympathetic fibers to the face and neck. Included among this group of twelve nerves are the optic nerve (vision), trigeminal nerve (sensation along the face), vagus nerve (pharynx and vocal cords). Evaluation of cranial nerve function is part of the standard neurologic exam.

Cystoscopy   A diagnostic procedure in which a special viewing device called a cystoscope is inserted into the urethra (a tubular structure that drains urine from the bladder) to examine the inside of the urinary bladder.

Cystostomy   A surgically created opening through the lower abdomen into the urinary bladder. A plastic tube inserted into the opening drains urine from the bladder into a plastic collection bag. This relatively simple procedure is done when a person requires an indwelling catheter to drain excess urine from the bladder but cannot, for some reason, have it pass through the urethral opening.

Decubitus   An ulcer (sore) of the skin resulting from pressure and lack of movement such as occurs when a person is bed- or wheelchair-bound. The ulcers occur most frequently in areas where the bone lies directly under the skin, such as elbow, hip, or over the coccyx (tailbone). A decubitus ulcer may become infected and cause general worsening of the person's health.

Deep tendon reflexes   The involuntary jerks that are normally produced at certain spots on a limb when the tendons are tapped with a hammer. Reflexes are tested as part of the standard neurologic exam.

Dementia   A generally profound and progressive loss of intellectual function, sometimes associated with personality change, that results from loss of brain substance and is sufficient to interfere with a person's normal functional activities.

Demyelination   A loss of myelin in the white matter of the central nervous system (brain, spinal cord).

DESD   *See* Detrusor-external sphincter dyssynergia.

Detrusor muscle   A muscle of the urinary bladder that contracts and causes the bladder to empty.

Detrusor-external sphincter dyssynergia (DESD)   *See* Combined (bladder) dysfunction.

Diplopia   Double vision, or the simultaneous awareness of two images of the same object that results from a failure of the two eyes to work in a coordinated fashion. Covering one eye will erase one of the images.

Disablement   As defined by the World Health Organization, a disability (resulting from an impairment) is a restriction or lack of ability to perform an activity in the manner or within the range considered normal for a human being.

Double-blind clinical study   A study in which none of the participants, including experimental subjects, examining doctors, attending nurses, or any other research staff, know who is taking the test drug and who is taking a control or placebo agent. The purpose of this research design is to avoid inadvertent bias of the test results. In all studies, procedures are designed to "break the blind" if medical circumstances require it.

Dysarthria   Poorly articulated speech resulting from dysfunction of the muscles controlling speech, usually caused by damage to the central nervous system or a peripheral motor nerve. The content and meaning of the spoken words remain normal.

Dysesthesia   Distorted or unpleasant sensations experienced by a person when the skin is touched, that are typically caused by abnormalities in the sensory pathways in the brain and spinal cord.

Dysmetria   A disturbance of coordination, caused by lesions in the cerebellum. A tendency to over- or underestimate the extent of motion needed to place an arm or leg in a certain position as, for example, in overreaching for an object.

Dysphagia   Difficulty in swallowing. It is a neurologic or neuromuscular symptom that may result in aspiration (whereby food or saliva enters the airway), slow swallowing (possibly resulting in inadequate nutrition), or both.

Dysphonia   Disorders of voice quality (including poor pitch control, hoarseness, breathiness, and hypernasality) caused by spasticity, weakness, and incoordination of muscles in the mouth and throat.

EAE   *See* Experimental allergic encephalomyelitis.

EEG   *See* Electroencephalography.

Electroencephalography (EEG)   A diagnostic procedure that records, via electrodes attached to various areas of the person's head, electrical activity generated by brain cells.

Electromyography (EMG)   Electromyography is a diagnostic procedure that records muscle electrical potentials through a needle or small plate electrodes. The test can also measure the ability of peripheral nerves to conduct impulses.

EMG   *See* Electromyography.

Erectile dysfunction   The inability to attain or retain a rigid penile erection.

Etiology   The study of all factors that may be involved in the development of a disease, including the patient's susceptibility, the nature of the disease-causing agent, and the way in which the person's body is invaded by the agent.

Euphoria   Unrealistic cheerfulness and optimism, accompanied by a lessening of critical faculties; generally considered to be a result of damage to the brain.

Evoked potentials (EPs)   EPs are recordings of the nervous system's electrical response to the stimulation of specific sensory pathways (e.g., visual, auditory, general sensory). In tests of evoked potentials, a person's recorded responses are displayed on an oscilloscope and analyzed on a computer that allows comparison with normal response times. Demyelination results in a slowing of response time. EPs can demonstrate lesions along specific nerve pathways whether or not the lesions are producing symptoms, thus making this test useful in confirming the diagnosis of MS. *See* Brainstem auditory evoked potential; Somatosensory evoked potential; Visual evoked potential.

Exacerbation   The appearance of new symptoms or the aggravation of old ones, lasting at least twenty-four hours (synonymous with attack, relapse, flare-up, or worsening); usually associated with inflammation and demyelination in the brain or spinal cord.

Experimental allergic encephalomyelitis (EAE)   Experimental allergic encephalomyelitis is an autoimmune disease resembling MS that has been induced in some genetically susceptible research animals. Before testing on humans, a potential treatment for MS may first be tested on laboratory animals with EAE in order to determine the treatment's efficacy and safety.

Extensor spasm   A symptom of spasticity in which the legs straighten suddenly into a stiff, extended position. These spasms, which typically last for several minutes, occur most commonly in bed at night or on rising from bed.

Failure to empty (bladder)   A type of neurogenic bladder dysfunction in MS resulting from demyelination in the voiding reflex center of the spinal cord. The bladder tends to overfill and become flaccid, resulting in symptoms of urinary urgency, hesitancy, dribbling, and incontinence.

Failure to store (bladder)   A type of neurogenic bladder dysfunction in MS resulting from demyelination of the pathways between the spinal cord and brain. Typically seen in a small, spastic bladder, storage failure can cause symptoms of urinary urgency, frequency, incontinence, and nocturia.

FDA   *See* Food and Drug Administration.

Finger-to-nose test   As a test of dysmetria and intention tremor, the person is asked, with eyes closed, to touch the tip of the nose with the tip of the index finger. This test is part of the standard neurologic exam.

Flaccid   A decrease in muscle tone resulting in weakened muscles and therefore loose, "floppy" limbs.

Flexor spasm   Involuntary, sometimes painful contractions of the flexor muscles, which pull the legs upward into a clenched position. These spasms, which last two to three seconds, are symptoms of spasticity. They often occur during sleep, but can also occur when the person is in a seated position.

Foley catheter   *See* Indwelling catheter.

Food and Drug Administration (FDA)   The U.S. federal agency that is responsible for enforcing governmental regulations pertaining to the manufacture and sale of food, drugs, and cosmetics. Its role is to prevent the sale of impure or dangerous substances. Any new drug that is proposed for the treatment of MS in the United States must be approved by the FDA.

Foot drop   A condition of weakness in the muscles of the foot and ankle, caused by poor nerve conduction, which interferes with a person's ability to flex the ankle and walk with a normal heel-toe pattern. The toes touch the ground before the heel, causing the person to trip or lose balance.

Frontal lobes   The largest lobes of the brain. The anterior (front) part of each of the cerebral hemispheres that make up the cerebrum. The back part of the frontal lobe is the motor cortex, which controls voluntary movement; the area of the frontal lobe that is further forward is concerned with learning, behavior, judgment, and personality.

Gadolinium   A chemical compound that can be administered to a person during magnetic resonance imaging to help distinguish between new lesions and old lesions.

Gadolinium-enhancing lesion   A lesion appearing on magnetic resonance imagery, following injection of the chemical compound gadolinium, that reveals a breakdown in the blood-brain barrier. This breakdown of the blood-brain barrier indicates either a newly active lesion or the re-activation of an old one. *See* Gadolinium.

Gastrocolic reflex A mass peristaltic (coordinated, rhythmic, smooth muscle contraction that acts to force food through the digestive tract) movement of the colon that often occurs fifteen to thirty minutes after ingesting a meal.

Gastrostomy *See* Percutaneous endoscopic gastrostomy.

Glucocorticoid hormones Steroid hormones that are produced by the adrenal glands in response to stimulation by adrenocorticotropic hormone (ACTH) from the pituitary. These hormones, which can also be manufactured synthetically (prednisone, prednisolone, methylprednisolone, betamethasone, dexamethasone), serve both an immunosuppressive and an anti-inflammatory role in the treatment of MS exacerbations: they damage or destroy certain types of T-lymphocytes that are involved in the overactive immune response, and interfere with the release of certain inflammation-producing enzymes.

Health care proxy *See* Advance (medical) directive.

Heel-knee-shin test A test of coordination in which the person is asked, with eyes closed, to place one heel on the opposite knee and slide it up and down the shin.

Helper T-lymphocytes White blood cells that are a major contributor to the immune system's inflammatory response against myelin.

Hemiparesis Weakness of one side of the body, including one arm and one leg.

Hemiplegia Paralysis of one side of the body, including one arm and one leg.

Hyperbaric oxygen A procedure in which the person breathes oxygen under greater than atmospheric pressure in a specially constructed chamber. Once thought to be a potential treatment for MS, it has been evaluated in several controlled, double-blind studies and found to be ineffective for this purpose.

Immune system A complex system of various types of cells that protects the body against disease-producing organisms and other foreign invaders.

Immunocompetent cells White blood cells (B- and T-lymphocytes and others) that defend against invading agents in the body.

Immunoglobulin   *See* Antibody.

Immunosuppression   In MS, a form of treatment that slows or inhibits the body's natural immune responses, including those directed against the body's own tissues. Examples of immunosuppressive treatments in MS include mitoxantrone, cyclosporine, methotrexate, and azathioprine.

Impairment   As defined by the World Health Organization, an impairment is any loss or abnormality of psychological, physiological, or anatomical structure or function. It represents a deviation from the person's usual biomedical state. An impairment is thus any loss of function directly resulting from injury or disease.

Incidence   The number of new cases of a disease in a specified population over a defined period of time.

Incontinence   Also called spontaneous voiding; the inability to control passage of urine or bowel movements.

Indwelling catheter   A type of catheter (*see* Catheter) that remains in the bladder on a temporary or permanent basis. It is used only when intermittent catheterization is not possible or is medically contraindicated. The most common type of indwelling catheter is a Foley catheter, which consists of a flexible rubber tube that is inserted in the bladder to allow the urine to flow into an external drainage bag. A small balloon, inflated after insertion, holds the Foley catheter in place.

Inflammation   A tissue's immunologic response to injury, characterized by mobilization of white blood cells and antibodies, swelling, and fluid accumulation.

Innervation The supply or conduction of nervous impulses to a muscle or body part.

Intention tremor   Rhythmic shaking that occurs in the course of a purposeful movement, such as reaching to pick something up or bringing an outstretched finger in to touch one's nose.

Interferon   A group of immune system proteins, produced and released by cells infected by a virus, which inhibit viral multiplication and modify the body's immune response. One of the interferons, interferon beta-1b (Betaseron®) was approved by the Food and Drug Administration in 1993 for treatment of relapsing-remitting MS. It was found in a clinical trial to reduce the frequency and severity of exacerbations by approximately 30 percent. A second interferon, interferon beta-1a (Avonex®) has also been shown to reduce the frequency and severity of MS exacerbations in people with relapsing-remitting disease, as well as to reduce the risk of clinically significant disease progression. Avonex® was approved for use in MS in 1996. Rebif®, also interferon beta-1a, has been approved for the treatment of relapsing-remitting MS in the U.S. and Canada. Interferon gamma is a naturally-occuring substance in the body that promotes inflammation and is thought to be involved in MS exacerbations. Once tried as a treatment for MS, it was found to make the disease worse. Interferon beta works to counteract the effects of interferon gamma.

Intermittent self-catheterization (ISC) A procedure in which the person periodically inserts a catheter into the urinary opening to drain urine from the bladder. ISC is used in the management of bladder dysfunction to drain urine that remains after voiding, prevent bladder distention, prevent kidney damage, and restore bladder function.

Internuclear ophthalmoplegia A disturbance of coordinated eye movements in which the eye turned outward to look toward the side develops nystagmus (rapid, involuntary movements) while the other eye simultaneously fails to turn completely inward. This neurologic sign, of which the person is usually unaware, can be detected during the neurologic exam.

Intrathecal space The space surrounding the brain and spinal cord that contains cerebrospinal fluid.

Intravenous Within a vein; often used in the context of an injection into a vein of medication dissolved in a liquid.

Lesion *See* Plaque.

Leukocyte White blood cell.

L'Hermitte's sign An abnormal sensation of electricity or "pins and needles" going down the spine into the arms and legs that occurs when the neck is bent forward so that the chin touches the chest.

Living will *See* Advance (medical) directive.

Loftstrand crutch A type of crutch with an attached holder for the forearm that provides extra support.

Lumbar puncture   A diagnostic procedure that uses a hollow needle (canula) to penetrate the spinal canal at the level of third–fourth or fourth–fifth lumbar vertebrae to remove cerebrospinal fluid for analysis. This procedure is used to examine the cerebrospinal fluid for changes in composition that are characteristic of MS (e.g., elevated white cell count, elevated protein content, the presence of oligoclonal bands).

Lymphocyte   A type of white blood cell that is part of the immune system. Lymphocytes can be subdivided into two main groups: B-lymphocytes, which originate in the bone marrow and produce antibodies; T-lymphocytes, which are produced in the bone marrow and mature in the thymus. Helper T-lymphocytes heighten the production of antibodies by B-lymphocytes; suppressor T-lymphocytes suppress B-lymphocyte activity and seem to be in short supply during an MS exacerbation.

Macrophage   A white blood cell with scavenger characteristics that has the ability to ingest and destroy foreign substances such as bacteria and cell debris.

Magnetic resonance imaging (MRI)   A diagnostic procedure that produces visual images of different body parts without the use of X-rays. Nuclei of atoms are influenced by a high frequency electromagnetic impulse inside a strong magnetic field. The nuclei then give off resonating signals that can produce pictures of parts of the body. An important diagnostic tool in MS, MRI makes it possible to visualize and count lesions in the white matter of the brain and spinal cord.

Marcus Gunn pupil   *See* Afferent pupillary defect.

Minimal Record of Disability (MRD)   A standardized method for quantifying the clinical status of a person with MS. The MRD is made up of five parts: demographic information; the Neurological Functional Systems (developed by John Kurtzke), which assign scores to clinical findings for each of the various neurologic systems in the brain and spinal cord (pyramidal, cerebellar, brainstem, sensory, visual, mental, bowel and bladder); the Disability Status Scale (developed by John Kurtzke), which gives a single composite score for the person's disease; the Incapacity Status Scale, which is an inventory of functional disabilities relating to activities of daily living; the Environmental Status Scale, which provides an assessment of social handicap resulting from chronic illness. The MRD has two main functions: to assist doctors and other professionals in planning and coordinating the care of persons with MS, and to provide a standardized means of recording repeated clinical evaluations of individuals for research purposes.

Monoclonal antibodies   Laboratory-produced antibodies, which can be programmed to react against a specific antigen in order to suppress the immune response.

Motor neurons   Nerve cells of the brain and spinal cord that enable movement of various parts of the body.

Motor point block   *See* Nerve block.

MRI   *See* Magnetic resonance imaging.

Muscle tone   A characteristic of a muscle brought about by the constant flow of nerve stimuli to that muscle, which describes its resistance to stretching. Abnormal muscle tone can be defined as: hypertonus (increased muscle tone, as in spasticity); hypotonus (reduced muscle tone); flaccid (paralysis); atony (loss of muscle tone). Muscle tone is evaluated as part of the standard neurologic exam in MS.

Myelin   A soft, white coating of nerve fibers in the central nervous system, composed of lipids (fats) and protein. Myelin serves as insulation and as an aid to efficient nerve fiber conduction. When myelin is damaged in MS, nerve fiber conduction is faulty or absent. Impaired bodily functions or altered sensations associated with those demyelinated nerve fibers are identified as symptoms of MS in various parts of the body.

Myelin basic protein   Proteins associated with the myelin of the central nervous system that may be found in higher than normal concentrations in the cerebrospinal fluid of individuals with MS and other diseases that damage myelin.

Myelitis   An inflammatory disease of the spinal cord. In transverse myelitis, the inflammation spreads across the tissue of the spinal cord, resulting in a loss of its normal function to transmit nerve impulses up and down, as though the spinal cord had been severed.

Myelogram   An X-ray procedure by which the spinal canal and the spinal cord can be visualized. It is performed in conjunction with a lumbar puncture and injection of a special X-ray contrast material into the spinal canal.

Nerve   A bundle of nerve fibers (axons). The fibers are either afferent (leading toward the brain and serving in the perception of sensory stimuli of the skin, joints, muscles, and inner organs) or efferent (leading away from the brain and mediating contractions of muscles or organs).

Nerve block   A procedure used to relieve otherwise intractable spasticity, including painful flexor spasms. An injection of phenol into the affected nerve interferes with the function of that nerve for up to three months, potentially increasing a person's comfort and mobility.

Nervous system   Includes all of the neural structures in the body: the central nervous system consists of the brain, spinal cord, and optic nerves; the peripheral nervous system consists of the nerve roots, nerve plexi, and nerves throughout the body.

Neuroendocrine   Refers to the relationship between the body's nervous system and endocrine system, whereby certain cells in the body release hormones in response to a neural stimulus.

Neurogenic   Related to activity of the nervous system, as in "neurogenic bladder."

Neurogenic bladder   Bladder dysfunction associated with neurologic malfunction in the spinal cord and characterized by a failure to empty, failure to store, or a combination of the two. Symptoms that result from these three types of dysfunction include urinary urgency, frequency, hesitancy, nocturia, and incontinence.

Neurologist   Physician who specializes in the diagnosis and treatment of conditions related to the nervous system.

Neurology   Study of the central, peripheral, and autonomic nervous system.

Neuron   The basic nerve cell of the nervous system. A neuron consists of a nucleus within a cell body and one or more processes (extensions) called dendrites and axons.

Neuropsychologist   A psychologist with specialized training in the evaluation of cognitive functions. Neuropsychologists use a battery of standardized tests to assess specific cognitive functions and identify areas of cognitive impairment. They also provide remediation for individuals with MS-related cognitive impairment. *See* Cognition and Cognitive impairment.

Nocturia   The need to urinate during the night.

Nystagmus   Rapid, involuntary movements of the eyes in the horizontal or, occasionally, the vertical direction.

Occupational therapist (OT)   Occupational therapists assess functioning in activities of everyday living, including dressing, bathing, grooming, meal preparation, writing, and driving, which are essential for independent living. In making treatment recommendations, the OT addresses (1) fatigue management, (2) upper body strength, movement, and coordination, (3) adaptations to the home and work environment, including both structural changes and specialized equipment for particular activities, and (4) compensatory strategies for impairments in thinking, sensation, or vision.

Oligoclonal bands   A diagnostic sign indicating abnormal levels of certain antibodies in the cerebrospinal fluid; seen in approximately 90 percent of people with multiple sclerosis, but not specific to MS.

Oligodendrocyte   A type of cell in the central nervous system that is responsible for making and supporting myelin.

Ophthalmoscope   An instrument designed for examination of the interior of the eye.

Optic atrophy   A wasting of the optic disc that results from partial or complete degeneration of optic nerve fibers and is associated with a loss of visual acuity.

Optic disc   The small blind spot on the surface of the retina where cells of the retina converge to form the optic nerve; the only part of the retina that is insensitive to light.

Optic neuritis   Inflammation or demyelination of the optic (visual) nerve with transient or permanent impairment of vision and occasionally pain.

Orthotic   Also called orthosis; a mechanical appliance such as a leg brace or splint that is specially designed to control, correct, or compensate for impaired limb function.

Orthotist   A person skilled in making mechanical appliances (orthotics) such as leg braces or splints that help to support limb function. *See* Orthotic.

Oscillopsia   Continuous, involuntary, and chaotic eye movements that result in a visual disturbance in which objects appear to be jumping or bouncing.

Osteoporosis   Decalcification of the bones, which can result from the lack of mobility experienced by wheelchair-bound individuals.

Paralysis   Inability to move a part of the body.

Paraparesis   A weakness but not total paralysis of the lower extremities (legs).

Paraplegia   Paralysis of both lower extremities (legs).

Paresis   Partial or incomplete paralysis of a part of the body.

Paresthesia   A spontaneously occurring sensation of burning, prickling, tingling, or creeping on the skin that may or may not be associated with any physical findings on neurologic examination.

Paroxysmal spasm   A sudden, uncontrolled limb contraction that occurs intermittently, lasts for a few moments, and then subsides.

Paroxysmal symptom   Any one of several symptoms that have sudden onset, apparently in response to some kind of movement or sensory stimulation, last for a few moments, and then subside. Paroxysmal symptoms tend to occur frequently in those individuals who have them, and follow a similar pattern from one episode to the next. Examples of paroxysmal symptoms include acute episodes of trigeminal neuralgia (sharp facial pain), tonic seizures (intense spasm of limb or limbs on one side of the body), dysarthria (slurred speech often accompanied by loss of balance and coordination), and various paresthesias (sensory disturbances ranging from tingling to severe pain).

PEG   *See* Percutaneous endoscopic gastrostomy.

Percutaneous endoscopic gastrostomy (PEG)   A PEG is a tube inserted into the stomach through the abdominal wall to provide food or other nutrients when eating by mouth is not possible. The tube is inserted in a bedside procedure using an endoscope to guide the tube through a small abdominal incision. An endoscope is a lighted instrument that allows the doctor to see inside the stomach.

Percutaneous rhizotomy   An outpatient surgical procedure used in the management of severe, intractable trigeminal neuralgia. The surgeon makes a tiny incision in the side of the person's face and blocks the function of the trigeminal nerve using laser surgery, cryosurgery (freezing), or cauterization.

Periventricular region   The area surrounding the four fluid-filled cavities within the brain. MS plaques are commonly found within this region.

Physiatrist   Physicians who specialize in physical medicine and rehabilitation of physical impairments.

Physical therapist (PT)   Physical therapists are trained to evaluate and improve movement and function of the body, with particular attention to physical mobility, balance, posture, fatigue, and pain. The physical therapy program typically involves (1) educating the person with MS about the physical problems caused by the disease, (2) designing an individualized exercise program to address the problems, and (3) enhancing mobility and energy conservation through the use of a variety of mobility aids and adaptive equipment.

Placebo   An inactive, non-drug compound that is designed to look just like the test drug. It is administered to control group subjects in double-blind clinical trials (in which neither the researchers nor the subjects know who is getting the drug and who is getting the placebo) as a means of assessing the benefits and liabilities of the test drug taken by experimental group subjects.

Placebo effect   An apparently beneficial result of therapy that occurs because of the patient's expectation that the therapy will help.

Plantar reflex   A reflex response obtained by drawing a pointed object along the outer border of the sole of the foot from the heel to the little toe. The normal flexor response is a bunching and downward movement of the toes. An upward movement of the big toe is called an extensor response, or Babinski reflex, which is a sensitive indicator of disease in the brain or spinal cord.

Plaque   An area of inflamed or demyelinated central nervous system tissue.

Plasma cell   A lymphocyte-like cell found in the bone marrow, connective tissue, and blood that is involved in the body's immune system. *See also* Lymphocyte.

Plasma exchange Plasma exchange involves removing blood from the person, mechanically separating the blood cells from the fluid plasma, mixing the blood cells with replacement plasma, and returning the blood mixture to the body. The rationale for plasma exchange is that the plasma contains immune factors that may stimulate disease activity. Substituting replacement plasma may dilute the strength of these potentially destructive immune factors. However, the detailed mechanisms involved are not yet clearly understood.

Plasmapharesis *See* plasma exchange

Position sense The ability to tell, with one's eyes closed, where fingers and toes are in space. Position sense is evaluated during the standard neurologic exam in MS.

Post-void residual test (PVR) The PVR test involves passing a catheter into the bladder following urination in order to drain and measure any urine that is left in the bladder after urination is completed. The PVR is a simple but effective technique for diagnosing bladder dysfunction in MS.

Postural tremor Rhythmic shaking that occurs when the muscles are tensed to hold an object or stay in a given position.

Power grading A measurement of muscle strength used to evaluate weakness or paralysis. Power is tested as part of the standard neurologic exam in MS.

Prevalence The number of all new and old cases of a disease in a defined population at a particular point in time.

Primary progressive MS A clinical course of MS characterized from the beginning by progressive disease, with no plateaus or remissions, or an occasional plateau and very short-lived, minor improvements.

Prognosis Prediction of the future course of the disease.

Progressive-relapsing MS A clinical course of MS that shows disease progression from the beginning, but with clear, acute relapses, with or without full recovery from those relapses along the way.

Prospective memory The ability to remember an event or commitment scheduled for the future. Thus, a person who agrees to meet or call someone at a given time on the following day must be able to remember the appointment when the time comes. People with MS-related memory impairment frequently report problems with this type of memory for upcoming appointments.

Pseudo-bulbar affect   *See* Affective release.

Pseudo-exacerbation   A temporary aggravation of disease symptoms, resulting from an elevation in body temperature or other stressor (e.g., an infection, severe fatigue, constipation), that disappears once the stressor is removed. A pseudo-exacerbation involves symptom flare-up rather than new disease activity or progression.

Pyramidal tracts   Motor nerve pathways in the brain and spinal cord that connect nerve cells in the brain to the motor cells located in the cranial, thoracic, and lumbar parts of the spinal cord. Damage to these tracts causes spastic paralysis or weakness.

Pyuria   The presence of pus in the urine, causing it to appear cloudy; indicative of bacterial infection in the urinary tract.

Quad cane   A cane that has a broad base on four short "feet," which provide extra stability.

Quadriplegia   The paralysis of both arms and both legs.

Recent memory   The ability to remember events, conversations, content of reading material or television programs from a short time ago, i.e., an hour or two ago or last night. People with MS-related memory impairment typically experience greatest difficulty remembering these types of things in the recent past.

Reflex   An involuntary response of the nervous system to a stimulus, such as the stretch reflex, which is elicited by tapping a tendon with a reflex hammer, resulting in a contraction. Increased, diminished, or absent reflexes can be indicative of neurologic damage, including MS, and are therefore tested as part of the standard neurologic exam.

Rehabilitation   Rehabilitation in MS involves the intermittent or ongoing use of multidisciplinary strategies (e.g., physiatry, physical terapy, occupational therapy, speech therapy) to promote functional independence, prevent unnecessary complications, and enhance overall quality of life. It is an active process directed toward helping the person recover and/or maintain the highest possible level of functioning and realize his or her optimal physical, mental, and social potential given any limitations that exist.   Rehabilitation is also an interactive, ongoing process of education and enablement in which people with MS and their care partners are active participants rather than passive recipients.

Relapsing-remitting MS   A clinical course of MS that is characterized by clearly defined, acute attacks with full or partial recovery and no disease progression between attacks.

Remission   A lessening in the severity of symptoms or their temporary disappearance during the course of the illness.

Remote memory   The ability to remember people or events from the distant past. People with MS tend to experience few, if any, problems with their remote memory.

Remyelination   The repair of damaged myelin. Myelin repair occurs spontaneously in MS but very slowly. Research is currently underway to find a way to speed the healing process.

Residual urine   Urine that remains in the bladder following urination.

Retrobulbar neuritis   *See* Optic neuritis.

Romberg's sign   The inability to maintain balance in a standing position with feet and legs drawn together and eyes closed.

Scanning speech   Abnormal speech characterized by staccato-like articulation that sounds clipped because the person unintentionally pauses between syllables and skips some of the sounds.

Sclerosis   Hardening of tissue. In MS, sclerosis is the body's replacement of lost myelin around CNS nerve cells with scar tissue.

Scotoma   A gap or blind spot in the visual field.

Secondary progressive MS   A clinical course of MS that initially is relapsing-remitting and then becomes progressive at a variable rate, possibly with an occasional relapse and minor remission.

Sensory   Related to bodily sensations such as pain, smell, taste, temperature, vision, hearing, acceleration, and position in space.

Sepsis   The presence of sufficient bacteria in the blood to cause illness.

Sign   An objective physical problem or abnormality identified by the physician during the neurologic examination. Neurologic signs may differ significantly from the symptoms reported by the patient because they are identifiable only with specific tests and may cause no overt symptoms. Common neurologic signs in multiple sclerosis include altered eye movements and other changes in the appearance or function of the visual system; altered reflexes; weakness; spasticity; circumscribed sensory changes.

Somatosensory evoked potential A test that measures the brain's electrical activity in response to repeated (mild) electrical stimulation of different parts of the body. Demyelination results in a slowing of response time. This test is useful in the diagnosis of MS because it can confirm the presence of a suspected lesion (area of demyelination) or identify the presence of an unsuspected lesion that has produced no symptoms.

Spasticity Abnormal increase in muscle tone, manifested as a spring-like resistance to moving or being moved.

Speech/language pathologist Speech/language pathologists specialize in the diagnosis and treatment of speech and swallowing disorders. A person with MS may be referred to a speech/language pathologist for help with either one or both of these problems. Because of their expertise with speech and language difficulties, these specialists also provide cognitive remediation for individuals with cognitive impairment.

Sphincter A circular band of muscle fibers that tightens or closes a natural opening of the body, such as the external anal sphincter, which closes the anus, and the internal and external urinary sphincters, which close the urinary canal.

Sphincterotomy A surgical enlargement of the urinary sphincter in a male whose spasticity is so severe that he cannot empty his bladder. Once the surgery is performed, the man loses urinary control and must wear an external, condom catheter to collect the urine. This procedure is seldom required in MS. It is performed only on males because urinary drainage problems in females might lead to skin breakdown.

Spinal tap *See* Lumbar puncture.

Spirometer An instrument used to assess lung function; it measures the volume and flow rate of inhaled and exhaled air.

Spontaneous voiding *See* Incontinence.

Stance ataxia   An inability to stand upright due to disturbed coordination of the involved muscles, which results in swaying and a tendency to fall in one or another direction.

Steroids   *See* ACTH; Corticosteroid; Glucocorticoid hormones.

Suppressor T-lymphocytes   White blood cells that act as part of the immune system and may be in short supply during an MS exacerbation.

Symptom   A subjectively perceived problem or complaint reported by the patient. In multiple sclerosis, common symptoms include visual problems, fatigue, sensory changes, weakness or paralysis of limbs, tremor, lack of coordination, poor balance, bladder or bowel changes, and psychological changes.

T-cell   A lymphocyte (white blood cell) that develops in the bone marrow, matures in the thymus, and works as part of the immune system in the body.

Tandem gait   A test of balance and coordination that involves alternately placing the heel of one foot directly against the toes of the other foot.

Tenotomy   An irreversible surgical procedure performed to cut severely contracted tendons attached to muscles that do not respond to any other type of spasticity control and are causing intractable pain and skin complications related to lack of physical movement.

Titubation   A form of tremor, resulting from demyelination in the cerebellum, that manifests itself primarily in the head and neck.

Tonic seizure   An intense spasm that lasts for a few minutes and affects one or both limbs on one side of the body. Like other types of paroxysmal symptoms in MS, these spasms occur abruptly and fairly frequently in those individuals who have them, and are similar from one brief episode to the next. The attacks may be triggered by movement or occur spontaneously. *See* Paroxysmal symptom.

Transcutaneous electric nerve stimulation (TENS)   TENS is a nonaddictive and noninvasive method of pain control that applies electric impulses to nerve endings via electrodes that are attached to a stimulator by flexible wires and placed on the skin. The electric impulses block the transmission of pain signals to the brain.

Transurethral resection A procedure to remove excess thickened tissue at the point of connection between the bladder and the urethra. This thickened tissue, which occasionally develops with the prolonged use of a Foley catheter, obstructs the flow of urine when the catheter is removed. This procedure is quite uncommon and is done mostly in males.

Transverse myelitis An acute attack of inflammatory demyelination that involves both sides of the spinal cord. The spinal cord loses its ability to transmit nerve impulses up and down. Paralysis and numbness are experienced in the legs and trunk below the level of the inflammation.

Trigeminal neuralgia Lightning-like, acute pain in the face caused by demyelination of nerve fibers at the site where the sensory (trigeminal) nerve root for that part of the face enters the brainstem.

Urethra Duct or tube that drains the urinary bladder.

Urinary frequency Feeling the urge to urinate even when urination has occurred very recently.

Urinary hesitancy The inability to void urine spontaneously even though the urge to do so is present.

Urinary incontinence *See* Incontinence.

Urinary sphincter The muscle closing the urethra, which in a state of flaccid paralysis causes urinary incontinence and in a state of spastic paralysis results in an inability to urinate.

Urinary urgency The inability to postpone urination once the need to void has been felt.

Urine culture and sensitivity (C & S) A diagnostic procedure to test for urinary tract infection and identify the appropriate treatment. Bacteria from a mid-stream urine sample is allowed to grow for three days in a laboratory medium and then tested for sensitivity to a variety of antibiotics.

Urologist A physician who specializes in the branch of medicine (urology) concerned with the anatomy, physiology, disorders, and care of the male and female urinary tract, as well as the male genital tract.

Urology A medical specialty that deals with disturbances of the urinary (male and female) and reproductive (male) organs.

Vertigo A dizzying sensation of the environment spinning, often accompanied by nausea and vomiting.

Vibration sense   The ability to feel vibrations against various parts of the body. Vibration sense is tested (with a tuning fork) as part of the sensory portion of the neurologic exam.

Videofluoroscopy   A radiographic study of a person's swallowing mechanism that is recorded on videotape. Videofluoroscopy shows the physiology of the pharynx, the location of the swallowing difficulty, and confirms whether or not food particles or fluids are being aspirated into the airway.

Visual acuity   Clarity of vision. Acuity is measured as a fraction of normal vision. 20/20 vision indicates an eye that sees at 20 feet what a normal eye should see at 20 feet; 20/400 vision indicates an eye that sees at 20 feet what a normal eye sees at 400 feet.

Visual evoked potential   A test in which the brain's electrical activity in response to visual stimuli (e.g., a flashing checkerboard) is recorded by an electroencephalograph and analyzed by computer. Demyelination results in a slowing of response time. Because this test is able to confirm the presence of a suspected brain lesion (area of demyelination) as well as identify the presence of an unsuspected lesion that has produced no symptoms, it is extremely useful in diagnosing MS. VEPs are abnormal in approximately 90 percent of people with MS.

Vocational rehabilitation (VR)   Vocational rehabilitation is a program of services designed to enable people with disabilities to become or remain employed. Originally mandated by the Rehabilitation Act of 1973, VR programs are carried out by individually created state agencies. In order to be eligible for VR, a person must have a physical or mental disability that results in a substantial handicap to employment. VR programs typically involve evaluation of the disability and need for adaptive equipment or mobility aids, vocational guidance, training, job-placement, and follow-up.

White matter   The part of the brain that contains myelinated nerve fibers and appears white, in contrast to the cortex of the brain, which contains nerve cell bodies and appears gray.

Appendix B

Medications Commonly Used in Multiple Sclerosis

The information contained in these sheets will help you to be more informed about the medications you are taking and therefore more able to discuss your questions and concerns with your physician. This information should never be used as a substitute for your own physician's instructions and recommendations.

The following guidelines apply to the use of any and all of the medications that you take:

◇ Make sure that your physician knows your medical history, including all medical conditions for which you are currently being treated and any allergies you have.

◇ Tell your physician if you are breast-feeding, currently pregnant, or planning to become pregnant in the near future.

◇ Make a list of all of the drugs you are currently taking—including both prescription and over-the-counter medications—and provide your physician with a copy for your medical chart.

◇ Take your medications only as your physician prescribes them for you. If you have questions about the recommended dosage, ask your physician.

◇ Unless otherwise instructed, store medications in a cool, dry place; exposure to heat or moisture may cause the medication to break down. Liquid medications that are stored in the refrigerator should not be allowed to freeze.

◇ Unless otherwise directed by your physician or pharmacist, the general instructions concerning a missed dose of medication are as follows: if you miss a dose, take it as soon as possible. However, if it is almost time for your next dose, skip the one you missed and go back to the regular dosing schedule. Do not double dose.

◇ Keep all medications out of the reach of children.

The following table lists all of the products described in this appendix. For each product, the table gives the generic or chemical name, the brand name, and the common usage in MS, as well as its availability in the United States and Canada. Products available without a prescription are so indicated.

GENERIC NAME	BRAND NAME[2]	USAGE IN MS
Alprostadil	Prostin VR	Erectile dysfunction
Alprostadil	Muse	Erectile dysfunction
Amantadine		Fatigue
Amitriptyline	Elavil	Pain (paresthesias)
Baclofen	Lioresal	Spasticity
Bisacodyl[1]	Dulcolax	Constipation
Carbamazepine	Tegretol	Pain (trigeminal neuralgia)
Ciprofloxacin	Cipro	Urinary tract infections
Clonazepam	Klonopin (US); Rivotril (Can)	Tremor; Pain; Spasticity
Diazepam	Valium	Spasticity (muscle spasms)
Docusate[1]	Colace	Constipation
Docusate mini enema[1]	Therevac Plus (US)	Constipation
Fluoxetine	Prozac	Depression; Fatigue
Gabapentin	Neurontin	Pain (dysesthesias; spasticity)
Glatiramer acetate	Copaxone	Disease modifying agent
Glycerin[1]	Sani-Supp suppository (US)	Constipation
Imipramine	Tofranil	Bladder dysfunction; Pain
Interferon beta-1a	Avonex	Disease modifying agent
Interferon beta-1a	Rebif (Canada)	Disease modifying agent

[1]Available without a prescription
[2]Available in both US and Canada unless otherwise noted

Interferon beta-1b	Betaseron	Disease modifying agent
Magnesium hydroxide[1]	Phillips' Milk of Magnesia	Constipation
Meclizine	Antivert (US); Bonamine (Can)	Nausea; Vomiting; Dizziness
Methenamine	Hiprex, Mandelamine (US); Hip-rex, Mandelamine (Can)	Urinary tract infections (preventative)
Methylprednisolone	Depo-Medrol	Acute exacerbations
Mineral oil[1]		Constipation
Nitrofurantoin	Macrodantin	Urinary tract infections
Nortriptyline	Pamelor (US); Aventyl (Can)	Pain (parasthesias)
Oxybutynin	Ditropan	Bladder dysfunction
Oxybutynin (extended release formula)	Ditropan XL	Bladder dysfunction
Papaverine		Erectile dysfunction
Paroxetine	Paxil	Depression
Pemoline	Cylert	Fatigue
Phenazopyridine	Pyridium	Urinary tract infections (symptom relief)
Phenytoin	Dilantin	Pain (dyesthesias)
Prednisone	Deltasone	Acute exacerbations
Propantheline bromide	Pro-Banthine	Bladder dysfunction
Psyllium hydrophilic mucilloid[1]	Metamucil	Constipation
Sertraline	Zoloft	Depression
Sildenafil	Viagra	Erectile dysfunction
Sodium phosphate[1]	Fleet Enema	Constipation
Sulfamethoxazole	Bactrim; Septra	Urinary tract infections
Tizanidine	Zanaflex	Spasticity
Tolterodine	Detrol (US)	Bladder dysfunction
Venlafaxine	Effexor	Depression

[1]Available without a prescription
[2]Available in both US and Canada unless otherwise noted

Chemical Name: Alprostadil (al-**pross**-ta-dill); also called Prostaglandin E1

Brand Name: Prostin VR (U.S. and Canada)

Generic Available: No

Description: Alprostadil belongs to a group of medicines called vasodilators, which cause blood vessels to expand, thereby increasing blood flow. When alprostadil is injected into the penis, it produces an erection by increasing blood flow to the penis.

Proper Usage

◇ Alprostadil should never be used as a sexual aid by men who are not impotent. If improperly used, this medication can cause permanent damage to the penis.

◇ Alprostadil is available by prescription and should be used only as directed by your physician, who will instruct you in the proper way to give yourself an injection so that it is simple and essentially pain-free.

◇ Alprostadil is sometimes used in combination with a medicine called phentolamine (Regitine—U.S.; Rogitine—Canada).

Precautions

◇ Do not use more of this medicine or use it more often than it has been prescribed for you. Using too much of this medicine will result in a condition called priapism, in which the erection lasts too long and does not resolve when it should. Permanent damage to the penis can occur if blood flow to the penis is cut off for too long a period of time.

Possible Side Effects

◇ Side effects that you should report to your physician so he or she can adjust the dosage or change the medication: pain at the injection site; burning or aching during erection.

◇ Rare side effects that require immediate attention: erection continuing for more than four hours. If you cannot be seen immediately by your physician, you should go to the emergency room for prompt treatment.

Chemical Name: Alprostadil (al-**pross**-ta-dill); also called Prostaglandin E1

Brand Name: MUSE (U.S. and Canada) [suppository form]

Generic Available: No

Description: Alprostadil belongs to a group of medicines called vasodilators, which cause blood vessels to expand, thereby increasing blood flow. MUSE is a semisolid pellet of medication in the form of a suppository. When the suppository is inserted into the urethra, it produces an erection by increasing blood flow to the penis.

Proper Usage

◇ Alprostadil should never be used as a sexual aid by men who are not impotent. If improperly used, this medication can cause permanent damage to the penis.

◇ Alprostadil is available by prescription and should be used only as directed by your physician, who will instruct you in the proper way to insert the suppository.

Precautions

◇ Do not use more of this medicine or use it more often than it has been prescribed for you. Using too much of this medicine will result in a condition called priapism, in which the erection lasts too long and does not resolve when it should. Permanent damage to the penis can occur if blood flow to the penis is cut off for too long a period of time.

Possible Side Effects

◇ Side effects that you should report to your physician so he or she can adjust the dosage or change the medication: pain at the injection site; burning or aching during erection.

◇ Rare side effects that require immediate attention: erection continuing for more than four hours. If you cannot be seen immediately by your physician, you should go to the emergency room for prompt treatment.

Chemical Name: Amantadine (a-**man**-ta-deen)
Brand Name: Symmetrel (U.S. and Canada)
Generic Available: Yes (U.S.)
Description: Amantadine is an antiviral medication used to prevent or treat certain influenza infections; it is also given as an
adjunct for the treatment of Parkinson's disease. It has been
demonstrated that this medication, through some unknown
mechanism, is sometimes effective in relieving fatigue in multiple sclerosis.

Proper Usage

◇ The usual dosage for the management of fatigue in MS is
100 to 200 mg daily, taken in the earlier part of the day in
order to avoid sleep disturbance. Doses in excess of 300 mg
daily usually cause livedo reticularis, a blotchy discoloration of the skin of the legs.

Precautions

The precautions listed here pertain to the use of this medication
as an antiviral or Parkinson's disease treatment. There are no
reports at this time concerning the precautions in the use of the
drug to treat fatigue in multiple sclerosis.

◇ Drinking alcoholic beverages while taking this medication
may cause increased side effects such as circulation problems, dizziness, lightheadedness, fainting, or confusion.
Do not drink alcohol while taking this medication.
◇ This medication may cause some people to become dizzy,
confused, or lightheaded, or to have blurred vision or trouble concentrating.
◇ Amantadine may cause dryness of the mouth and throat. If
your mouth continues to feel dry for more than two weeks,
check with your physician or dentist since continuing dryness may increase the risk of dental disease.
◇ This medication may cause purplish red, net-like, blotchy
spots on the skin. This problem occurs more often in
females and usually occurs on the legs and/or feet after
amantadine has been taken regularly for a month or more.
The blotchy spots usually go away within two to twelve
weeks after you stop taking the medication.

◇ Studies of the effects of amantadine in pregnancy have not been done in humans. Studies in some animals have shown that amantadine is harmful to the fetus and causes birth defects.

◇ Amantadine passes into breast milk. However, the effect of amantadine in newborn babies and infants is not known.

Possible Side Effects

The side effects listed here pertain to the use of amantadine as an antiviral or Parkinson's disease treatment. There are no reports at the present time of the side effects associated with the use of this drug in the treatment of MS-related fatigue.

◇ Side effects that may go away as your body adjusts to the medication and do not require medical attention unless they continue or are bothersome: difficulty concentrating; dizziness; headache; irritability; loss of appetite; nausea; nervousness; purplish red, net-like, blotchy spots on skin; trouble sleeping or nightmares; constipation*; dryness of the mouth; vomiting.

◇ Rare side effects that should be reported as soon as possible to your physician: blurred vision*; confusion; difficult urination*; fainting; hallucinations; convulsions; unusual difficulty in coordination*; irritation and swelling of the eye; mental depression; skin rash; swelling of feet or lower legs; unexplained shortness of breath.

*Since it may be difficult to distinguish between certain common symptoms of MS and some side effects of amantadine, be sure to consult your health care professional if an abrupt change of this type continues for more than a few days.

Chemical Name: Amitriptyline (a-mee-**trip**-ti-leen)
Brand Name: Elavil (U.S. and Canada)
Generic Available: Yes (U.S. and Canada)
Description: Amitriptyline is a tricyclic antidepressant used to treat mental depression. In multiple sclerosis, it is frequently used to treat painful paresthesias in the arms and legs (e.g., burning sensations, pins and needles, stabbing pains) caused by damage to the pain regulating pathways of the brain and spinal cord.
Note: Other tricyclic antidepressants are also used for the management of neurologic pain symptoms. Clomipramine (Anafranil—U.S. and Canada), desipramine (Norpramin—U.S. and Canada), doxepin (Sinequan—U.S. and Canada), imipramine (Tofranil—U.S. and Canada), nortriptyline (Pamelor—U.S.; Aventyl—Canada), trimipramine (U.S. and Canada). While each of these medications is given in different dosage levels, the precautions and side effects listed for amitriptyline apply to these other tricyclic medications as well.

Precautions

◇ Amitriptyline adds to the effects of alcohol and other central nervous system depressants (e.g., antihistamines, sedatives, tranquilizers, prescription pain medications, seizure medications, muscle relaxants, sleeping medications), possibly causing drowsiness. Be sure that your physician knows if you are taking these or other medications.

◇ This medication causes dryness of the mouth. Because continuing dryness of the mouth may increase the risk of dental disease, alert your dentist that you are taking amitriptyline.

◇ This medication may cause your skin to be more sensitive to sunlight than it is normally. Even brief exposure to sunlight may cause a skin rash, itching, redness or other discoloration of the skin, or severe sunburn.

◇ This medication may affect blood sugar levels of diabetic individuals. If you notice a change in the results of your blood or urine sugar tests, check with your physician.

◇ Do not stop taking this medication without consulting your physician. The physician may want you to reduce the amount you are taking gradually in order to reduce the possibility of withdrawal symptoms such as headache, nausea, and/or an overall feeling of discomfort.

◇ Studies of amitriptyline have not been done in pregnant women. There have been reports of newborns suffering from muscle spasms and heart, breathing, and urinary problems when their mothers had taken tricyclic antidepressants immediately before delivery. Studies in animals have indicated the possibility of unwanted effects in the fetus.

◇ Tricyclics pass into breast milk. Only doxepin (Sinequan) has been reported to cause drowsiness in the nursing baby.

Possible Side Effects

◇ Side effects that may go away as your body adjusts to the medication and do not require medical attention unless they continue for more than two weeks or are bothersome: dryness of mouth; constipation*; increased appetite and weight gain; dizziness; drowsiness*; decreased sexual ability*; headache; nausea; unusual tiredness or weakness*; unpleasant taste; diarrhea; heartburn; increased sweating; vomiting.

◇ Uncommon side effects that should be reported to your physician as soon as possible: blurred vision*; confusion or delirium; difficulty speaking or swallowing*; eye pain*; fainting; hallucinations; loss of balance control*; nervousness or restlessness; problems urinating*; shakiness or trembling; stiffness of arms and legs*.

◇ Rare side effects that should be reported to your physician as soon as possible: anxiety; breast enlargement in males and females; hair loss; inappropriate secretion of milk in females; increased sensitivity to sunlight; irritability; muscle twitching; red or brownish spots on the skin; buzzing or other unexplained sounds in the ears; skin rash, itching; sore throat and fever; swelling of face and tongue; weakness*; yellow skin.

◇ Symptoms of acute overdose: confusion; convulsions; severe drowsiness*; enlarged pupils; unusual heartbeat; fever; hallucinations; restlessness and agitation; shortness of breath; unusual tiredness or weakness; vomiting.

---

*Since it may be difficult to distinguish between certain common symptoms of MS and some side effects of amitriptyline, be sure to consult your health care professional if an abrupt change of this type occurs.

Chemical Name: Baclofen (**bak**-loe-fen)

Brand Name: Lioresal (no longer available in the U.S.)

Generic Available: Yes (U.S. and Canada)

Description: Baclofen acts on the central nervous system to relieve spasms, cramping, and tightness of muscles caused by spasticity in multiple sclerosis. It is usually administered orally in pill form. Recently, an intrathecal delivery system (via a surgically implanted pump) has been approved for those individuals with significant spasticity who cannot tolerate a sufficiently high dose of the oral form of the medication.

Proper Usage

◇ People with MS are usually started on an initial dose of 5 mg every six to eight hours. If necessary, the amount is increased by 5 mg per dose every five days until symptoms improve. The goal of treatment is to find a dosage level that relieves spasticity without causing excessive weakness or fatigue. The effective dose may vary from 15 mg to 160 mg per day or more.

Precautions

◇ If you are taking more than 30 mg daily, do not stop taking this medication suddenly. Stopping high doses of this medication abruptly can cause convulsions, hallucinations, increases in muscle spasms or cramping, mental changes, or unusual nervousness or restlessness. Consult your physician about how to reduce the dosage gradually before stopping the medication completely.

◇ This drug adds to the effects of alcohol and other CNS depressants (such as antihistamines, sedatives, tranquilizers, prescription pain medications, seizure medications, other muscle relaxants), possibly causing drowsiness. Be sure that your physician knows if you are taking these or other medications.

◇ Studies of birth defects with baclofen have not been done with humans. Studies in animals have shown that baclofen, when given in doses several times higher than the amount given to humans, increases the chance of hernias, incomplete or slow development of bones in the fetus, and lower birth weight.

◇ Baclofen passes into the breast milk of nursing mothers but has not been reported to cause problems in nursing infants.

Possible Side Effects

◇ Side effects that typically go away as your body adjusts to the medication and do not require medical attention unless they continue for several weeks or are bothersome: drowsiness or unusual tiredness*; increased weakness*; dizziness or lightheadedness; confusion; unusual constipation*; new or unusual bladder symptoms*; trouble sleeping; unusual unsteadiness or clumsiness*.

◇ Unusual side effects that require immediate medical attention: fainting; hallucinations; severe mood changes; skin rash or itching.

◇ Symptoms of overdose: sudden onset of blurred or double vision*; convulsions; shortness of breath or troubled breathing; vomiting.

---

*Since it may be difficult to distinguish between certain common symptoms of MS and some side effects of baclofen, be sure to consult your health care professional if an abrupt change of this type occurs.

Chemical Name: Bisacodyl (bis-a-**koe**-dill)

Brand Name: Dulcolax—tablet or suppository (U.S.); Bisaco-lax—tablet or suppository (Canada)

Generic Available: Yes (U.S. and Canada)

Description: Bisacodyl is an over-the-counter stimulant laxative that can be used in either oral or suppository form. Stimulant laxatives encourage bowel movements by increasing the muscle contractions in the intestinal wall that propel the stool mass. Although stimulant laxatives are popular for self-treatment, they are more likely to cause side effects than other types of laxatives.

Proper Usage

◇ Laxatives are to be used to provide short-term relief only, unless otherwise directed by the nurse or physician who is helping you to manage your bowel symptoms. A regimen that includes a healthy diet containing roughage (whole grain breads and cereals, bran, fruit, and green, leafy vegetables), six to eight full glasses of liquids each day, and some form of daily exercise is most important in stimulating healthy bowel function.

◇ If your physician has recommended this laxative for management of constipation, follow his or her recommendations for its use. If you are treating yourself for constipation, follow the directions on the package insert.

◇ The tablet form of this laxative is usually taken on an empty stomach in order to speed results. The tablets are coated to allow them to work properly without causing stomach irritation or upset. Do not chew or crush the tablets or take them within an hour of drinking milk or taking an antacid.

◇ A bedtime dose usually produces results the following morning. Be sure to consult your physician if you experience problems or do not get relief within a week.

Precautions

◇ Do not take any laxative if you have signs of appendicitis or inflamed bowel (e.g., stomach or lower abdominal pain, cramping, bloating, soreness, nausea, or vomiting). Check with your physician as soon as possible.

◇ Do not take any laxative for more than one week unless you have been told to do so by your physician. Many people tend to overuse laxatives, which often leads to dependence on the laxative action to produce a bowel movement. Discuss the use of laxatives with your health care professional in order to ensure that the laxative is used effectively as part of a comprehensive, healthy bowel management regimen.

◇ Do not take any laxative within two hours of taking other medication because the desired effectiveness of the other medication may be reduced.

◇ If you are pregnant, discuss with your physician the most appropriate type of laxative for you to use.

◇ Some laxatives pass into breast milk. Although it is unlikely to cause problems for a nursing infant, be sure to let your physician know if you are using a laxative and breast-feeding at the same time.

Possible Side Effects

◇ Side effects that may go away as your body adjusts to the medication and do not require medical attention unless they persist or are bothersome: belching; cramping; diarrhea; nausea.

◇ Unusual side effects that should be reported to your physician as soon as possible: confusion; irregular heartbeat; muscle cramps; skin rash, unusual tiredness or weakness.

Chemical Name: Carbamazepine (kar-ba-**maz**-e-peen)
Brand Name: Tegretol (U.S. and Canada)
Generic Available: Yes (U.S.)
Description: Carbamazepine is used to relieve shock-like pain, such as the facial pain caused by trigeminal neuralgia (tic douloureux).

Proper Usage

◇ It is very important that you take this medicine exactly as directed by your physician in order to obtain the best results and lessen the chance of serious side effects.

◇ Carbamazepine is not an ordinary pain reliever. It should be used only when your physician prescribes it for certain types of pain. Do not take this medication for other aches or pains.

◇ If you miss a dose of this medication, take it as soon as possible. If it is almost time for your next dose, skip the missed dose and go back to your regular dosing schedule. Do not double dose. If you miss more than one dose in a day, check with your physician.

◇ It is very important that your physician check your progress at regular intervals. Your physician may want to have certain tests done to see if you are receiving the correct amount of medication or to check for certain side effects of which you might be unaware.

Precautions

◇ Carbamazepine adds to the effects of alcohol and other central nervous system depressants that may cause drowsiness (e.g., antihistamines, sedatives, tranquilizers, prescription pain medications, seizure medications, muscle relaxants). Be sure that your physician knows if you are taking these or other medications.

◇ Some people who take carbamazepine may become more sensitive to sunlight than they are normally. Exposure to sunlight, even for brief periods of time, may cause a skin rash, itching, redness or other discoloration of the skin, or severe sunburn.

◇ Oral contraceptives (birth control pills) that contain estrogen may not work properly while you are taking carbamazepine. You should use an additional or alternative form of birth control while taking this drug.

◇ Carbamazepine affects the urine sugar levels of diabetic patients. If you notice a change in the results of your urine sugar tests, check with your physician.

◇ Before having any medical tests or any kind of surgical, dental, or emergency treatment, be sure to let the health care professional know that you are taking this medication.

◇ Carbamazepine has not been studied in pregnant women. There have been reports of babies having low birth weight, small head size, skull and facial defects, underdeveloped fingernails, and delays in growth when their mothers had taken carbamazepine in high doses during pregnancy. Studies in animals have shown that carbamazepine causes birth defects when given in large doses.

◇ Carbamazepine passes into breast milk, and the baby may receive enough of it to cause unwanted effects. In animal studies, carbamazepine has affected the growth and appearance of nursing babies.

Possible Side Effects

◇ Side effects that typically go away as your body adjusts to the medication and do not require medical attention unless they continue for several weeks or are bothersome: clumsiness or unsteadiness*; mild dizziness*; mild drowsiness*; lightheadedness; mild nausea or vomiting; aching joints or muscles; constipation*; diarrhea; dryness of mouth; skin sensitivity to sunlight; irritation of mouth or tongue; loss or appetite; loss of hair; muscle or abdominal cramps; sexual problems in males*.

◇ Check with your physician as soon as possible if any of the following side effects occur: blurred or double vision*; confusion; agitation; severe diarrhea, nausea, or vomiting; skin rash or hives; unusual drowsiness; chest pain; difficulty speaking or slurred speech*; fainting; frequent urination*; unusual heartbeat; mental depression or other mood or emotional changes; unusual numbness, tingling, pain, or weakness in hands or feet*; ringing or buzzing in ears; sudden decrease in urination; swelling of face, hands, feet, or lower legs; trembling; uncontrolled body movements; visual hallucinations.

◇ Check with your physician immediately if any of the following occur: black tarry stools or blood in urine or stools; bone or joint pain; cough or hoarseness; darkening of urine; nosebleeds or other unusual bleeding or bruising; painful or difficult urination; tenderness, swelling, or bluish color in leg or foot; pale stools; pinpoint red spots on skin; shortness of breath or cough; sores, ulcers, or white spots on lips or in the mouth; sore throat, chills, and fever; swollen glands; unusual tiredness or weakness*; wheezing, tightness in chest; yellow eyes or skin.

◇ Symptoms of overdose that require immediate attention: unusual clumsiness or unsteadiness*; severe dizziness or fainting; fast or irregular heartbeat; unusually high or low blood pressure; irregular or shallow breathing; severe nausea or vomiting; trembling, twitching, and abnormal body movements.

---

*Since it may be difficult to distinguish between certain common symptoms of MS and some side effects of carbamazepine, be sure to consult your health care professional if an abrupt change of this type occurs.

Chemical Name: Ciprofloxacin (sip-roe-**flox**-a-sin) combination
Brand Name: Cipro (U.S. and Canada)
Generic Available: No
Description: Ciprofloxacin is one of a group of antibiotics (fluo-
roquinolones) used to kill bacterial infection in many parts of
the body. It is used in multiple sclerosis primarily to treat urinary tract infections.

Proper Usage

◇ This medication is best taken with a full glass (eight
ounces) of water. Additional water should be taken each
day to help prevent some unwanted effects.

◇ Ciprofloxacin may be taken with meals or on an empty
stomach.

◇ Finish the full course of treatment prescribed by your
physician. Even if your symptoms disappear after a few
days, stopping this medication prematurely may result in a
return of the symptoms.

◇ This medication works most effectively when it is maintained at a constant level in your blood or urine. To help
keep the amount constant, do not miss a dose. It is best to
take the doses at evenly spaced times during the day and
night.

Precautions

◇ This medication may cause some people to become dizzy,
lightheaded, drowsy, or less alert.

◇ If you are taking antacids that contain aluminum or magnesium, be sure to take them at least two hours before or
after you take ciprofloxacin. These antacids may prevent
the ciprofloxacin from working properly.

◇ This medication may cause your skin to become more sensitive to sunlight. Stay out of direct sunlight during the
midday hours, wear protective clothing, and apply a sun
block product that has a skin protection factor (SPF) of at
least 15.

◇ Studies of birth defects have not been done in humans.
This medication is not recommended during pregnancy
since antibiotics of this type have been reported to cause
bone development problems in young animals.

◇ Some of the antibiotics in this group are known to pass into human breast milk. Since they have been reported to cause bone development problems in young animals, breast-feeding is not recommended during treatment with this medication.

Possible Side Effects

◇ Side effects that may go away as your body adjusts to the medication and do not require medical attention unless they continue or are bothersome: abdominal or stomach pain; diarrhea; dizziness; drowsiness*; headache; light-headedness; nausea or vomiting; nervousness; trouble sleeping.

◇ Rare side effects that should be reported to your physician immediately: agitation; confusion; fever; hallucinations; peeling of the skin; shakiness or tremors*; shortness of breath; skin rash; itching; swelling of face or neck.

*Since it may be difficult to distinguish between certain common symptoms of MS and some side effects of ciprofloxacin, be sure to consult your health care professional if an abrupt change of this type occurs.

Chemical Name: Clonazepam (kloe-**na**-ze-pam)

Brand Name: Klonopin (U.S.); Rivotril; Syn-Clonazepam (Canada)

Generic Available: No

Description: Clonazepam is a benzodiazepine that belongs to the group of medications called central nervous system depressants, which slow down the nervous system. Although clonazepam is used for a variety of medical conditions, it is used in multiple sclerosis primarily for the treatment of tremor, pain, and spasticity.

Proper Usage

◇ Keep this medication out of the reach of children. An overdose of this medication may be especially dangerous for children.

Precautions

◇ During the first few months taking clonazepam, your physician should check your progress at regular visits to make sure that this medicine does not cause unwanted effects.

◇ Take this medication only as directed by your physician; do not increase the dose without a prescription to do so.

◇ Clonazepam adds to the effects of alcohol and other central nervous system depressants (e.g., antihistamines, sedatives, tranquilizers, prescription pain medications, seizure medications, muscle relaxants, sleeping medications). Consult your physician before taking any of these CNS depressants while you are taking clonazepam. Taking an overdose of this medication or taking it with alcohol or other CNS depressants may lead to unconsciousness and possibly death.

◇ Stopping this medication suddenly may cause withdrawal side effects. Reduce the amount gradually before stopping completely.

◇ Clonazepam frequently causes people to become drowsy, dizzy, lightheaded, clumsy, or unsteady. Even if taken at bedtime, it may cause some people to feel drowsy or less alert on awakening.

◇ Studies in animals have shown that clonazepam can cause birth defects or other problems, including death of the animal fetus.

◇ Overuse of clonazepam during pregnancy may cause the baby to become dependent on it, leading to withdrawal side effects after birth. The use of clonazepam, especially during the last weeks of pregnancy, may cause breathing problems, muscle weakness, difficulty in feeding, and body temperature problems in the newborn infant.

◇ Clonazepam may pass into breast milk and cause drowsiness, slow heartbeat, shortness of breath, or troubled breathing in nursing babies.

Possible Side Effects

◇ Side effects that may go away during treatment as your body adjusts to the medication and do not require medical attention unless they continue for several weeks or are bothersome: drowsiness or tiredness; clumsiness or unsteadiness*; dizziness or lightheadedness; slurred speech*; abdominal cramps or pain; blurred vision or other changes in vision*; changes in sexual drive or performance*; gastrointestinal changes, including constipation* or diarrhea; dryness of mouth; fast or pounding heartbeat; muscle spasm*; trouble with urination*; trembling.

◇ Unusual side effects that should be discussed as soon as possible with your physician: behavior problems, including difficulty concentrating and outbursts of anger; confusion or mental depression; convulsions; hallucinations; low blood pressure; muscle weakness; skin rash or itching; sore throat, fever, chills; unusual bleeding or bruising; unusual excitement or irritability.

◇ Symptoms of overdose that require immediate emergency help: continuing confusion; severe drowsiness; shakiness; slowed heartbeat; shortness of breath; slow reflexes; continuing slurred speech*; staggering*; unusual severe weakness*.

---

*Since it may be difficult to distinguish between certain common symptoms of MS and some side effects of clonazepam, be sure to consult your health care professional if an abrupt change of this type occurs.

Chemical Name: Desmopressin (des-moe-**press**-in)
Brand Name: DDAVP Nasal Spray (U.S. and Canada)
Generic Available: No
Description: Desmopressin is a hormone used as a nasal spray. The hormone works on the kidneys to control frequent urination.

Proper Usage

◇ Keep this medication in the refrigerator but do not allow it to freeze.

Precautions

◇ Let your physician know if you have heart disease, blood vessel disease, or high blood pressure. Desmopressin can cause an increase in blood pressure.

◇ Studies have not been done in pregnant women. It has been used before and during pregnancy to treat diabetes mellitus and has not been shown to cause birth defects.

◇ Desmopressin passes into breast milk but has not been reported to cause problems in nursing infants.

Possible Side Effects

◇ Side effects that typically go away as your body adjusts to the medication and do not require medical attention unless they continue for several weeks or are bothersome: runny or stuffy nose; abdominal or stomach cramps; flushing of the skin; headache; nausea; pain in the vulva.

◇ Unusual side effects that require immediate medical attention: confusion; convulsions; unusual drowsiness[*]; continuing headache; rapid weight gain; markedly decreased urination.

[*]Since it may be difficult to distinguish between certain common symptoms of MS and some side effects of desmopressin, be sure to consult your health care professional if an abrupt change of this type occurs.

Chemical Name: Diazepam (dye-**az**-e-pam)

Brand Name: Valium (U.S. and Canada)

Generic Available: Yes (U.S.)

Description: Diazepam is a benzodiazepine that belongs to the group of medicines called central nervous system depressants, which slow down the nervous system. Although diazepam is used for a variety of medical conditions, it is used in multiple sclerosis primarily for the relief of muscle spasms and spasticity.

Proper Usage

◇ Keep this medication out of the reach of children. An overdose of this medication may be especially dangerous for children.

Precautions

◇ Your physician should check your progress at regular visits to make sure that this medication does not cause unwanted effects.

◇ Take diazepam only as directed by your physician; do not increase the dose without a prescription to do so.

◇ Diazepam adds to the effects of alcohol and other central nervous system depressants (e.g., antihistamines, sedatives, tranquilizers, prescription pain medications, seizure medications, muscle relaxants, sleeping medications). Consult your physician before taking any of these CNS depressants while you are taking diazepam. Taking an overdose of this medication or taking it with alcohol or other CNS depressants may lead to unconsciousness and possibly death.

◇ Stopping this medication suddenly may cause withdrawal side effects. Reduce the amount gradually before stopping completely.

◇ Diazepam may cause some people to become drowsy, dizzy, lightheaded, clumsy, or unsteady. Even if taken at bedtime, it may cause some people to feel drowsy or less alert on awakening.

◇ The use of diazepam during the first three months of pregnancy has been reported to increase the chance of birth defects.

◇ Overuse of diazepam during pregnancy may cause the baby to become dependent on the medicine, leading to withdrawal side effects after birth. The use of diazepam, especially during the last weeks of pregnancy, may cause breathing problems, muscle weakness, difficulty in feeding, and body temperature problems in the newborn infant. When diazepam is given in high doses (especially by injection) within fifteen hours before delivery, it may cause breathing problems, muscle weakness, difficulty in feeding, and body temperature problems in the newborn infant.

◇ Diazepam may pass into breast milk and cause drowsiness, slow heartbeat, shortness of breath, or troubled breathing in nursing babies.

Possible Side Effects

◇ Side effects that may go away during treatment as your body adjusts to the medication and do not require medical attention unless they continue for several weeks or are bothersome: clumsiness or unsteadiness*; dizziness or lightheadedness; slurred speech*; abdominal cramps or pain; blurred vision or other changes in vision*; changes in sexual drive or performance*; constipation*; diarrhea; dryness of mouth; fast or pounding heartbeat; muscle spasm*; trouble with urination*; trembling*; unusual tiredness or weakness*.

◇ Unusual side effects that should be discussed with your physician as soon as possible: behavior problems, including difficulty concentrating and outbursts of anger; confusion or mental depression; convulsions; hallucinations; low blood pressure; muscle weakness*; skin rash or itching; sore throat, fever, chills; unusual bleeding or bruising; unusual excitement or irritability.

◇ Symptoms of overdose that require immediate emergency help: continuing confusion; unusually severe drowsiness; shakiness; slowed heartbeat; shortness of breath; slow reflexes; continuing slurred speech; staggering; unusually severe weakness*.

*Since it may be difficult to distinguish between certain common symptoms of MS and some side effects of diazepam, be sure to consult your health care professional if an abrupt change of this type occurs.

Chemical Name: Docusate (**doe**-koo-sate)

Brand Name: Colace (U.S. and Canada)

Generic Available: Yes (U.S. and Canada)

Description: Docusate is an over-the-counter stool softener (emollient) that helps liquids to mix into dry, hardened stool, making the stool easier to pass.

Proper Usage

◇ Laxatives are to be used to provide short-term relief only, unless otherwise directed by the nurse or physician who is helping you to manage your bowel symptoms. A regimen that includes a healthy diet containing roughage (whole grain breads and cereals, bran, fruit, and green, leafy vegetables), six to eight full glasses of liquids each day, and some form of daily exercise is most important in stimulating healthy bowel function.

◇ If your physician has recommended this laxative for management of constipation, follow his or her recommendations for its use. If you are treating yourself for constipation, follow the directions on the package insert.

◇ Results usually occur one to two days after the first dose; some individuals may not get results for three to five days. Be sure to consult your physician if you experience problems or do not get relief within a week.

Precautions

◇ Do not take any type of laxative if you have signs of appendicitis or inflamed bowel (e.g., stomach or lower abdominal pain, cramping, bloating, soreness, nausea, or vomiting). Check with your physician as soon as possible.

◇ Do not take any laxative for more than one week unless you have been told to do so by your physician. Many people tend to overuse laxatives, which often leads to dependence on the laxative action to produce a bowel movement. Discuss the use of laxatives with your health care professional in order to ensure that the laxative is used effectively as part of a comprehensive, healthy bowel management regimen.

◇ Do not take mineral oil within two hours of taking docusate. The docusate may increase the amount of mineral oil that is absorbed by the body.

◇ Do not take any laxative within two hours of taking another medication because the desired effectiveness of the other medication may be reduced.

◇ If you are pregnant, discuss with your physician the most appropriate type of laxative for you to use.

◇ Some laxatives pass into breast milk. Although it is unlikely to cause problems for a nursing infant, be sure to let your physician know if you are using a laxative and breast-feeding at the same time.

Possible Side Effects

◇ Side effects that may go away as your body adjusts to the medication and do not require medical attention unless they persist or are bothersome: stomach and/or intestinal cramping.

◇ Unusual side effect that should be reported to your physician as soon as possible: skin rash.

Chemical Name: Docusate (**doe**-koo-sate) mini enema
Brand Name: Therevac Plus (U.S.)
Generic Available: No
Description: Therevac Plus is an over-the counter stool softener
   (emollient) that comes in a plastic, single-dose, two-inch
   ampule for insertion into the rectum. It works to produce
   bowel movements in a short time by helping liquids to mix
   into dry, hardened stool, making the stool easier to pass. The
   small size of this enema makes it easy to use without compromising its effectiveness.

Proper Usage

◇ Laxatives are to be used to provide short-term relief only,
   unless otherwise directed by the nurse or physician who is
   helping you to manage your bowel symptoms. A regimen
   that includes a healthy diet containing roughage (whole
   grain breads and cereals, bran, fruit, and green, leafy vegetables), 6 to 8 full glasses of liquids each day, and some
   form of daily exercise, is most important in stimulating
   healthy bowel function.

◇ If your physician has recommended this laxative for management of constipation, follow his or her recommendations for its use. If you are treating yourself for constipation, follow the directions on the package insert.

◇ Results usually occur fifteen minutes to one hour after
   insertion. Be sure to consult your physician if you experience problems or do not get relief within a day or two.

Precautions

◇ Do not use any type of laxative if you have signs of appendicitis or inflamed bowel (e.g., stomach or lower abdominal pain, cramping, bloating, soreness, nausea, or vomiting). Check with your physician as soon as possible.

◇ Do not take any laxative for more than one week unless you
   have been told to do so by your physician. Many people
   tend to overuse laxatives, which often leads to dependence
   on the laxative action to produce a bowel movement. Discuss the use of laxatives with your health care professional in order to ensure that the laxative is used effectively as

part of a comprehensive, healthy bowel management regimen.

◇ If you are pregnant, discuss with your physician the most appropriate type of laxative for you to use.

Possible Side Effects

◇ Side effect that may go away as your body adjusts to the medication and does not require medical attention unless it persists or is bothersome: skin irritation surrounding the rectal area.

◇ Less common side effects that should be reported to your physician: rectal bleeding, blistering, burning, itching, or pain.

Chemical Name: Fluoxetine (floo-**ox**-uh-teen)

Brand Name: Prozac (U.S. and Canada)

Generic Available: No

Description: Fluoxetine is used to treat mental depression. It is also used occasionally to treat MS fatigue.

Proper Usage

◇ This medication should be taken in the morning when used to treat depression because it can interfere with sleep. If it upsets your stomach, you may take it with food.

Precautions

◇ It may take four to six weeks for you to feel the beneficial effects of this medication.

◇ Your physician should monitor your progress at regularly scheduled visits in order to adjust the dose and help reduce any side effects.

◇ There have been suggestions that the use of fluoxetine may be related to increased thoughts about suicide in a very small number of individuals. More study is needed to determine if the medicine causes this effect. If you have concerns about this, be sure to discuss them with your physician.

◇ Fluoxetine adds to the effects of alcohol and other central nervous system depressants (e.g., antihistamines, sedatives, tranquilizers, sleeping medicine, prescription pain medicine, barbiturates, seizure medication, muscle relaxants). Be sure that your physician knows if you are taking these or any other medications.

◇ This medication affects the blood sugar levels of diabetic individuals. Check with your physician if you notice any changes in your blood or urine sugar tests.

◇ Dizziness or lightheadedness may occur, especially when you get up from a lying or sitting position. Change positions slowly to help alleviate this problem. If the problem continues or gets worse, consult your physician.

◇ Fluoxetine may cause dryness of the mouth. If your mouth continues to feel dry for more than two weeks, check with your physician or dentist. Continuing dryness of the mouth may increase the chance of dental disease.

◇ Studies have not been done in pregnant women. Fluoxetine has not been shown to cause birth defects or other problems in animal studies.

◇ Fluoxetine passes into breast milk and may cause unwanted effects, such as vomiting, watery stools, crying, and sleep problems in nursing babies. You may want to discuss alternative medications with your physician.

Possible Side Effects

◇ Side effects that may go away as your body adjusts to the medication and do not require medical attention unless they continue for several weeks or are bothersome: decreased sexual drive or ability*; anxiety and nervousness; diarrhea; drowsiness*; headache; trouble sleeping; abnormal dreams; change in vision*; chest pain; decreased appetite; decrease in concentration; dizziness; dry mouth; fast or irregular heartbeat; frequent urination*; menstrual pain; tiredness or weakness*; tremor*; vomiting.

◇ Unusual side effects that should be discussed with your physician as soon as possible: chills or fever; joint or muscle pain; skin rash; hives or itching; trouble breathing.

◇ Symptoms of overdose that require immediate medical attention: agitation and restlessness; convulsions; severe nausea and vomiting; unusual excitement.

---

*Since it may be difficult to distinguish between certain common symptoms of MS and some side effects of fluoxetine, be sure to consult your health care professional if an abrupt change of this type occurs.

Chemical Name: Gabapentin (ga-ba-**pen**-tin)
Brand Name: Neurontin (U.S.)
Generic Available: No
Description: Gabapentin is an antiepileptic used to control some types of seizures in epilepsy. It is used in multiple sclerosis to control dysesthesias (pain caused by MS lesions) and the pain caused by spasticity.

Proper Usage:

◇ Gabapentin may be taken with or without food. You must wait two hours after taking an antacid to take gabapentin.

◇ If gabapentin is taken three times a day, do not allow more than 12 hours to elapse between any two doses.

◇ If you miss a dose of this medication, take it as soon as possible. However, if it is almost time for your next dose, skip the missed dose the go back to your regular dosing schedule. Do not double dose.

Precautions:

◇ This medicine will add to the effects of alcohol and other central nervous system depressants that may cause drowsiness (e.g., antihistamines, sedatives, tranquilizers, prescription pain medications, seizure medications, muscle relaxants). Be sure that your physician knows if you are taking these or any other medications.

◇ Before having any medical tests, or surgical, dental, or emergency treatment of any kind, be sure to let the health care professional know that you are taking this medication.

◇ Consult your physician before stopping this medication because stopping abruptly may result in seizures. Depending on the dose you are taking, your physician may want you to decrease your dose gradually in order to avoid seizures.

◇ Gabapentin has not been studied in pregnant women. However, animal studies have shown possible bone and kidney problems in offspring. If you are pregnant or planning to become pregnant, discuss this with your physician before starting this medication.

◇ It is not known whether gabapentin passes into breast milk. Women who wish to breast-feed should consult with their physician.

Possible Side Effects:

◇ *Side effects that typically go away as your body adjusts to the medication and do not require medical attention unless they continue for several weeks or are bothersome:* blurred or double vision;* dizziness; drowsiness, muscle ache; swelling of hands or legs; tremor;* unusual tiredness;* weakness;* diarrhea, frequent urination;* indigestion; low blood pressure; slurred speech;* sleep difficulty; weakness .*

◇ *Check with your doctor as soon as possible if any of the following side effects occur:* clumsiness or unsteadiness;* continuous, uncontrolled eye movements; depression; mood changes; memory problems;* hoarseness; lower back pain; painful or difficult urination.

◇ *Symptoms of overdose requiring immediate attention:* double vision;* severe diarrhea, dizziness; drowsiness; slurred speech.*

*Since it may be difficult to distinguish certain symptoms of MS from some of the side effects of gabapentin, consult your health care professional if an abrupt change of this type occurs.

Chemical Name: Glatiramer Acetate (gla-**teer**-a-mer **ass**-i-tate)
Brand Name: Copaxone (U.S. and Canada)
Generic Available: No
Description: Glatiramer acetate is a synthetic protein that simulates myelin basic protein, a component of the myelin that insulates nerve fibers in the brain and spinal cord. Through a mechanism that is not completely understood, this drug seems to block myelin-damaging T cells by acting as a myelin decoy. In a two-year randomized, double-blind, controlled trial involving 251 ambulatory patients with relapsing-remitting MS, those taking the drug had a 29 percent reduction in annual relapse rate compared with control subjects who were given a placebo. An extension of this two-year trial, which confirmed the ability of glatiramer acetate to reduce the frequency of relapses in patients with relapsing-remitting MS, will be continued to year 10.

Proper Usage:

◇ Glatiramer acetate is injected subcutaneously (between the fat layer just under the skin and the muscles beneath) once a day. A physician or nurse will instruct you in the preparation of the medication for injection and the injection procedure itself, using a specially designed set of training materials. Do not attempt to inject yourself until you are sure that you understand the procedures.

◇ Glatiramer acetate should be kept refrigerated at all times. If refrigeration is not available, the drug may be safely stored at room temperature for up to seven days.

◇ Do not reuse needles or syringes. Dispose of the syringes as directed by your physician and keep them out of the reach of children.

◇ Because injection-site reactions (swelling, redness, discoloration, or pain) are relatively common, it is recommended that the sites be rotated according to a schedule provided for you by your physician. Do not use any one site more than once per week.

◇ Before you have a Papanicolaou (Pap) test, tell your doctor or nurse that you are taking this medication. The results of the test may be affected by glatiramer acetate.

Precautions:

◇ Do not change the dose or dosing schedule of this medication without consulting your physician.

◇ Glatiramer acetate has not been studied in pregnant women. Therefore, it should not be used during pregnancy or by any woman who is trying to become pregnant. If you are pregnant or planning to become pregnant, discuss this with your physician before starting the medication. If you become pregnant while on the medication, inform your physician.

◇ It is not known whether glatiramer acetate passes into breast milk. Nursing women should discuss the use of this medication with their physician.

Possible Side Effects:

◇ *Side effects that generally resolve on their own and do not require medical attention unless they continue for several weeks or are bothersome:* injection-site reactions (e.g., swelling, the development of a hardened lump, redness, tenderness, increased warmth of the skin, itching at the site of the injection); runny nose; tremor;* unusual tiredness or weakness;* weight gain.

◇ *Unusual side effects that should be discussed as soon as possible with your doctor:* hives (an itchy, blotchy swelling of the skin) or severe pain at the injection site.

◇ *Possible immediate post-injection reaction:* Approximately 13 percent of individuals using Copaxone will experience, at one time or another, a transient (very temporary) reaction immediately after injecting glatiramer acetate. This reaction, which usually occurs only once, includes flushing or chest tightness with heart palpitations, anxiety, and difficulty breathing. During the clinical trials, these reactions occurred very rarely, usually within minutes of an injection. They lasted approximately 15 minutes and resolved without further problem.

---

*Since it may be difficult to distinguish certain symptoms of MS from some of the side effects of glatiramer acetate, consult your health care professional if an abrupt change of this type occurs.

Chemical Name: Glycerin (**gli**-ser-in)

Brand Name: Sani-Supp suppository (U.S.)

Generic Available: Yes (U.S. and Canada)

Description: A glycerin suppository is a hyperosmotic laxative that draws water into the bowel from surrounding body tissues. This water helps to soften the stool mass and promote bowel action.

Proper Usage

◇ Laxatives are to be used to provide short-term relief only, unless otherwise directed by the nurse or physician who is helping you to manage your bowel symptoms. A regimen that includes a healthy diet containing roughage (whole grain breads and cereals, bran, fruit, and green, leafy vegetables), six to eight full glasses of liquids each day, and some form of daily exercise is most important in stimulating healthy bowel function.

◇ If your physician has recommended this laxative for management of constipation, follow his or her recommendations for its use. If you are treating yourself for constipation, follow the directions on the package insert.

◇ If the suppository is too soft to insert, refrigerate it for thirty minutes or hold it under cold water before removing the foil wrapper.

◇ Glycerin suppositories often produce results within fifteen minutes to one hour. Be sure to consult your physician if you experience problems or do not get relief within a week.

Precautions

◇ Do not take any type of laxative if you have signs of appendicitis or inflamed bowel (e.g., stomach or lower abdominal pain, cramping, bloating, soreness, nausea, or vomiting). Check with your physician as soon as possible.

◇ Do not take any laxative for more than one week unless you have been told to do so by your physician. Many people tend to overuse laxatives, which often leads to dependence on the laxative action to produce a bowel movement. Discuss the use of laxatives with your health care professional in order to ensure that the laxative is used effectively as part of a comprehensive, healthy bowel management regimen.

◇ If you are pregnant, discuss with your physician the most appropriate type of laxative for you to use.

◇ Use only water to moisten the suppository prior to insertion in the rectum. Do not lubricate the suppository with mineral oil or petroleum jelly, which might affect the way the suppository works.

Possible Side Effects

◇ Side effects that may go away as your body adjusts to the medication and do not require medical attention unless they persist or are bothersome: skin irritation around the rectal area.

◇ Less common side effects that should be reported to your physician as soon as possible: rectal bleeding; blistering, or itching.

Chemical Name: Imipramine (im-**ip**-ra-meen)

Brand Name: Tofranil (U.S. and Canada)

Generic Available: Yes (U.S. and Canada)

Description: Imipramine is a tricyclic antidepressant used to treat mental depression. Its primary use in multiple sclerosis is to treat bladder symptoms, including urinary frequency and incontinence. Imipramine is also prescribed occasionally for the management of neurologic pain in MS.

Proper Usage

◇ To lessen stomach upset, take this medication with food, even for a daily bedtime dose, unless your physician has told you to take it on an empty stomach.

Precautions

◇ Imipramine adds to the effects of alcohol and other central nervous system depressants (e.g., antihistamines, sedatives, tranquilizers, prescription pain medications, seizure medications, muscle relaxants, sleeping medications), possibly causing drowsiness. Be sure that your physician knows if you are taking these or any other medications.

◇ This medication causes dryness of the mouth. Because continuing dryness of the mouth can increase the risk of dental disease, alert your dentist if you are taking imipramine.

◇ Imipramine may cause your skin to be more sensitive to sunlight than it is normally. Even brief exposure to sunlight may cause a skin rash, itching, redness or other discoloration of the skin, or severe sunburn. Stay out of the sun during the midday hours. Wear protective clothing and a sun block that has a skin protection factor (SPF) of at least 15.

◇ This medication may affect blood sugar levels of diabetic individuals. If you notice a change in the results of your blood or urine sugar tests, check with your physician.

◇ Do not stop taking imipramine without consulting your physician. The physician may want you to reduce the amount you are taking gradually in order to reduce the possibility of withdrawal symptoms such as headache, nausea, and/or an overall feeling of discomfort.

◇ Studies of imipramine have not been done in pregnant women. There have been reports of newborns suffering

from muscle spasms and heart, breathing, and urinary problems when their mothers had taken tricyclic antidepressants immediately before delivery. Studies in animals have
indicated the possibility of unwanted effects in the fetus.

◇ Imipramine passes into breast milk but has not been
reported to have any effect on the nursing infant.

Possible Side Effects

◇ Side effects that may go away as your body adjusts to the
medication and do not require medical attention unless
they continue for more than two weeks or are bothersome:
dizziness; drowsiness*; headache; decreased sexual
ability*; increased appetite; nausea; unusual tiredness or
weakness*; unpleasant taste; diarrhea; heartburn; increased
sweating; vomiting.

◇ Uncommon side effects that should be reported to your
physician as soon as possible: blurred vision*; confusion or
delirium; constipation*; difficulty speaking or swallowing;
eye pain*; fainting; fast or irregular heartbeat; hallucinations; loss of balance control*; nervousness or restlessness;
problems urinating*; shakiness or trembling; stiffness of
arms and legs*.

◇ Rare side effects that should be reported to your physician
as soon as possible: anxiety; breast enlargement in males
and females; hair loss; inappropriate secretion of milk in
females; increased sensitivity to sunlight; irritability; muscle twitching; red or brownish spots on the skin; buzzing or
other unexplained sounds in the ears; skin rash; itching;
sore throat and fever; swelling of face and tongue; weakness*; yellow skin.

◇ Symptoms of acute overdose: confusion; convulsions;
severe drowsiness*; enlarged pupils; unusual heartbeat;
fever; hallucinations; restlessness and agitation; shortness
of breath; unusual tiredness or weakness*; vomiting.

---

*Since it may be difficult to distinguish between certain common
symptoms of MS and some side effects of imipramine, be sure to consult your health care professional if an abrupt change of this type
occurs.

Chemical Name: Interferon beta-1a

Brand Name: Avonex (U.S.—approval in Canada is pending)

Generic Available: No

Description: Avonex is a medication manufactured by a biotechnological process from one of the naturally occurring interferons (a type of protein). It is made up of exactly the same amino
   acids (major components of proteins) as the natural interferon
   beta found in the human body. In a clinical trial of 380 ambulatory patients with relapsing-remitting MS, those taking the
   currently recommended dose of the medication had a reduced
   risk of disability progression, experienced fewer exacerbations, and showed a reduction in number and size of active
   lesions in the brain (as shown on MRI) when compared with
   the group taking a placebo.

Proper Usage

◇ Avonex is given as a once-a-week intramuscular (IM) injection, usually in the large muscles of the thigh, upper arm, or
   hip. If your physician decides that you or a care partner can
   safely administer the injection, you will be taught how to
   reconstitute the medication (mix the sterile powder with the
   sterile water that is packaged with it) and instructed in safe
   and proper IM injection procedures. If you are unable to self-
   inject, and have no family member or friend available to do
   the injections, the injections will be given by your physician
   or nurse. Do not attempt to mix the medication or inject yourself until you are sure that you understand the procedures.

◇ Avonex must be kept cold. Be sure to store it in a refrigerator both before and after the medication is mixed for injection. Do not expose the medication to high temperatures
   (in a glove compartment or on a window sill, for example)
   and do not allow it to freeze. Once the medication has been
   mixed for use, it is recommended that you administer the
   injection as soon as possible; the reconstituted powder
   should not be used once it has been stored in the refrigerator longer than six hours.

◇ Do not reuse needles or syringes. Dispose of the syringes as
   directed by your physician and keep them out of the reach
   of children.

◇ Since flu-like symptoms are a fairly common side effect
   during the initial weeks of treatment, it is recommended

that the injection be given at bedtime. Taking aceta-minophen (Tylenol®) or ibuprofen (Advil®) immediately prior to each injection and during the 24 hours following the injection will also help to relieve the flu-like symptoms.

Precautions

◇ Avonex should not be used during pregnancy or by any woman who is trying to become pregnant. Women taking Avonex should use birth control measures at all times. If you want to become pregnant while being treated with Avonex, discuss the matter with your physician. If you become pregnant while using Avonex, stop the treatment and contact your physician.

◇ There was no increase in depression reported by people receiving Avonex in the clinical trial. However, since depression and suicidal thoughts are known to occur with some frequency in MS, and depression and suicidal thoughts have been reported with high doses of various interferon products, it is recommended that individuals with a history of severe depressive disorder be closely monitored while taking Avonex.

◇ Prior to starting treatment with Avonex, alert your physician if you have any prior history of a seizure disorder.

◇ Prior to starting treatment with Avonex, alert your physician if you have any history of cardiac disease, including angina, congestive heart failure, or arrhythmia.

Possible Side Effects

◇ Common side effects include flu-like symptoms (fatigue, chills, fever, muscle aches, and sweating). Most of these symptoms will tend to disappear after the initial few weeks of treatment. If they continue, become more severe, or cause you significant discomfort, be sure to talk them over with your physician.

◇ Symptoms of depression, including ongoing sadness, anxiety, loss of interest in daily activities, irritability, low self-esteem, guilt, poor concentration, indecisiveness, confusion, and eating and sleep disturbances, should be reported promptly to your doctor.

Avonex Support Line: 800-456-2255

Chemical Name: Interferon beta-1a

Brand Name: Rebif (Canada)

Please note: This drug is not currently available in the United States (see chapter 3).

Generic Available: No

Description: Rebif is a medication manufactured by a biotechnological process from one of the naturally occurring interferons (a type of protein). It is made up of exactly the same amino acids (major components of proteins) as the natural interferon beta found in the human body. A clinical trial of 560 ambulatory patients with relapsing-remitting MS compared three groups—those receiving 66mcg per week, those receiving 132mcg three times a week, and those receiving placebo. Over the two-year study, the two experimental groups demonstrated a lower relapse rate, prolonged time to first relapse, a higher proportion of relapse-free patients, a lower number of active lesions on MRI, and delay in progression of disability, when compared to the placebo group. Rebif is available at both dosage levels in pre-filled syringes ready for subcutaneous injection. The drug is also available at both dosage levels in a sterile powder to be mixed with a diluent.

Proper Usage

◇ Rebif is given three times a week subcutaneously (between the fat layer just under the skin and the muscles beneath). The physician or nurse will instruct you in the preparation of the medication for injection and/or the injection procedure itself, using a specially designed set of training materials. Do not attempt to inject yourself until you are sure that you understand the procedures.

◇ When starting treatment, it is recommended that 20% of the total dose be given during the first two weeks of therapy, 50% of the total dose be given in weeks three and four, and the full dose be given from the fifth week onward, in order reduce the severity of side effects.

◇ Rebif, in both the pre-mixed and powder forms, must be kept refrigerated. Do not expose the medication to high temperatures (in a glove compartment or on a window sill, for example) and do not allow it to freeze.

◇ Do not reuse needles or syringes. Dispose of the syringes as directed by your physician and keep them out of the reach of children.

◇ Since flu-like symptoms are a fairly common side effect during the initial weeks of treatment, it is recommended that the injection be given at bedtime. Taking acetaminophen (Tylenol®) or ibuprofen (Advil®) immediately prior to each injection and during the 24 hours following the injection will also help to relieve the flu-like symptoms.

Precautions

◇ Rebif should not be used during pregnancy or breast-feeding, or by any woman who is trying to become pregnant. Women taking Rebif should use birth control measures at all times. If you want to become pregnant while being treated with Rebif, discuss the matter with your physician. If you become pregnant while using Rebif, stop the treatment and contact your physician.

◇ There was no increase in depression reported by people receiving Rebif in the clinical trial. However, since depression and suicidal thoughts are known to occur with some frequency in MS, and depression and suicidal thoughts have been reported with high doses of various interferon products, it is recommended that individuals with a history of severe depressive disorder be closely monitored while taking Rebif.

Possible Side Effects

◇ Common side effects include flu-like symptoms (fatigue, chills, fever, muscle aches, and sweating) and injection site reactions (swelling, redness, discoloration, and pain). Most of these symptoms tend to disappear over time. If they continue, become more severe, or cause significant discomfort, be sure to talk them over with your physician. Contact your physician if the injection sites become inflamed, hardened, or lumpy, and do not inject into any area that has become hardened or lumpy.

◇ Most of these symptoms will tend to disappear after the initial few weeks of treatment. If they continue, become more severe, or cause you significant discomfort, be sure to talk them over with your physician.

◇ Symptoms of depression, including ongoing sadness, anxiety, loss of interest in daily activities, irritability, low self-esteem, guilt, poor concentration, indecisiveness, confusion, and eating and sleep disturbances, should be reported promptly to your doctor.

Chemical Name: Interferon beta-1b
Brand Name: Betaseron (U.S. and Canada)
Generic Available: No
Description: Betaseron is a medication manufactured by a biotechnological process from one of the naturally occurring interferons (a type of protein). In a clinical trial of 372 ambulatory patients with relapsing-remitting MS, those taking the currently recommended dose of the medication experienced fewer exacerbations, a longer time between exacerbations, and exacerbations that were generally less severe than those of patients taking a lower dose of the medication or a placebo. Additionally, patients on interferon beta-1b had no increase in total lesion area, as shown on MRI, in contrast to the placebo group, which had a significant increase.

Proper Usage

◇ Betaseron is injected subcutaneously (between the fat layer just under the skin and the muscles beneath) every other day. The physician or nurse will instruct you in the preparation of the medication for injection and the injection procedure itself, using a specially designed set of training materials. Do not attempt to inject yourself until you are sure that you understand the procedures.

◇ Betaseron must be kept cold. Be sure to store it in a refrigerator before and after the medication is mixed for injection.

◇ Do not reuse needles or syringes. Dispose of the syringes as directed by your physician and keep them out of the reach of children.

◇ Since flu-like symptoms are a common side effect associated with at least the initial weeks of taking Betaseron, it is recommended that the medication be taken at bedtime. Taking acetaminophen (Tylenol®) or ibuprofen (Advil®) thirty minutes before each injection will also help to relieve the flu-like symptoms.

◇ Because injection site reactions (swelling, redness, discoloration, or pain) are relatively common, it is recommended that the sites be rotated according to a schedule provided for you by your physician.

Precautions

◇ Betaseron should not be used during pregnancy or by any woman who is trying to become pregnant. Women taking Betaseron should use birth control measures at all times.

◇ During the clinical trial of interferon beta-1b, there were four suicide attempts and one completed suicide among those taking interferon beta-1b. Although there is no evidence that the suicide attempts were related to the medication itself, it is recommended that individuals with a history of severe depressive disorder be closely monitored while taking Betaseron.

Possible Side Effects

◇ Common side effects include flu-like symptoms (fatigue, chills, fever, muscle aches, and sweating) and injection site reactions (swelling, redness, discoloration, and pain). Most of these symptoms tend to disappear over time. If they continue, become more severe, or cause significant discomfort, be sure to talk them over with your physician. Contact your physician if the injection sites become inflamed, hardened, or lumpy, and do not inject into any area that has become hardened or lumpy.

◇ Depression, including suicide attempts, has been reported by patients taking Betaseron. Common symptoms of depression are sadness, anxiety, loss of interest in daily activities, irritability, low self-esteem, guilt, poor concentration, indecisiveness, confusion, and eating and sleep disturbances. If you experience any of these symptoms for longer than a day or two, contact your physician promptly.

Betaseron Customer Service: 800-788-1467

Chemical Name: Magnesium hydroxide (mag-**nee**-zhum hye-**drox**-ide)

Brand Name: Phillips' Milk of Magnesia (available in granule form in Canada, in wafer form in the U.S., and in powder or effervescent powder in the U.S. and Canada) is one of several brands of bulk-forming laxative that are available over-the-counter.

Generic Available: No

Description: Magnesium hydroxide is an over-the-counter hyperosmotic laxative of the saline type that encourages bowel movements by drawing water into the bowel from surrounding body tissue. Saline hyperosmotic laxatives (often called "salts") are used for rapid emptying of the lower intestine and bowel. They are not to be used for the long-term management of constipation.

Proper Usage

◇ Laxatives are to be used to provide short-term relief only, unless otherwise directed by the nurse or physician who is helping you to manage your bowel symptoms. A regimen that includes a healthy diet containing roughage (whole grain breads and cereals, bran, fruit, and green, leafy vegetables), six to eight full glasses of liquids each day, and some form of daily exercise is most important in stimulating healthy bowel function.

◇ If your physician has recommended this laxative for management of constipation, follow his or her recommendations for its use. If you are treating yourself for constipation, follow the directions on the package insert. Results are often obtained ninety minutes to three hours after taking a hyperosmotic laxative. Be sure to consult your physician if you experience problems or do not get relief within a week.

◇ Each dose should be taken with eight ounces or more of cold water or fruit juice. A second glass of water or juice with each dose is often recommended to prevent dehydration. If concerns about loss of bladder control keep you from drinking this amount of water, talk it over with the nurse or physician who is helping you manage your bowel and bladder symptoms.

Precautions

◇ Do not take any type of laxative if you have signs of appendicitis or inflamed bowel (e.g., stomach or lower abdominal pain, cramping, bloating, soreness, nausea, or vomiting). Check with your physician as soon as possible.

◇ Do not take any laxative for more than one week unless you have been told to do so by your physician. Many people tend to overuse laxatives, which often leads to dependence on the laxative action to produce a bowel movement. Discuss the use of laxatives with your health care professional in order to ensure that the laxative is used effectively as part of a comprehensive, healthy bowel management regimen.

◇ Do not take any laxative within two hours of taking another medication because the desired effectiveness of the other medication may be reduced.

◇ Although laxatives are commonly used during pregnancy, some types are better than others. If you are pregnant, consult your physician about the best laxative for you to use.

◇ Some laxatives pass into breast milk. Although it is unlikely to cause problems for a nursing infant, be sure to let your physician know if you are using a laxative and breast-feeding at the same time.

Possible Side Effects

◇ Side effects that may go away as your body adjusts to the medication and do not require medical attention unless they continue or are bothersome: cramping; diarrhea; gas; increased thirst.

◇ Unusual side effects that should be reported to your physician as soon as possible: confusion; dizziness; irregular heartbeat; muscle cramps, unusual tiredness or weakness[*].

---

[*]Since it may be difficult to distinguish between certain common symptoms of MS and some side effects of magnesium hydroxide, be sure to consult your health care professional if an abrupt change of this type occurs.

Chemical Name: Meclizine (**mek**-li-zeen)
Brand Name: Antivert (U.S.); Bonamine (Canada)
Generic Available: Yes (U.S.)
Description: Meclizine is used to prevent and treat nausea, vomiting, and dizziness.

Precautions

◇ This drug adds to the effects of alcohol and other central nervous system depressants (e.g., antihistamines, sedatives, tranquilizers, prescriptions pain medications, seizure medications, muscle relaxants, sleeping medications), possibly causing drowsiness. Be sure that your physician knows if you are taking these or any other medications.

◇ Meclizine may cause dryness of the mouth. If dryness continues for more than two weeks, speak to your physician or dentist since continuing dryness of the mouth may increase the risk of dental disease.

◇ This medication has not been shown to cause birth defects or other problems in humans. Studies in animals have shown that meclizine given in doses many times the usual human dose causes birth defects such as cleft palate.

◇ Although meclizine passes into breast milk, it has not been reported to cause problems in nursing babies. However, since this medication tends to decrease bodily secretions, it is possible that the flow of breast milk may be reduced in some women.

Possible Side Effects

◇ Side effects that typically go away as your body adjusts to the medication and do not require medical attention unless they continue for more than two weeks or are bothersome: drowsiness*; blurred vision*; constipation*; difficult or painful urination; dizziness; dryness of mouth, nose, and throat; fast heartbeat; headache; loss of appetite; nervousness or restlessness; trouble sleeping; skin rash; upset stomach.

*Since it may be difficult to distinguish between certain common symptoms of MS and some side effects of meclizine, be sure to consult your health care professional if an abrupt change of this type occurs.

Chemical Name: Methenamine (meth-**en**-a-meen)

Brand Name: Hiprex; Mandelamine (U.S.); Hip-Rex; Mandelamine (Canada)

Generic Available: No

Description: Methenamine is an anti-infective medication that
is used to help prevent infections of the urinary tract. It is usually prescribed on a long-term basis for individuals with a history of repeated or chronic urinary tract infections.

Proper Usage

◇ Before you start taking this medication, check your urine
with phenaphthazine paper or another test to see if it is
acidic. Your urine must be acidic (pH 5.5 or below) for this
medicine to work properly. Consult your health care professional about possible changes in your diet if necessary
to increase the acidity of your urine (e.g., avoiding citrus
fruits and juices, milk and other dairy products, antacids;
eating more protein and foods such as cranberries and
cranberry juice with added vitamin C, prunes, or plums).

Precautions

◇ The effects of methenamine in pregnancy have not been
studied in either humans or animals. Individual case
reports have not shown that this medication causes birth
defects or other problems in humans.

◇ Methenamine passes into breast milk but has not been
reported to cause problems in nursing infants.

Possible Side Effects

◇ Side effects that typically go away as your body adjusts to
the medication and do not require medical attention unless
they continue or are bothersome: nausea; vomiting.

◇ Unusual side effects that should be reported immediately
to your physician: skin rash.

Chemical Name: Methylprednisolone (meth-ill-pred-**niss**-oh-lone)

Brand Name: Depo-Medrol (U.S. and Canada)

Generic Available: Yes (U.S. and Canada)

Description: Methylprednisolone is one of a group of cortico-steroids (cortisone-like medications) that are used to relieve inflammation in different parts of the body. Corticosteroids are used in MS for the management of acute exacerbations because they have the capacity to close the damaged blood-brain barrier and reduce inflammation in the central nervous system. Although methylprednisolone is among the most commonly used corticosteroids in MS, it is only one of several possibilities. Other commonly used corticosteroids include dexamethazone, prednisone, betamethasone, and pred-nisolone. The following information pertains to all of the various corticosteroids.

Proper Usage

◇ Most neurologists treating MS believe that high-dose corti-costeroids given intravenously are the most effective treat-ment for an exacerbation, although the exact protocol for the drug's use may differ somewhat from one treating physician to another. Patients generally receive a four-day course of treatment (either in the hospital or as an outpa-tient), with doses of the medication spread throughout the day. This high-dose, intravenous steroid treatment is then typically followed by a gradually tapering dose of an oral corticosteroid (see Prednisone).

Precautions

◇ Since corticosteroids can stimulate the appetite and increase water retention, it is advisable to follow a low-salt and/or potassium-rich diet and watch your caloric intake. Your physician will make specific dietary recommenda-tions for you.

◇ Corticosteroids can lower your resistance to infection and make any infection that you get more difficult to treat. Con-tact your physician if you notice any sign of infection, such as sore throat, fever, coughing, or sneezing.

◇ Avoid close contact with anyone who has chicken pox or measles. Tell your physician right away if you think you have been exposed to either of these illnesses. Do not have any immunizations after you stop taking this medication until you have consulted your physician. People living in your home should not have the oral polio vaccine while you are being treated with corticosteroids since they might pass the polio virus on to you.

◇ Corticosteroids may affect the blood sugar levels of diabetic patients. If you notice a change in your blood or urine sugar tests, be sure to speak to your physician.

◇ The risk of birth defects for women taking corticosteroids is not known. Overuse of corticosteroids during pregnancy may slow the growth of the infant after birth. Animal studies have demonstrated that corticosteroids cause birth defects.

◇ Corticosteroids pass into breast milk and may slow the infant's growth. If you are nursing or plan to nurse, be sure to discuss this with your physician. It may be necessary for you to stop nursing while taking this medication.

◇ Corticosteroids may produce mood changes and/or mood swings of varying intensity. These mood alterations can vary from relatively mild to extremely intense, and can vary in a single individual from one course of treatment to another. Neither the patient nor the physician can predict with any certainty whether the corticosteroids are likely to precipitate these mood alterations. If you have a history of mood disorders (depression or bipolar disorder, for example), be sure to share this information with your physician. If you begin to experience mood changes or swings that feel unmanageable, contact your physician so that a decision can be made about whether or not you need an additional medication to help you until the mood alterations subside.

Possible Side Effects

◇ Side effects that may go away as your body adjusts to the medication and do not require medical attention unless they continue or are bothersome: increased appetite; indigestion; nervousness or restlessness; trouble sleeping; headache; increased sweating; unusual increase in hair growth on body or face.

◇ Less common side effects that should be reported as soon as possible to your physician: severe mood changes or mood swings; decreased or blurred vision*; frequent urination*.

◇ Additional side effects that can result from the prolonged use of corticosteroids and should be reported to your physician: acne or other skin problems; swelling of the face; swelling of the feet or lower legs; rapid weight gain; pain in the hips or other joints (caused by bone cell degeneration); bloody or black, tarry stools; elevated blood pressure; markedly increased thirst (with increased urination indicative of diabetes mellitus); menstrual irregularities; unusual bruising of the skin; thin, shiny skin; hair loss; muscle cramps or pain. Once you stop this medication after taking it for a long period of time, it may take several months for your body to readjust.

---

*Since it may be difficult to distinguish between certain common symptoms of MS and some side effects of methylprednisolone, be sure to consult your health care professional if an abrupt change of this type occurs.

Chemical Name: Mineral oil

Mineral oil is available in a variety of brands in the U.S. and Canada.

Generic Available: Yes

Description: Mineral oil is a lubricant laxative that is taken by mouth. It encourages bowel movements by coating the bowel and the stool with a waterproof film that helps to retain moisture in the stool.

Proper Usage

◇ Laxatives are to be used to provide short-term relief only, unless otherwise directed by the nurse or physician who is helping you to manage your bowel symptoms. A regimen that includes a healthy diet containing roughage (whole grain breads and cereals, bran, fruit, and green, leafy vegetables), six to eight full glasses of liquids each day, and some form of daily exercise is most important in stimulating healthy bowel function.

◇ If your physician has recommended this type of laxative for management of constipation, follow his or her recommendations for its use. If you are treating yourself for constipation, follow the directions on the package insert. Mineral oil is usually taken at bedtime because it takes six to eight hours to produce results. Be sure to consult your physician if you experience problems or do not get relief within a week.

◇ Mineral oil should not be taken within two hours of mealtime because the mineral oil may interfere with food digestion and the absorption of important nutrients.

◇ Mineral oil should not be taken within two hours of taking a stool softener (see Docusate) because the stool softener may increase the amount of mineral oil that is absorbed by the body.

Precautions

◇ Do not take any type of laxative if you have signs of appendicitis or inflamed bowel (e.g., stomach or lower abdominal pain, cramping, bloating, soreness, nausea, or vomiting). Check with your physician as soon as possible.

◇ Do not take any laxative for more than one week unless you have been told to do so by your physician. Many people tend to overuse laxative products, which often leads to dependence on the laxative action to produce a bowel movement. Discuss the use of laxatives with your health care professional in order to ensure that the laxative is used effectively as part of a comprehensive, healthy bowel management regimen.

◇ Mineral oil should not be used very often or for long periods of time. Its gradual build-up in body tissues can cause problems, and may interfere with the body's absorption of important nutrients and vitamins A, D, E, and K.

◇ Do not take any laxative within two hours of taking another medication because the desired effectiveness of the other medication may be reduced.

◇ Mineral oil should not be used during pregnancy because it may interfere with absorption of nutrients in the mother and, if used for prolonged periods, cause severe bleeding in the newborn infant.

◇ Be sure to let your physician know if you are using a laxative and breast-feeding at the same time.

Possible Side Effects

◇ Uncommon side effect that usually does not need medical attention: skin irritation around the rectal area.

Chemical Name: Nitrofurantoin (nye-troe-fyoor-**an**-toyn)
Brand Name: Macrodantin (U.S. and Canada)
Generic Available: No
Description: Nitrofurantoin is an *anti-infective* that is used primarily to treat urinary tract infections.

Proper Usage:

◇ Nitrofurantoin should be taken with food or milk to lessen stomach upset and to promote your body's absorption of the medication.

◇ Finish the full course of treatment prescribed by your doctor and avoid missing doses. Even if your symptoms disappear after a few days, stopping this medication prematurely may result in a return of the symptoms.

◇ If you miss a dose of this medication, take it as soon as possible. If, however, it is almost time for your next dose, skip the missed dose and go back to your regular dosing schedule. Do not double dose.

◇ The use of nitrofurantoin may cause your urine to become rust-yellow or brownish. This change does not require medical treatment and does not need to be reported to your physician.

Precautions:

◇ Nitrofurantoin can interact with, or alter the action of, a variety of other medications you may be taking. It is very important to let your physician know about all the medications you are taking so that necessary substitutions or dosage adjustments can be made.

◇ If you will be taking this medication over an extended period of time, your doctor will need to check your progress at regular visits. If your symptoms do not improve within a few days, or become worse, consult your physician.

◇ Individuals with diabetes may find that this medication alters the results of some urine sugar tests. Consult with your physician before changing your diet or the dose of your diabetes medicine.

◇ Certain medical conditions may affect the use of nitrofurantoin. Be sure to alert your physician about any medical conditions you have, especially glucose-6-phosphate dehydrogenase (G6PD) deficiency, kidney disease, or lung disease.

◇ Because nitrofurantoin may cause problems in infants, it should not be used by a woman who is within a week or two of her delivery date, or during labor and delivery.

◇ Nitrofurantoin passes into breast milk in small amounts and may cause problems in nursing babies (especially those with glucose-6-phosphate dehydrogenase (G6PD) deficiency).

Possible Side Effects:

◇ *Side effects that may go away as your body adjusts to the medication and do not require medical attention unless they continue or are bothersome:* abdominal or stomach pain; diarrhea, loss of appetite, nausea, or vomiting.

◇ *Rare side effects that should be reported to your doctor immediately:* chest pain; chills; cough; fever; trouble breathing; dizziness; headache; numbness, tingling, or burning of face or mouth;* unusual weakness or tiredness;* itching; joint pain; skin rash; yellow eyes or skin.

---

*Since it may be difficult to distinguish between certain common symptoms of MS and some side effects of nitrofurantoin, be sure to consult your health care professional if an abrupt change of this type occurs.

Chemical Name: Nortriptyline (nor-**trip**-ti-leen)
Brand Name: Pamelor (U.S.) Aventyl (Canada)
Generic Available: Yes (U.S.)
Description: Nortriptyline is a tricyclic antidepressant used to treat mental depression. In multiple sclerosis, it is frequently used to treat painful parsthesias in the arms and legs (e.g., burning sensations, pins and needles, stabbing pains) caused by damage to the pain regulating pathways of the brain and spinal cord.
Note: Other tricyclic antidepressants are also used for the management of neurologic pain symptoms: amitriptyline (Elavil—U.S. and Canada), clomipramine (Anafranil—U.S. and Canada), desipramine (Norpramin—U.S. and Canada), doxepin (Sinequan—U.S. and Canada), imipramine (Tofranil—U.S. and Canada), and trimipramine (U.S. and Canada). Although each of these medications is given in different dosage levels, the precautions and side effects listed here for nortriptyline apply to these other tricyclic medications as well.

Precautions:

◇ Nortriptyline will add to the effects of alcohol and other central nervous system depressants (e.g., antihistamines, sedatives, tranquilizers, prescription pain medications, seizure medications, muscle relaxants, sleeping medications), possibly causing drowsiness. Be sure that your physician knows if you are taking these or any other medications.

◇ This medication causes dryness of the mouth. Because continuing dryness of the mouth may increase the risk of dental disease, alert your dentist that you are taking nortriptyline.

◇ This medication may cause your skin to be more sensitive to sunlight than it normally is. Even brief exposure to sunlight may cause a rash, itching, redness or other discoloration of the skin, or severe sunburn.

◇ This medication may affect blood sugar levels of diabetic individuals. If you notice a change in the results of your blood or urine sugar tests, check with your doctor.

◇ Do not stop taking this medication without consulting your doctor. The doctor may want you to reduce the amount you are taking gradually in order to reduce the possibility of withdrawal symptoms such as headache, nausea, and/or an overall feeling of discomfort.

◇ Studies of nortriptyline have not been done in pregnant women. However, there have been reports of newborns suffering from muscle spasms and heart, breathing, and urinary problems when their mothers had taken tricyclic antidepressants immediately before delivery. Studies in animals have indicated the possibility of unwanted affects on the fetus.

◇ Tricyclics pass into breast milk. Only doxepin (Sinequan) has been reported to cause drowsiness in the nursing baby.

Possible Side Effects:

◇ *Side effects that may go away as your body adjusts to the medication and do not require medical attention unless they continue for more than two weeks or are bothersome:* dryness of mouth; constipation;* increased appetite and weight gain; dizziness; drowsiness;* decreased sexual ability;* headache; nausea; unusual tiredness or weakness;* unpleasant taste; diarrhea; heartburn; increased sweating; vomiting.

◇ *Uncommon side effects that should be reported to the doctor as soon as possible:* blurred vision;* confusion or delirium; difficulty speaking or swallowing;* eye pain;* fainting; hallucinations; loss of balance control;* nervousness or restlessness; problems urinating;* shakiness or trembling; stiffness of arms and legs.*

◇ *Rare side effects that should be reported to the doctor as soon as possible:* anxiety; breast enlargement in males and females; hair loss; inappropriate secretion of milk in females; increased sensitivity to sunlight; irritability; muscle twitching; red or brownish spots on the skin; buzzing or other unexplained sounds in the ears; rash, itching; sore throat and fever; swelling of face and tongue; weakness*; yellow skin.

◇ *Symptoms of acute overdose:* confusion; convulsions; severe drowsiness;* enlarged pupils; unusual heartbeat; fever; hallucinations; restlessness and agitation; shortness of breath; unusual tiredness or weakness; vomiting.

---

*Since it may be difficult to distinguish between certain common symptoms of MS and some side effects of nortriptyline, be sure to consult your health care professional if an abrupt change of this type occurs.

Chemical Name: Oxybutynin (ox-i-**byoo**-ti-nin) chloride—
extended release

Brand Name: Ditropan XL (U.S. and Canada)

Generic Available: No

Description: This form of oxybutynin is an extended-release
antispasmodic that is formulated to help decrease muscle
spasms of the bladder and the frequent urge to urinate caused
by these spasms.

Proper Usage

◇ The tablet is to be swallowed whole, once a day, with liquids. It can be taken with or with or without food. Because
the medication is contained within a nonabsorbable shell
that is designed to release the drug at a controlled rate, the
tablet should not be chewed, crushed, or divided. The
shell is routinely eliminated from the body in the stool.

Precautions

◇ This medication adds to the effects of alcohol and other
central nervous system depressants (such as antihistamines, sedatives, tranquilizers, prescription pain medications, seizure medications, muscle relaxants). Be sure that
your physician knows if you are taking these or any other
medications.

◇ Oxybytynin, like all anticholinergic medications, can
induce drowsiness and/or blurred vision.

◇ Oxybutynin, like all anticholinergic medications, can
cause heat prostration (fever and heat stroke due to
decreased sweating) when taken in very hot weather.

◇ Oxybutynin may cause drying of the mouth. Since continuing dryness of the mouth can increase the risk of dental
disease, alert your dentist if you are taking oxybutynin.

◇ Oxybutynin has not been studied in pregnant women. It
has not been shown to cause birth defects or other problems in animal studies. Do not take this medication while
pregnant unless specifically instructed to do so by your
physician.

◇ This medication has not been reported to cause problems
in nursing babies. However, since it tends to decrease body
secretions, oxybutynin may reduce the flow of breast milk.

Do not take this medication while nursing without discussing it with your physician.

Possible Side Effects

◇ Side effects that typically go away as your body adjusts to the medication and do not require medical attention unless they continue for a few weeks or are bothersome: constipation*; decreased sweating; unusual drowsiness*; dryness of mouth, nose, throat; blurred vision*; decreased flow of breast milk; difficulty swallowing*; headache; increased light sensitivity; nausea or vomiting; unusual tiredness or weakness*

◇ Less common side effects that should be reported immediately to your physician include: urinary retention*, dehydration, cardiac arrhythmia.

*Since it may be difficult to distinguish between certain common symptoms of MS and some side effects of oxybutynin, be sure to consult your health care professional if an abrupt change of this type occurs.

Chemical Name: Oxybutynin (ox-i-**byoo**-ti-nin)
Brand Name: Ditropan (U.S. and Canada)
Generic Available: Yes (U.S.)
Description: Oxybutynin is an antispasmodic that helps decrease muscle spasms of the bladder and the frequent urge to urinate caused by these spasms.

Proper Usage

◇ This medication is usually taken with water on an empty stomach, but your physician may want you to take it with food or milk to lessen stomach upset.

Precautions

◇ This medication adds to the effects of alcohol and other central nervous system depressants (such as antihistamines, sedatives, tranquilizers, prescription pain medications, seizure medications, muscle relaxants). Be sure that your physician knows if you are taking these or any other medications.

◇ This medication may cause your eyes to become more sensitive to light.

◇ Oxybutynin may cause drying of the mouth. Since continuing dryness of the mouth can increase the risk of dental disease, alert your dentist if you are taking oxybutynin.

◇ Oxybutynin has not been studied in pregnant women. It has not been shown to cause birth defects or other problems in animal studies.

◇ This medication has not been reported to cause problems in nursing babies. However, since it tends to decrease body secretions, oxybutynin may reduce the flow of breast milk.

Possible Side Effects

◇ Side effects that typically go away as your body adjusts to the medication and do not require medical attention unless they continue for a few weeks or are bothersome: constipation*; decreased sweating; unusual drowsiness*; dryness of mouth, nose, throat; blurred vision*; decreased flow of breast milk; decreased sexual ability*; difficulty swallowing*; headache; increased light sensitivity; nausea or vomiting; trouble sleeping; unusual tiredness or weakness*.

◇ Less common side effects that should be reported to your physician immediately: difficulty in urination[*].

[*]Since it may be difficult to distinguish between certain common symptoms of MS and some side effects of oxybutynin, be sure to consult your health care professional if an abrupt change of this type occurs.

Chemical Name: Papaverine (pa-**pav**-er-een)

Brand Name: None

Generic Available: Yes (U.S. and Canada)

Description: Papaverine belongs to a group of medicines called vasodilators, which cause blood vessels to expand, thereby increasing blood flow. Papaverine is used in MS to treat erectile dysfunction. When papaverine is injected into the penis, it produces an erection by increasing blood flow to the penis.

Proper Usage

◇ Papaverine should never be used as a sexual aid by men who are not impotent. If improperly used, this medication can cause permanent damage to the penis.

◇ Papaverine is available by prescription and should be used only as directed by your physician, who will instruct you in the proper way to give yourself an injection so that it is simple and essentially pain-free.

Precautions

◇ Do not use more of this medication or use it more often than it has been prescribed for you. Using too much of this medicine will result in a condition called priapism, in which the erection lasts too long and does not resolve when it should. Permanent damage to the penis can occur if blood flow to the penis is cut off for too long a period of time.

◇ Examine your penis regularly for possible lumps near the injection sites or for curvature of the penis. These may be signs that unwanted tissue is growing (called fibrosis), which should be examined by your physician.

Possible Side Effects

◇ Side effects that you should report to your physician so that he or she can adjust the dosage or change the medication: bruising at the injection site; mild burning along the penis; difficulty ejaculating; swelling at the injection site.

◇ Rare side effects that require immediate treatment: erection continuing for more than four hours. If you cannot be seen immediately by your physician, you should go to the emergency room for prompt treatment.

Chemical Name: Paroxetine (pa-**rox**-uh-teen)
Brand Name: Paxil (U.S. and Canada)
Generic Available: No
Description: Paroxetine is used to treat mental depression.

Proper Usage

◇ Paroxetine may be taken with or without food, on an empty or full stomach.

Precautions

◇ It may take up to four weeks or longer for you to feel the beneficial effects of this medication.

◇ Your physician should monitor your progress at regularly scheduled visits in order to adjust the dose and help reduce any side effects.

◇ This medication could add to the effects of alcohol and other central nervous system depressants (e.g., antihistamines, sedatives, tranquilizers, sleeping medicine, prescription pain medicine, barbiturates, seizure medication, muscle relaxants). Be sure that your physician knows if you are taking these or any other medications.

◇ Paroxetine may cause dryness of the mouth. If your mouth continues to feel dry for more than two weeks, check with your physician or dentist. Continuing dryness of the mouth may increase the risk of dental disease.

◇ This medication may cause you to become drowsy.

◇ Studies have not been done in pregnant women. Studies in animals have shown that paroxetine may cause miscarriages and decreased survival rates when given in doses that are many times higher than the human dose.

◇ Paroxetine passes into breast milk but has not been shown to cause any problems in nursing infants.

Possible Side Effects

◇ Side effects that typically go away as your body adjusts to the medication and do not require medical attention unless they continue for several weeks or are bothersome: decrease in sexual drive or ability*; headache; nausea; problems urinating*; decreased or increased appetite; unusual tiredness or weakness*; tremor*; trouble sleeping;

anxiety; agitation; nervousness or restlessness; changes in vision, including blurred vision[*]; fast or irregular heartbeat; tingling, burning, or prickly sensations[*]; vomiting.

◇ Unusual side effects that should be discussed with your physician as soon as possible: agitation; lightheadedness or fainting; muscle pain or weakness; skin rash; mood or behavior changes.

---

[*]Since it may be difficult to distinguish between certain common symptoms of MS and some side effects of paroxetine, be sure to consult your health care professional if an abrupt change of this type occurs.

Chemical Name: Pemoline (**pem**-oh-leen)
Brand Name: Cylert (U.S. and Canada)
Generic Available: No
Description: Pemoline is a mild central nervous system stimulant that has been used primarily to treat children with attention deficit hyperactivity disorder and adults with narcolepsy. It is used in multiple sclerosis to relieve certain types of fatigue.

Proper Usage

◇ As directed by the Food and Drug Administration, Abbott Laboratories, the manufacturer of Cylert, has recommended evaluation of liver function prior to starting this medication, followed by bi-weekly liver function evaluations while the drug is being used. [Note: No liver failure has been reported in anyone with MS; however, extra care should be taken when this medication is used in combination with other drugs that may potentially harm the liver, e.g., the interferons, or carbamazepine (Tegretol®).] The Medical Advisory Board of the National MS Society recognizes the issues raised by the FDA, but also supports the clear benefit of pemoline for many individuals with MS and associated non-exertional fatigue.

◇ The usual starting dose for the treatment of fatigue in MS is 18.75 mg each morning for one week. If necessary, in order to manage the fatigue, the dosage can be gradually increased in increments of 18.75 mg and spread out over the early part of the day. In order to maximize the medication's effectiveness and minimize sleep disturbance, it should all be taken before mid-afternoon. The maximum dose of this medication is not known. Some individuals feel jittery or uncomfortable taking more than the minimum dose; others tolerate higher doses without discomfort. Typically, the drug is not prescribed at levels over 100–140 mgs per day for MS-related fatigue.

Precautions

◇ Pemoline can increase hypertension. It should not be taken if you have angina and/or known coronary artery disease.

◇ If you are taking pemoline in large doses for a long time, do not stop taking it without consulting your physician. Your physician may want you to reduce the amount you are taking gradually.

◇ This drug may interact with the effects of alcohol and other central nervous system depressants (e.g., antihistamines, sedatives, tranquilizers, prescription pain medications, seizure medications, muscle relaxants, sleeping medications). Be sure your physician knows if you are taking these or any other medications.

◇ Pemoline may cause some people to become dizzy or less alert than they are normally.

◇ If you have been using this medicine for a long time and think you may have become mentally or physically dependent on it, check with your physician. Some signs of dependence on pemoline are a strong desire or need to continue taking the medicine; a need to increase the dose to receive the effects of the medicine; withdrawal side effects such as mental depression, unusual behavior, unusual tiredness* or weakness* after the medication is stopped.

◇ Pemoline has not been shown to cause birth defects or other problems in humans. Studies in animals given large doses of pemoline have shown that it causes an increase in stillbirths and decreased survival of the offspring.

◇ It is not known if pemoline is excreted in breast milk.

Possible Side Effects

Side effects of this medication have not been studied in adults. Side effects that have been reported by some adults in clinical practice include insomnia; elevated heart rate; nervousness; agitation; loss of appetite and weight loss; gastrointestinal upset, including constipation and diarrhea; hallucinations.

---

*Since it may be difficult to distinguish between certain common symptoms of MS and some side effects of pemoline, be sure to consult your health care professional if an abrupt change of this type occurs.

Chemical Name: Phenazopyridine (fen-az-oh-**peer**-i-deen)
Brand Name: Pyridium (U.S. and Canada)
Generic Available: Yes (U.S.)
Description: Phenazopyridine is used to relieve the pain, burning, and discomfort caused by urinary tract infections. It is not an antibiotic and will not cure the infection itself. This medication is available in the U.S. only with a prescription; it is available in Canada without a prescription. The medication comes in tablet form.

Precautions

◇ The medication causes the urine to turn reddish orange. This effect is harmless and goes away after you stop taking phenazopyridine.

◇ It is best not to wear soft contact lenses while taking this medication; phenazopyridine may cause permanent discoloration or staining of soft lenses.

◇ Check with your physician if symptoms such as bloody urine, difficult or painful urination, frequent urge to urinate, or sudden decrease in the amount of urine appear or become worse while you are taking this medication.

◇ Phenazopyridine has not been studied in pregnant women. It has not been shown to cause birth defects in animal studies.

◇ It is not known whether this medication passes into breast milk. It has not been reported to cause problems in nursing babies.

Possible Side Effects

◇ Uncommon side effects that typically go away as your body adjusts to the medication and do not require medical attention unless they continue or are bothersome: dizziness; headache; indigestion; stomach cramps or pain.

◇ Unusual side effects that should be reported to your physician: blue or blue-purple color of skin; fever and confusion; shortness of breath; skin rash; sudden decrease in amount of urine; swelling of face, fingers, feet and/or lower legs; unusual weakness or tiredness*; weight gain; yellow eyes or skin.

*Since it may be difficult to distinguish between certain common symptoms of MS and some side effects of phenazopyridine, be sure to consult your health care professional if an abrupt change of this type occurs.

Chemical Name: Phenytoin (**fen**-i-toyn)

Brand Name: Dilantin (U.S. and Canada)

Generic Available: Yes (U.S.)

Description: Phenytoin is one of a group of hydantoin anticonvulsants that are used most commonly in the management of seizures in epilepsy. It is used in MS to manage painful dysesthesias (most commonly trigeminal neuralgia) caused by abnormalities in the sensory pathways in the brain and spinal cord.

Precautions

◇ This drug may interact with the effects of alcohol and other central nervous system depressants (e.g., antihistamines, sedatives, tranquilizers, certain prescription pain medications, seizure medications, muscle relaxants, sleeping medications). Be sure your physician knows if you are taking these or any other medications.

◇ Oral contraceptives (birth control pills) that contain estrogen may not be as effective if taken in conjunction with phenytoin. Consult with your physician about using a different or additional form of birth control to avoid unplanned pregnancies.

◇ This medication may affect the blood sugar levels of diabetic individuals. Check with your physician if you notice any change in the results of your blood or urine sugar level tests while taking phenytoin.

◇ Antacids or medicines for diarrhea can reduce the effectiveness of phenytoin. Do not take any of these medications within two to three hours of the phenytoin.

◇ Before having any type of dental treatment or surgery, be sure to inform your physician or dentist if you are taking phenytoin. Medications commonly used during surgical and dental treatments can increase the side effects of phenytoin.

◇ There have been reports of increased birth defects when hydantoin anticonvulsants were used for seizure control during pregnancy. It is not definitely known whether these medications were the cause of the problem. Be sure to tell your physician if you are pregnant or considering becoming pregnant.

◇ Phenytoin passes into breast milk in small amounts.

Possible Side Effects

◇ Side effects that may go away as your body adjusts to the medication and do not require medical attention unless they continue or are bothersome: constipation*; mild dizziness*; mild drowsiness*.

◇ Side effects that should be reported to your physician: bleeding or enlarged gums; confusion; enlarged glands in the neck or underarms; mood or mental changes*; muscle weakness or pain*; skin rash or itching; slurred speech or stuttering; trembling; unusual nervousness or irritability.

◇ Symptoms of overdose that require immediate attention: sudden blurred or double vision*; sudden severe clumsiness or unsteadiness*; sudden severe dizziness or drowsiness*; staggering walk*; severe confusion or disorientation.

*Since it may be difficult to distinguish between certain common symptoms of MS and some side effects of phenytoin, be sure to consult your health care professional if an abrupt change of this type occurs.

Chemical Name: Prednisone (**pred**-ni-sone)

Brand Name: Deltasone (U.S. and Canada)

Generic Available: Yes (U.S. and Canada)

Description: Prednisone is one of a group of corticosteroids (cortisone-like medicines) that are used to relieve inflammation in different parts of the body. Corticosteroids are used in MS for the management of acute exacerbations because they have the capacity to close the damaged blood-brain barrier and reduce inflammation in the central nervous system. Although prednisone is among the most commonly used corticosteroids in MS, it is only one of several different possibilities. Other commonly used corticosteroids include dexamethasone; prednisone; betamethasone; and prednisolone. The following information pertains to all of the various corticosteroids.

Proper Usage

◇ Most neurologists treating MS believe that high-dose corticosteroids given intravenously are the most effective treatment for an MS exacerbation, although the exact protocol for the drug's use may differ somewhat from one treating physician to another. Patients generally receive a four-day course of treatment (either in the hospital or as an outpatient), with doses of the medication spread throughout the day (see Methylprednisolone). The high-dose, intravenous dose is typically followed by a gradually tapering dose of an oral corticosteroid (usually ranging in length from ten days to five or six weeks). Prednisone is commonly used for this oral taper. Oral prednisone may also be used instead of the high-dose, intravenous treatment if the intravenous treatment is not desired or is medically contraindicated.

Precautions

◇ This medication can cause indigestion and stomach discomfort. Always take it with a meal and/or a glass or milk. Your physician may prescribe an antacid for you to take with this medication.

◇ Take this medication exactly as prescribed by your physician. Do not stop taking it abruptly; your physician will give you a schedule that gradually tapers the dose before you stop it completely.

◇ Since corticosteroids can stimulate the appetite and increase water retention, it is advisable to follow a low-salt and/or a potassium-rich diet and watch your caloric intake.

◇ Corticosteroids can lower your resistance to infection and make any infection that you get more difficult to treat. Contact your physician if you notice any sign of infection, such as sore throat, fever, coughing, or sneezing.

◇ Avoid close contact with anyone who has chicken pox or measles. Tell your physician immediately if you think you have been exposed to either of these illnesses. Do not have any immunizations after you stop taking this medication until you have consulted your physician. People living in your home should not have the oral polio vaccine while you are being treated with corticosteroids since they might pass the polio virus on to you.

◇ Corticosteroids may affect the blood sugar levels of diabetic patients. If you notice a change in your blood or urine sugar tests, be sure to discuss it with your physician.

◇ The risk of birth defects in women taking corticosteroids during pregnancy has not been studied. Overuse of corticosteroids during pregnancy may slow the growth of the infant after birth. Animal studies have demonstrated that corticosteroids cause birth defects.

◇ Corticosteroids pass into breast milk and may slow the infant's growth. If you are nursing or plan to nurse, be sure to discuss this with your physician. It may be necessary for you to stop nursing while taking this medication.

◇ Corticosteroids can produce mood changes and/or mood swings of varying intensity. These mood alterations can vary from relatively mild to extremely intense, and can vary in a single individual from one course of treatment to another. Neither the patient nor the physician can predict with any certainty whether the corticosteroids are likely to precipitate these mood alterations. If you have a history of mood disorders (depression or bipolar disorder, for example), be sure to share this information with your physician. If you begin to experience unmanageable mood changes or swings while taking corticosteroids, contact your physician so that a decision can be made whether or not you need an additional medication to help you until the mood alterations subside.

Possible Side Effects

◇ Side effects that may go away as your body adjusts to the medication and do not require medical attention unless they continue or are bothersome: increased appetite; indigestion; nervousness or restlessness; trouble sleeping; headache; increased sweating; unusual increase in hair growth on body or face.

◇ Less common side effects that should be reported as soon as possible to your physician: severe mood changes or mood swings; decreased or blurred vision[*]; frequent urination[*].

◇ Additional side effects that can result from the prolonged use of corticosteroids and should be reported to your physician: acne or other skin problems; swelling of the face; swelling of the feet or lower legs; rapid weight gain; pain in the hips or other joints (caused by bone cell degeneration); bloody or black, tarry stools; elevated blood pressure; markedly increased thirst (with increased urination indicative of diabetes mellitus); menstrual irregularities; unusual bruising of the skin; thin, shiny skin; hair loss; muscle cramps or pain. Once you stop this medication after taking it for a long period of time, it may take several months for your body to readjust.

---

[*]Since it may be difficult to distinguish between certain common symptoms of MS and some side effects of prednisone, be sure to consult your health care professional if an abrupt change of this type occurs.

Chemical Name: Propantheline (proe-**pan**-the-leen) bromide
Brand Name: Pro-Banthine (U.S. and Canada)
Generic Available: Yes (U.S.)
Description: Propantheline is one of a group of antispasmodic/anticholinergic medications used to relieve cramps or spasms of the stomach, intestines, and bladder. Propantheline is used in the management of neurogenic bladder symptoms to control urination.

Proper Usage

◇ Take this medicine thirty minutes to one hour before meals unless otherwise directed by your physician.

Precautions

◇ Do not stop this medication abruptly. Stop gradually to avoid possible vomiting, sweating, and dizziness.
◇ Anticholinergic medications such as propantheline can cause blurred vision and light sensitivity. Make sure you know how you react to this medication before driving.
◇ Anticholinergic medications may cause dryness of the mouth. If your mouth continues to feel dry for more than two weeks, check with your dentist. Continuing dryness of the mouth may increase the chance of dental disease.
◇ No studies of the effects of this drug in pregnancy have been done in either humans or animals.
◇ Anticholinergic medications have not been reported to cause problems in nursing babies. The flow of breast milk may be reduced in some women.
◇ Be sure that your physician knows if you are taking a tricyclic antidepressant or any other anticholinergic medication. Taking propantheline with any of these may increase the anticholinergic effects, resulting in urinary retention.

Possible Side Effects

◇ Side effects that typically go away as your body adjusts to the medication and do not require medical attention unless they continue for several weeks or are bothersome: constipation*; decreased sweating; dryness of mouth, nose, and throat; bloated feeling; blurred vision*; difficulty swallowing.

◇ Unusual side effects that require immediate medical attention: inability to urinate; confusion; dizziness*; eye pain*; skin rash or hives.

◇ Symptoms of overdose that require immediate emergency attention: unusual blurred vision*; unusual clumsiness or unsteadiness*; unusual dizziness; unusually severe drowsiness*; seizures; hallucinations; confusion; shortness of breath; unusual slurred speech*; nervousness; unusual warmth, dryness, and flushing of skin.

*Since it may be difficult to distinguish between certain common symptoms of MS and some side effects of propantheline, be sure to consult your health care professional if an abrupt change of this type occurs.

Chemical Name: Psyllium hydrophilic mucilloid (**sill**-i-yum hye-droe-**fill**-ik **myoo**-sill-oid)

Brand Name: Metamucil (available in granule form in Canada, in wafer form in the U.S., and in powder or effervescent powder in the U.S. and Canada) is one of several available brands of bulk-forming laxative.

Generic Available: No

Description: Psyllium hydrophilic mucilloid is a bulk-forming oral laxative. This type of laxative is not digested by the body; it absorbs liquids from the intestines and swells to form a soft, bulky stool. The bowel is then stimulated normally by the presence of the bulky stool.

Proper Usage

◇ Laxatives are to be used to provide short-term relief only, unless otherwise directed by the nurse or physician who is helping you to manage your bowel symptoms. A regimen that includes a healthy diet containing roughage (whole grain breads and cereals, bran, fruit, and green, leafy vegetables), six to eight full glasses of liquids each day, and some form of daily exercise is most important in stimulating healthy bowel function.

◇ If your physician has recommended this laxative for management of constipation, follow his or her recommendations for its use. If you are treating yourself for constipation, follow the directions on the package insert. Results are often obtained in twelve hours but may take as long as two or three days. Be sure to consult your physician if you experience problems or do not get relief within a week.

◇ In order for this type of bulk-forming laxative to work effectively without causing intestinal blockage, it is advisable to drink six to eight glasses (eight ounces) of water each day. Each dose of the laxative should be taken with eight ounces of cold water or fruit juice. If concerns about loss of bladder control keep you from drinking this amount of water, discuss it with the nurse or physician who is helping you manage your bowel and bladder symptoms.

Precautions

◇ Do not take any type of laxative if you have signs of appendicitis or inflamed bowel (e.g., stomach or lower abdominal pain, cramping, bloating, soreness, nausea, or vomiting). Check with your physician as soon as possible.

◇ Do not take any laxative for more than one week unless you have been told to do so by your physician. Many people tend to overuse laxatives, which often leads to dependence on the laxative action to produce a bowel movement. Discuss the use of laxatives with your health care professional in order to ensure that the laxative is used effectively as part of a comprehensive, healthy bowel management regimen.

◇ Do not take any laxative within two hours of taking another medication because the desired effectiveness of the other medication may be reduced.

◇ Bulk-forming laxatives are commonly used during pregnancy. Some of them contain a large amount of sodium or sugars, which may have possible unwanted effects such as increasing blood pressure or causing fluid retention. Look for those that contain lower sodium and sugar.

◇ Some laxatives pass into breast milk. Although it is unlikely to cause problems for a nursing infant, be sure to let your physician know if you are using a laxative and breast-feeding at the same time.

Possible Side Effects:

◇ Check with your physician as soon as possible if you experience any of the following: difficulty breathing; intestinal blockage; skin rash or itching; swallowing difficulty (feelings of lump in the throat).

Chemical Name: Sertraline (**ser**-tra-leen)
Brand Name: Zoloft (U.S. and Canada)
Generic Available: No
Description: Sertraline is used to treat mental depression.

Proper Usage

This medication should always be taken at the same time in relation to meals and snacks to make sure that it is absorbed in the same way. Because sertraline may be given to different individuals at different times of the day, you and your physician should discuss what to do about any missed doses.

Precautions

◇ It may take four to six weeks for you to feel the beneficial effects of this medication.

◇ Your physician should monitor your progress at regularly scheduled visits in order to adjust the dose and help reduce any side effects.

◇ This medication could add to the effects of alcohol and other central nervous system depressants (e.g., antihistamines, sedatives, tranquilizers, sleeping medicine, prescription pain medicine, barbiturates, seizure medication, muscle relaxants). Be sure that your physician knows if you are taking these or any other medications.

◇ Sertraline may cause dryness of the mouth. If your mouth continues to feel dry for more than two weeks, check with your physician or dentist. Continuing dryness of the mouth may increase the risk of dental disease.

◇ This medication may cause drowsiness.

◇ Studies have not been done in pregnant women. Studies in animals have shown that sertraline may cause delayed development and decreased survival rates of offspring when given in doses many times the usual human dose.

◇ It is not known if sertraline passes into breast milk.

Possible Side Effects

◇ Side effects that typically go away as your body adjusts to the medication and do not require medical attention unless they continue for several weeks or are bothersome:

decreased appetite or weight loss; decrease sexual drive or ability*; drowsiness*; dryness of mouth; headache; nausea; stomach or abdominal cramps; tiredness or weakness*; tremor*; trouble sleeping; anxiety; agitation; nervousness or restlessness; changes in vision including blurred vision*; constipation*; fast or irregular heartbeat; flushing of skin; increased appetite; vomiting.

◇ Unusual side effects that should be discussed with your physician as soon as possible: fast talking and excited feelings or actions that are out of control; fever; skin rash; hives; itching.

---

*Since it may be difficult to distinguish between certain common symptoms of MS and some side effects of sertraline, be sure to consult your health care professional if an abrupt change of this type occurs.

Chemical Name: Sildenafil (sil-**den**-a-fil)

Brand Name: Viagra (U.S.)

Generic Available: No

Description: Sildenafil belongs to a group of medicines that delay the action of enzymes called phosphodiesterases, which may interfere with erectile function. Sildenafil is used to treat men with erectile dysfunction (also called sexual impotence) because it helps to maintain an erection that is produced when the penis is stroked. *Without physical stimulation of the penis, sildenafil will not work to cause an erection.* Sildenafil is not indicated for use in women.

Proper Usage:

◇ Sildenafil begins to work approximately 30 minutes after it is taken. The medication continues to work for up to four hours, although the effect is usually less after two hours.

◇ Sildenafil is available by prescription and should be used only as directed by your physician. The dose of this medication will be different for different patients. Do not take more of this medication than has been prescribed for you.

Precautions:

◇ Sildenafil can interact with, or interfere with the action of, other medications you may be taking. Be sure to inform your physician of all other medications you are taking so that appropriate substitutions or dosage adjustments can be made. Sildenafil should not be used by men who are using nitrates such as nitroglycerin (e.g., Nitrostat or Transderm-Nitro) to lower their blood pressure; sildenafil may cause the blood pressure to drop too far.

◇ The presence of certain medical problems may interfere with the use of sildenafil. Be sure to inform your doctor if you have any of the following medical problems: an abnormality of the penis (including a curved penis or birth defect); bleeding problems; retinitis pigmentosa; any conditions causing thickened blood or slower blood flow (e.g., leukemia, multiple myeloma, polycythemia, sickle cell disease, or thrombocythemia); a history of priapism (erection lasting longer than six hours); heart or blood disease; severe kidney problems; severe liver problems.

◇ Sildenafil has not been studied in combination with other medications that are used in the treatment of erectile dysfunction. At the present time, it is not recommended that these drugs be used together.

Possible Side Effects:

◇ *Side effects that you should report to your physician so that he or she can adjust the dosage or change the medication:*flushing; headache; nasal congestion, stomach discomfort after meals; diarrhea.

◇ *Rare side effects that should be discussed with your physician:* abnormal vision (e.g., blurred vision,* seeing shades of colors differently than before, sensitivity to light); bladder pain; cloudy or bloody urine; dizziness, increased frequency of urination; painful urination.

Note: There are a variety of other possible side effects that have not yet been definitely shown to be caused by sildenafil. Therefore, if you notice any other effects that cause you concern, be sure to talk them over with your doctor.

Chemical Name: Sodium phosphate
Brand Name: Fleet Enema (U.S. and Canada)
Generic Available: No
Description: Sodium phosphate enemas are available over-the-counter.

Proper Usage

◇ Rectal enemas are to be used to provide short-term relief only, unless otherwise directed by the nurse or physician who is helping you to manage your bowel symptoms. A regimen that includes a healthy diet containing roughage (whole grain breads and cereals, bran, fruit, and green, leafy vegetables), six to eight full glasses of liquids each day, and some form of daily exercise is most important in stimulating healthy bowel function.

◇ If your physician has recommended this rectal laxative for management of constipation, follow his or her recommendations for its use. If you are treating yourself for constipation, follow the directions on the package insert.

◇ Results usually occur within two to five minutes. Be sure to consult your physician if you notice rectal bleeding, blistering, pain, burning, itching, or other signs of irritation that was not present before you began using a sodium phosphate enema.

Precautions

◇ Do not use any type of laxative if you have signs of appendicitis or inflamed bowel (e.g., stomach or lower abdominal pain, cramping, bloating, soreness, nausea, or vomiting). Check with your physician as soon as possible.

◇ Do not use any laxative for more than one week unless you have been told to do so by your physician. Many people tend to overuse laxatives, which often leads to dependence on the laxative action to produce a bowel movement. Discuss the use of laxatives with your health care professional in order to ensure that the laxative is used effectively as part of a comprehensive, healthy bowel management regimen.

◇ If you are pregnant, discuss with your physician the most appropriate type of laxative for you to use.

Possible Side Effects

◇ Side effect that may go away as your body adjusts to the medication and does not require medical attention unless it persists or is bothersome: skin irritation in the rectal area.

◇ Unusual side effects that should be reported to your physician as soon as possible: rectal bleeding, blistering, burning, itching.

Chemical Name: Sulfamethoxazole (sul-fa-meth-**ox**-a-zole) and trimethoprim (try-**meth**-oh-prim) combination

Brand Name: Bactrim; Septra (U.S. and Canada)

Generic Available: Yes (U.S.)

Description: Sulfamethoxazole and trimethoprim combination is used in multiple sclerosis to treat (and sometimes to prevent) urinary tract infections.

Proper Usage

◇ This medication is best taken with a full glass (eight ounces) of water. Additional water should be taken each day to help prevent unwanted effects.

◇ Finish the full course of treatment prescribed by your physician. Even if your symptoms disappear after a few days, stopping this medication prematurely may result in a return of the symptoms.

◇ This medication works most effectively when it is maintained at a constant level in your blood or urine. To help keep the amount constant, do not miss any doses. It is best to take the doses at evenly spaced times during the day and night. For maximum effectiveness, four doses per day would be spaced at six-hour intervals.

Precautions

◇ This medication may cause dizziness.

◇ If taken for a long time, sulfamethoxazole and trimethoprim combination may cause blood problems. It is very important that your physician monitor your progress at regular visits.

◇ This medication can cause changes in the blood, possibly resulting in a greater chance of certain infections, slow healing, and bleeding of the gums. Be careful with the use of your toothbrush, dental floss, and toothpicks. Delay dental work until your blood counts are completely normal. Check with your dentist if you have questions about oral hygiene during treatment.

◇ This medication may cause your skin to become more sensitive to sunlight. Stay out of direct sunlight during the midday hours, wear protective clothing, and apply a sun block product that has a skin protection factor (SPF) of at least 15.

◇ Sulfamethoxazole and trimethoprim combination has not been reported to cause birth defects or other problems in humans. Studies in mice, rats, and rabbits have shown that some sulfonamides cause birth defects, including cleft palate and bone problems. Studies in rabbits have also shown that trimethoprim causes birth defects, as well as a decrease in the number of successful pregnancies.

◇ Sulfamethoxazole and trimethoprim pass into breast milk. This medication is not recommended for use during breast-feeding. It may cause liver problems, anemia, and other problems in nursing babies.

Possible Side Effects

◇ Side effects that may go away as your body adjusts to the medication and do not require medical attention unless they continue or are bothersome: diarrhea; dizziness; headache; loss of appetite; nausea or vomiting.

◇ Less common side effects that should be reported to your physician immediately: itching; skin rash; aching of muscles and joints; difficulty in swallowing; pale skin; redness, blistering, peeling, or loosening of skin; sore throat and fever; unusual bleeding or bruising; unusual tiredness or weakness*; yellow eyes or skin.

---

*Since it may be difficult to distinguish between certain common symptoms of MS and some side effects of sulfamethoxazole, be sure to consult your health care professional if an abrupt change of this type occurs.

Chemical Name: Tizanidine hydrochloride (tye-**zan**-i-deen)
Brand Name: Zanaflex (U.S. and Canada)
Generic Available: No
Description: Tizanidine is used in multiple sclerosis to treat the
   increased muscle tone associated with spasticity. Although it
   does not provide a cure for the problems, it is designed to
   relieve the spasms, cramping, and tightness of muscles.

Proper Usage:

◇ Tizanidine is a short-acting drug for the management of
   spasticity. Its peak effectiveness occurs one to two hours
   after dosing and is finished between three to six hours after
   dosing. Therefore, your physician will prescribe a dosing
   schedule that provides maximal relief during activities and
   periods of time of greatest importance to you.

◇ In order to minimize unwanted side effects of this medication, your physician will start you on a low dose and gradually increase it until a well-tolerated and effective level is
   reached.

◇ Studies of tizanidine have not been done in pregnant
   women. Animal studies, using doses significantly higher
   than those prescribed for humans, have resulted in damage
   to the offspring. If you are pregnant or planning to become
   pregnant, discuss this with your physician before starting
   this medication.

◇ It is not known whether tizanidine passes into the breast
   milk. Women should not take this medication while nursing unless told to do so by their physician.

Precautions:

◇ Oral contraceptives (birth control pills) may slow the
   release of tizanidine from the body; women using birth
   control pills should inform their physician so that the dose
   level of tizanidine can be reduced accordingly.

◇ This medication may cause blurred vision,* dizziness, or
   drowsiness in some people.

◇ This drug will add to the effects of alcohol and other central nervous system depressants (such as antihistamines,
   sedatives, tranquilizers, prescription pain medications,
   seizure medications, other muscle relaxants), possibly

causing drowsiness. Be sure that your physician knows if you are taking these or any other medications.

Possible Side Effects:

◇ Common side effects that may go away as your body adjusts to the medication and do not require medical attention unless they continue for more than two weeks or are bothersome: dryness of mouth; sleepiness or sedation; weakness,* fatigue,* and or tiredness;* dizziness or light-headedness, especially when getting up from a sitting or lying position; increase in muscle spasms, cramps, or tightness; back pain.

◇ *Common side effects that should be reported to the doctor as soon as possible:* burning, prickling, or tingling sensation;* diarrhea; fainting; fever; loss of appetite; nausea; nervousness; pain or burning during urination; sores on skin; stomach pain; vomiting; yellow eyes or skin; blurred vision.*

---

*Since it may be difficult to distinguish between certain common symptoms of MS and some side effects of tizanidine, be sure to consult your health care professional if an abrupt change of this type occurs.

Chemical Name: Tolterodine (tole-**tare**-oh-deen)
Brand Name: Detrol (U.S.)
Generic Available: (No)
Description: Tolterodine is an *antispasmodic* that is used to treat bladder spasms causing urinary frequency, urgency, or urge incontinence.

Proper Usage:

◇ Take only the amount of this medication that has been prescribed for you by your doctor; taking more than the prescribed amount may cause adverse effects.

◇ If you miss a dose of this medication, take it as soon as possible. If, however, it is almost time for your next dose, skip the missed dose and go back to your regular schedule. Do not double dose.

Precautions:

◇ Individuals with any of the following medical problems should not take this medication: gastric retention, urinary retention, or narrow angle or uncontrolled glaucoma. Tolterodine can aggravate each of these conditions.

◇ Tolterodine may cause dizziness or drowsiness; use caution when driving or doing any activities that require alertness.

◇ Tolterodine may cause drying of the mouth. Because continued dryness of the mouth may increase the risk of dental disease, alert your dentist if you are taking this medication.

◇ This medication may interact with fluoxetine (Prozac) in such a way as to increase the effect of tolterodine. If you are taking fluoxetine, your physician may start you at a lower dose of tolterodine, gradually raising it to the standard dose if necessary.

◇ This medication has not been studied in pregnant women. However, it has been shown in animal studies to result in increased embryo deaths, reduced birth weight, and increased incidence of fetal abnormalities. If you are pregnant or planning to become pregnant, do not start this medication before you have discussed it with your physician.

◇ It is not known whether tolterodine passes into breast milk. Because tolterodine is known to pass into the milk of nursing animals, causing temporary reduction in weight gain in the offspring, women should stop taking this drug as long as they are nursing.

Possible Side Effects:

◇ *Side effects that will typically go away as your body adjusts to the medication and do not require medical attention unless they continue for a few weeks or are bothersome:* dry mouth; dizziness; headache; fatigue;* gastrointestinal symptoms, including abdominal pain, constipation,* or diarrhea; difficult urination.

◇ *Less common side effects that should be reported to your physician immediately:* abnormal vision, including difficulty adjusting to distances; urinary tract infection.

◇ *Symptoms of overdose:* severe central anticholinergic effects, including blurred vision;* clumsiness or unsteadiness;* confusion; seizures; severe diarrhea, excessive watering of the mouth; increasing muscle weakness (especially in the arms, neck, shoulders, and tongue); muscle cramps or twitching; severe nausea or vomiting; shortness of breath, slow heartbeat; slurred speech;* unusual irritability, nervousness, or restlessness; unusual tiredness or weakness.*

---

*Since it may be difficult to distinguish between certain common symptoms of MS and some side effects of tolterodine, be sure to consult your health care professional if an abrupt change of this type occurs.

Chemical Name: Venlafaxine (ven-la-**fax**-een)
Brand Name: Effexor (U.S. and Canada)
Generic Available: No
Description: Venlafaxine is used to treat mental depression.

Dosage and Proper Usage:

◇ Unless your physician has instructed otherwise, this medication should be taken with food or on a full stomach to reduce the chances of stomach upset.

◇ If you miss a dose of this medication, take it as soon as possible. If, however, it is within two hours of your next dose, skip the missed dose and return to your regular schedule. Do not double dose.

Precautions:

◇ It may take 4 to 6 weeks for you to feel the beneficial effects of this medication.

◇ Your physician should monitor your progress at regularly scheduled visits in order to adjust the dose and help reduce any side effects.

◇ Do not stop taking this medication without consulting your physician. The doctor may want you to reduce the amount you are taking gradually in order to decrease unwanted side effects.

◇ This medication could add to the effects of alcohol and other central nervous system depressants (e.g., antihistamines, sedatives, tranquilizers, sleeping medicine, prescription pain medicine, barbiturates, seizure medication, muscle relaxants). Be sure that your doctor knows if you are taking these or any other medications.

◇ Venlafaxine may cause dryness of the mouth. If your mouth continues to feel dry for more than two weeks, check with your physician or dentist. Continuing dryness of the mouth may increase the risk of dental disease.

◇ This medication may cause you to become drowsy or to have double vision

◇ Venlafaxine may cause dizziness, lightheadedness, or fainting, especially when you stand from a sitting or lying position. If rising slowly from a sitting or lying position does not relieve the problem, consult your physician.

◇ Studies have not been done in pregnant women. However, studies in animals have shown that venlafaxine may cause decreased survival rates of offspring when given in doses that are many times the usual dose for humans. If you are pregnant or planning to become pregnant, do not start this medication before you have discussed it with your physician.

◇ It is not known whether venlafaxine passes into breast milk. Mothers who are taking this medication and wish to breast-feed should discuss this with their doctor.

Possible Side Effects:

◇ *Side effects that will typically go away as your body adjusts to the medication and do not require medical attention unless they continue for several weeks or are bothersome:* abnormal dreams; anxiety or nervousness; constipation,* dizziness, drowsiness,* dryness of mouth, tingling or burning sensations,* decreased appetite, nausea, stomach or abdominal cramps; trouble sleeping; tiredness;* tremor.*

◇ *Unusual side effects that should be discussed with the doctor as soon as possible:* changes in vision or double vision;* changes in sexual desire or ability;* headache, chest pain; fast heartbeat; itching or skin rash; mood or mental changes; problems with urination;* menstrual changes; uncontrolled excitability; high blood pressure.

◇ *Symptoms of overdose include:* extreme drowsiness, tiredness, or weakness.*

*Since it may be difficult to distinguish between certain common symptoms of MS and some side effects of venlafaxine, be sure to consult your health care professional if an abrupt change of this type occurs.

National Multiple Sclerosis Society Consensus Statement

In September, 1998, the National Multiple Sclerosis Society's medical advisors approved a statement regarding early intervention and access to therapy for patients with relapsing-remitting multiple sclerosis. The statement addresses the three immunomodulating agents approved for use in the U.S. It does not address Rebif®, which is approved in Canada and Europe, but has not yet been approved for use in the U.S.

Recommendations

The Medical Advisory Board of the National Multiple Sclerosis Society has adopted the following recommendations regarding use of the current MS disease-modifying agents—Betaseron® (beta interferon 1-b), Avonex® (beta interferon 1-a), and Copaxone® (glatiramer acetate):

◇ Initiation of therapy is advised as soon as possible following a definite diagnosis of MS and determination of a relapsing course.

◇ Patients' access to medication should not be limited by the frequency of relapses, age or level of disability.

◇ Treatment is not to be stopped during evaluation for continuing treatment.

◇ Therapy is to be continued indefinitely, unless there is clear lack of benefit, intolerable side effects, new data that reveals other reasons for cessation, or better therapy is available.

◇ All three agents should be included in formularies and covered by third party payors so that physicians and patients may determine the most appropriate agent on an individual basis.

◇ Movement from one immunomodulating drug to another should be permitted.

◇ Most concurrent medical conditions do not contraindicate use of any of these therapies.

Rationale

The management of multiple sclerosis has been substantially advanced by the availability of the disease-modifying agents interferon beta-1a (Avonex®) and -1b (Betaseron®), and glatiramer acetate (Copaxone®). A number of positive outcomes have been demonstrated in people with relapsing-remitting disease, including reduction in the frequency and severity of relapses and reduction of brain lesion development by all three agents as evidenced by magnetic resonance imaging (MRI). There is also early indication of slowed progression of disability. As a result, the U.S. Food and Drug Administration (FDA) has approved the use of these drugs by individuals identified as having relapsing-remitting MS. In addition, preliminary data from European studies of interferon beta-1b support the use of that agent in secondary progressive disease.

After several tears of experience with the beta interferons, and more recently with glatiramer acetate, it is the consensus of researchers and clinicians with expertise in MS that these agents reduce future disability and improve quality of life for many individuals with MS. The National MS Society Medical Advisory Board strongly supports early intervention with one of these agents. Recent studies . . . confirm that early relapses can cause permanent axonal damage as well as destruction of the myelin sheath. Thus, even early relapses that appear benign and leave no apparent impairments in their wake can have permanent neurologic consequences. Furthermore, repeat MRI studies of individuals who are clinically in remission have demonstrated the presence of ongoing brain lesion development and atrophy. It is for these reasons that the Medical Advisory Board has issued its recommendations for early intervention.

If a copy of the entire document is desired, please call 1-800-FIGHT-MS, and select option 1, or call 1-212-986-3240 and ask for the Information Resource Center.

Appendix D

Additional Readings

NOTE: Your local chapter of the National Multiple Sclerosis Society has a complete collection of booklets and articles about all aspects of MS research, treatments, and management. Call 1-800-FIGHT MS to be connected to the chapter nearest you. Chapter personnel are available to answer your questions and send you information on any MS-related topics that are of interest to you.

Barrett, S, Jarvis, WT (eds.). (1993). *The Health Robbers: A Close Look at Quackery in America.* Buffalo: Prometheus Books.

Bondo BE. (1995). *Tax Options and Strategies: A State-by-State Guide for Persons with Disabilities, Senior Citizens, Veterans, and Their Families.* New York: Demos.

Burstein, E. (1994). *Legwork: An Inspiring Journey Through a Chronic Illness.* New York: Simon & Schuster.

Cassileth, BR. (1998). *The Alternative Medicine Handbook.* New York: W.W. Norton & Co.

Cohen, MD. (1996). *Dirty Details: The Days and Nights of a Well Spouse.* Philadelphia: Temple University Press.

Cooke, M, Putman, E. (1996). *Ways You Can Help: Creative, Practical Suggestions for Family and Friends of Patients and Caregivers.* New York: Warner Books.

Cristall, B. (1992). *Coping When a Parent has Multiple Sclerosis.* New York: Rosen Publishing [written for teens].

Enders A, Hall M. (1990). *Assistive Technology Sourcebook.* Washington, D.C.: Resna Press.

Giffels JJ. (1996). *Clinical Trials: What You Should Know Before Volunteering to Be a Research Subject.* New York: Demos.

Halligan F. (1995). *The Art of Coping.* New York: Crossroad.

Halper, J, Holland, J.(eds.). (1996). *Comprehensive Nursing Care in Multiple Sclerosis.* New York: Demos.

Hecker H. (1995). *Travel for the Disabled: A Handbook of Travel Resources and 500 Worldwide Access Guides.* Vancouver, WA: Twin Peaks Press.

Holland, N., Halper, J. (eds.) (1998). *Multiple Sclerosis: A Self-Care Guide to Wellness.* Washington, D.C.: Paralyzed Veterans of America.

Holland, N, Murray, TJ, Reingold, SC. (1996). *Multiple Sclerosis: A Guide for the Newly Diagnosed.* New York: Demos.

James JL. (1993). *One Particular Harbor: The Outrageous True Adventures of One Woman with Multiple Sclerosis Living in the Alaskan Wilderness.* Chicago: Noble Press.

Kalb RC. (1998). *Multiple Sclerosis: A Guide for Families.* New York: Demos Medical Publishing.

Koplowitz, A., Celizic, M. (1997). *The Winning Spirit: Lessons Learned in Last Place.* New York: Doubleday.

Kraft GH, Catanzaro M. (2000). *Living with Multiple Sclerosis: A Wellness Approach* (2nd ed.). New York: Demos Medical Publishing.

Kroll K, Klein EL. (1995). *Enabling Romance: A Guide to Love, Sex, and Relationships for the Disabled.* Bethesda, MD: Woodbine House.

Lechtenberg R. (1995). *Multiple Sclerosis Fact Book* (2nd ed.). Philadelphia: Davis.

LeMaistre J. (1994). *Beyond Rage: Mastering Unavoidable Health Changes.* Dillon, CO: Alpine Guild.

Lunt S. (1982). *A Handbook for the Disabled: Ideas and Inventions for Easier Living.* New York: Charles Scribner's Sons.

MacFarlane EB, Burstein P. (1994). *Legwork: An Inspiring Journey Through a Chronic Illness.* New York: Charles Scribner's Sons.

Mairs, N. (1998). *Waist-High in the World: A Life Among the Nondisabled.* Beacon Press.

Mendelsohn SB. (1996). *Tax Options and Strategies for People with Disabilities* (2nd ed.). New York: Demos.

Perkins, L, Perkins, S. (1999). *Multiple Sclerosis: Your Legal Rights* (2nd ed.). New York: Demos Medical Publishing.

Pitzele SK. (1986). *We Are Not Alone: Learning to Live with Chronic Illness.* New York: Workman.

Pitzele SK. (1988). *One More Day: Daily Meditations for the Chronically Ill.* Minneapolis: Hazelden.

Rao S (ed.) (1990). *Neurobehavioral Aspects of Multiple Sclerosis.* New York: Oxford.

Register C. (1987). *Living with Chronic Illness: Days of Patience and Passion.* New York: Free Press.

Resources for Rehabilitation (1993a). *Meeting the Needs of Employees with Disabilities.* Lexington, MA: Resources for Rehabilitation.

Resources for Rehabilitation (1993b). *Resources for People with Disabilities and Chronic Conditions.* Lexington, MA: Resources for Rehabilitation.

Resources for Rehabilitation (1994). *A Woman's Guide to Coping with Disability.* Lexington, MA: Resources for Rehabilitation.

Resources for Rehabilitation (1996). *Living with Low Vision: A Resource Guide for People with Sight Loss.* Lexington, MA: Resources for Rehabilitation.

Rogers J, Matsumura M. (1990). *Mother to Be: A Guide to Pregnancy and Birth for Women with Disabilities.* New York: Demos.

Rosner LJ, Ross S. (1992). *Multiple Sclerosis: New Hope and Practical Guidelines for People with MS and Their Families.* New York: Prentice Hall.

Rumrill, P.D., Jr. (ed.). (1996). *Employment Issues and Multiple Sclerosis.* New York: Demos.

Russell LM, Grant AE, Joseph SM, Fee RW. (1993). *Planning for the Future: Providing a Meaningful Life for a Child with a Disability After Your Death* (2nd ed.). Evanston, IL: American Publishing.

Schapiro RT. (1998). *Symptom Management in Multiple Sclerosis* (3rd ed.). New York: Demos Medical Publishing.

Schwarz, SP. (1999). *300 Tips for Making Life with Multiple Sclerosis Easier.* New York: Demos Medical Publishing.

Shapiro, JP. (1993). *No Pity.* New York: Time Books.

Sherkin-Langer, F. (1995). *When Mommy Is Sick.* St. Louis: Fern Publications (P.O. Box 16893, St. Louis, MO 63105; fax: 314-994-0052. [Recommended for children ages 2–8]

Sherman, JR. *The Caregiver Survival Series.* [includes Coping with Caregiver Worries, Preventing Caregiver Burnout, Creative Caregiving, Positive Caregiver Attitudes, and The Magic of Humor in Caregiving. Golden Valley, MN: Pathways Books (Tel: 800-958-3378; Internet: HYPERLINK http://www.caregiver911.com).

Shrout RN. (1991). *Resource Directory for the Disabled.* New York: Oxford.

Shuman R, Schwartz J. (1988). *Understanding Multiple Sclerosis.* Riverside, NJ: Macmillan.

Sibley WA. (1996). *Therapeutic Claims in Multiple Sclerosis* (4th ed.). New York: Demos.

Stolman MD. (1994). *A Guide to Legal Rights for People With Disabilities.* New York: Demos.

Stone, K. (1997). *Awakening to Disability: Nothing About Us Without Us.* Volcano, CA: Volcano Press (P.O. Box 270, Volcano, CA 95689; Tel: 800-879-9636).

Strong M. (1997). *For the Well Spouse of the Chronically Ill* (3rd rev.). Mainstay, NY: Little, Brown.

Tyler, VE. (1998). *The Honest Herbal* (4th ed.). New York: Haworth Press.

Webster B. (1989). *All of a Piece: A Life with Multiple Sclerosis.* Baltimore: Johns Hopkins.

Wells, SM. (1998). *A Delicate Balance: Living Successfully with Chronic Illness.* New York: Plenum Press.

Wolf J. (1987). *Mastering Multiple Sclerosis: A Guide to Management.* Rutland, VT: Academy Books.

Wolf J, Miles M, Pickett K. (1993). *Vignettes: Stories from Lives with Multiple Sclerosis.* Rutland, VT: Academy Books.

Wolf J. (1991). *Fall Down Seven Times, Get Up Eight.* Rutland, VT: Academy Books.

Wright LM, Leahey M. (1987). *Families and Chronic Illness.* Philadelphia: Spring House.

Younger V, Sardegna J. (1994). *A Guide to Independence for the Visually Impaired and Their Families.* New York: Demos.

Zola IK. (1982). *Missing Pieces: A Chronicle of Living with a Disability.* Philadelphia: Temple University Press.

National Multiple Sclerosis Society Publications (212-986-3240; 800-344-4867)

Booklets

- ◇ *Living with MS* (ES 0087)
- ◇ *What Everyone Should Know About Multiple Sclerosis* (ER 100)
- ◇ *Things I Wish Someone Had Told Me: Practical Thoughts for People Newly Diagnosed with Multiple Sclerosis* (ES 6028)
- ◇ *Research Directions in Multiple Sclerosis* (ES 6017)
- ◇ *ADA and People with MS* (ECS 6021)
- ◇ *Enhancing Productivity On Your Job: The Win-Win Approach* (ES 6025)
- ◇ *A Guide for Caregivers* ES 6010)
- ◇ *Exercise as Part of Everyday Life* (ES 6008)
- ◇ *Clear Thinking About Alternative Therapies* (ECS 6038)
- ◇ *Choosing a Pharmacy Service* (ECS 6032)
- ◇ *Managing MS Through Rehabilitation* (ECS 6022)
- ◇ *Food for Thought: MS and Nutrition* (ES 6020)
- ◇ *Multiple Sclerosis and Your Emotions* (ES 6007)
- ◇ *Taming Stress in Multiple Sclerosis* (ES 6034)
- ◇ *At Home with MS: Adapting Your Environment* (ECS 6035)
- ◇ *Solving Cognitive Problems* (ECS 6029)
- ◇ *Controlling Bladder Problems in MS* (ES 0039)
- ◇ *Understanding Bowel Problems in MS* (ECS 6036)
- ◇ *PLAINTALK: A Booklet About MS for Families* (ECS 55)
- ◇ *Someone You Know Has MS: A Book for Families* (ES 0045)
- ◇ *At Our House*—a coloring book for children ages 3–5 (contains very basic facts as well as an afterword for parents on how to talk to young children about MS) (ECS 6033)
- ◇ *When a Parent Has MS: A Teenager's Guide* (ECS 6024)
- ◇ *Controlling Spasticity* (ECS 6037)

Materials Available in Spanish:

◇ *Hacia una Comprension de los Problemas de la Vejiga en la Esclerosis Multiple*

◇ *Lo qué Todo el Mundo Debe Saber sobre la Esclerosis Multiple*

◇ *Qué es la Esclerosis Multiple?*

◇ *Qué le Interesa Conocer sobre la Esclerosis Multiple?*

◇ *Sobre la Conservacion de Energia*

◇ *Sobre la Fatiga*

◇ *Sobre las Problemas Sexuales que no Mencionan los Medicos*

◇ *Sobre el Diagnostico: Atando Los Cabos de una Larga Historia*

Other MS Society Publications

◇ *The History of Multiple Sclerosis* (reprint)—Loren Rolak, M.D.

◇ *Facts and Issues* (reprints of articles that originally appeared in the National MS Society magazine, *Inside MS,* covering such topics as diagnosis, disclosure, pregnancy, pain, fatigue, energy management, gait problems, sexuality, depression, hiring home help, computer adaptations, genes and MS susceptibility, complementary therapies, etc.)

◇ *Inside MS*—a 32-page magazine for people living with MS published three times yearly

◇ *Inside MS Bulletin*—an 8-page newsletter for donors and friends (published three times a year)

◇ *Knowledge is Power*—a series of articles for individuals newly diagnosed with MS

◇ *Living Well with MS*—a series of workbooks written for, and by, people who have been living with MS for some time.

◇ *Monograph Series* (1995)

—*Families Affected by Multiple Sclerosis: Disease Impacts and Coping Strategies*—Rosalind C. Kalb, Ph.D.

—*Long-Term Care and Multiple Sclerosis*—Debra Frankel, M.S., O.T.R.

—*Employment and Multiple Sclerosis*—Nicholas G. LaRocca, Ph.D.

—*Economic Costs of Multiple Sclerosis: How Much and Who Pays*—Carol Harvey, Ph.D.

—*Utilization and Perceptions of Healthcare Services by People with MS*—Leon Sternfeld, M.D., Ph.D., M.P.H.

Canadian Multiple Sclerosis Society Publication (416-922-6065)

◇ *Coping with Fatigue in MS Takes Understanding and Planning*—Alexander Burnfield, M.B., M.R.C. Psych.

Eastern Paralyzed Veterans Association Publications (800-444-0120)

◇ *Understanding the Americans with Disabilities Act* (English and Spanish)

◇ *The ADA: Resource Information Guide* (bibliography of books and videotapes)

◇ *Air Carrier Access* (defines the Air Carrier Access Act and gives information about air travel for wheelchair users)

◇ *Accessible Building Design* (a description of the essential components of an accessible building, including dimensions)

◇ *Planning for Access: A Guide for Planning and Modifying Your Home*

◇ *Programs of EPVA* (a summary of 15 programs designed to improve the lives of spinal cord injured veterans and people with disabilities)

General Publications

◇ *Access to Travel*—A quarterly magazine published by the Society for the Advancement of Travel for the Handicapped—SATH—a nonprofit organization that works to create a barrier-free environment throughout the travel and tourism industry (347 Fifth Avenue, Suite 610, New York, NY 10016; 212-447-7284)

◇ *An Approach to Barrier Free Design*—A magazine available from A Positive Approach, Inc., a nonprofit organization that services individuals with disabilities (P.O. Box 910, Millville, NJ 08322; 609-451-4777)

◇ *Handicapped Americans Reports*—a biweekly newsletter that reports disability-related events and issues, published by Capital Publications, Inc. (1300 N. 17th Street, Arlington, VA 22209; 703-528-1100)

◇ *Mainstream*—A monthly magazine available from Exploding Myths, Inc. (2973 Beech Street, San Diego, CA 92101; 619-234-3138)

◇ *Multiple Sclerosis Quarterly Report*—A quarterly publication with articles on medical management, living with MS, and summaries of research on the cause and treatment of MS, available on a subscription basis from Demos Medical Publishing (386 Park Avenue South, Suite 201, New York, NY 10016; 800-532-8663)

◇ *New Mobility*—A monthly magazine available from Miramar Communications (23815 Stuart Ranch Road, P.O. Box 8987, Malibu, CA 90265; 800-543-4116)

◇ *A Positive Approach*—A magazine available from A Positive Approach, Inc., a nonprofit organization that services individuals with disabilities (P.O. Box 910, Millville, NJ 08322; 609-451-4777)

◇ *Real Living with MS*—A monthly newsletter available by subscription from the Cobb Group (9420 Bunsen Parkway, Louisville, KY 40220; 800-223-8720)

◇ *Take Care*—A quarterly newsletter for caregivers published by the National Family Caregivers Association (9621 East Bexhill Drive, Kensington, MD 20895; 301-942-6430)

◇ *The Very Special Traveler*—A bimonthly newsletter for people with disabilities who travel, published by Beverly Nelson (The Very Special Traveler, P.O. Box 756, New Windsor, MD 21776-9016; 410-635-2881)

◇ *We Magazine*—subscription magazine published six times a year (Tel: 800-WEMAG26; website: www.wemagazine.com).

◇ *"We're Accessible": News for Disabled Travelers*—A newsletter from British Colombia for world travelers with disabilities (Lynne Atkinson, 32-1675 Cypress St., Vancouver, B.C. V6J3L4; 604-731-2197)

Appendix **E**

Resources

There is a vast array of resources available to help you in your efforts to meet the challenges of multiple sclerosis. This list is by no means a complete one; it is designed as a starting point in your efforts to identify the resources you need. Each resource that you investigate will lead you to others and they, in turn, will lead you to even more.

Information Sources

Clearinghouse on Disability Information, Communications and Information Services, Office of Special Education and Rehabilitative Services, U.S. Department of Education, Switzer Building, 330 C Street, S.W., Washington, D.C. 20202; tel: 202-205-8241; Internet: www.ed.gov/offices/OSER. Created by the Rehabilitation Act of 1973, the Clearinghouse responds to inquiries about federal laws, services, and programs for individuals of all ages with disabilities.

Disability Rights Education and Defense Fund, Inc. (DREDF) (2212 Sixth Street, Berkeley, CA 94710; tel: 610-644-2555; 800-466-4232; Internet: www.dredf.org). DREDF is a national law and policy center dedicated to furthering the civil rights of people with disabilities. The Center provides assistance, information, and referrals on disability rights laws; legal representation in cases involving civil rights; and education/training for legislators, policy makers, and law students.

Easter Seals/March of Dimes National Council (90 Eglinton Avenue East, Suite 511, Toronto, Ontario M4P 2Y3, Canada; tel: 416-932-8382). The Council is a federation of regional and provincial groups serving individuals with disabilities throughout Canada. It operates an information service and publishes a newsletter and a quarterly journal.

Inglis House (2600 Belmont Avenue, Philadelphia, PA 19131; tel: 215-878-5600). A national information exchange network specializing in long-term facilities for mentally alert persons with physical disabilities.

National Health Information Center (P.O. Box 1133, Washington, D.C. 20013; tel: 800-336-4797; Internet: nhic-nt.health.org). The Center maintains a library and a database of health-related organizations. It also provides referrals related to health issues for consumers and professionals.

President's Committee on Employment of People with Disabilities (1331 F Street, N.W., Washington, D.C. 20004-1107; tel: 202-376-6200; Internet: www.info@pcepd.gov). The Committee publishes employment-related brochures for individuals with disabilities and their employers, and provides the Job Accommodation Network (tel: 800-526-7234).

Electronic Information Sources

There are many sources of information available free through the Internet on the World Wide Web. If you are an experienced "net surfer," switch to your favorite search facility and enter the key words "MS" or "multiple sclerosis." This will generally give you a listing of dozens of web sites that pertain to MS. Keep in mind, however, that the World Wide Web is a free and open medium; while many of the web sites have excellent and useful information, others may contain highly unusual and inaccurate information. Following is a list of some recommended MS sites available through the Internet. Each of these will provide links to other sites.

ABLEDATA
Information on Assistive Technology
http://www.abledata.com/

Allsup, Inc
Assists Individuals Applying for Social Security Disability Benefits
http://www.allsupinc.com/

Apple Computer Disability Resources
http://www.apple.com/education/k12/disability/

The Ares-Serono Group/Rebif®
http://www.serono.com/ms/

Berlex/Betaseron®
http://www.betaseron.com/

Biogen/Avonex®
http://www.biogen.com/

CenterWatch Clinical Trials Listing Service™
http://www.centerwatch.com/

CLAMS—Computer Literate Advocates for Multiple Sclerosis
http://www.clams.org/

The Consortium of Multiple Sclerosis Centers
http://www.mscare.org/

IBM Special Needs Systems
http://www.austin.ibm.com/sns/

Immunex/Novantrone®
http://www.MSknowledge.com

Infosci
Selected Links on MS
http://www.infosci.org/

International Federation of Multiple Sclerosis Societies/The World of Multiple Sclerosis
http://www.nmss.org/

The International Journal of MS Care
http://www.mscare.com/

Medicare Information
http://www.hcfa.gov/medicare/medicare.htm

Microsoft Accessibility Technology for Everyone
http://www.microsoft.com/enable/

MS Crossroads
Personal Website of Aapo Halko, Ph.D., mathematician with
MS in Finland
http://www.helsinki.fi/~ahalko/ms.html

The Multiple Sclerosis Information Gateway
Schering AG, Berlin, Germany
http://www.ms-gateway.com/

The Multiple Sclerosis Society of Canada
http://www.mssoc.ca/

The Myelin Project
http://www.myelin.org/

The National Family Caregivers Association
http://www.nfcacares.org/

The National Institute of Neruological Disorders and Stroke
http://www.ninds.nih.gov/

The National Library of Medicine
http://www.nlm.nih.gov/

The National Multiple Sclerosis Society
http://www.nmss.org/

The National Organization for Rare Disorders
http://www.rarediseases.org/

NARIC—The National Rehabilitation Information Center
http://www.naric.com/

Teva Marion Partners/Copaxone
http://www.tevamarionpartners.com/

Resource Materials

Assistive Technology Sourcebook. (Written by A. Enders and M.
   Hall, published by Resna Press, Washington, D.C. 1990).
The Complete Directory for People with Chronic Illness,
   1998–1999, (published by Grey House Publishing, Inc., Pock-

et Knife Square, P.O. Box 1866, Lakeville, CT 06039; tel: 800-562-2139; fax: 860-435-3004; e-mail: www.greyhouse.com).

The Complete Directory for People with Disabilities, 1999–2000 (published by Grey House Publishing, Inc., Pocket Knife Square, P.O. Box 1866, Lakeville, CT 06039; tel: 800-562-2139; fax: 860-435-3004; e-mail: www.greyhouse.com).

Complete Drug Reference. (Compiled by United States Pharmacopoeia, published by Consumer Report Books, A division of Consumers Union, Yonkers, NY.). This comprehensive, readable, and easy-to-use drug reference includes almost every prescription and non-prescription medication available in the United States and Canada. A new edition is published yearly.

Complete Guide to Prescription and Non-Prescription Drugs. (Written by H. Winter Griffith, M.D., published by The Body Press/Perigee, 200 Madison Avenue, New York, NY 10016, 1995).

Directory of National Information Sources on Disabilities. (Published by the National Institute on Disability and Rehabilitation Research, Washington, D.C. 1994-1995. Vols. I and II).

Dressing Tips and Clothing Resources for Making Life Easier. (Written by Shelly Peterman Schwarz, c/o Real Living with MS, 1111 Bethlehem Pike, P.O. Box 908, Springhouse, PA 19477).

Exceptional Parent: Parenting Your Child or Young Adult with a Disability. A magazine for families and professionals. (Exceptional Parent, P.O. Box 3000, Dept. EP, Denville, NJ 07834; tel: 800-247-8080). A monthly magazine that celebrated its 25th anniversary by producing the 1996 Resource Guide, which includes ten directories with more than one thousand resources in the United States and Canada. This is a very useful directory for adults with disabilities as well.

Guide to Catalogs for People with Disabilities, Their Families and Their Friends. (EKA Publications, Inc., 9151 Hampton Overlook, Capital Heights, MD 20743; tel: 800-386-5367).

Parenting with a Disability. (Through the Looking Glass, 2198 Sixth Street, Suite 100, Berkeley, CA 94710; tel: 510-848-1112; 800-644-2666; Internet: www.lookingglass.org).

Resource Directory for the Disabled. (Written by R.N. Shrout, published by Facts-on-File, 460 Park Avenue South, New York, NY 10016; 1991). A resource directory that includes associations and organizations, government agencies, libraries and research centers, publications, and products of all types for disabled individuals.

Agencies and Organizations

Consortium of Multiple Sclerosis Centers (CMSC) (c/o Gimbel MS Center at Holy Name Hospital, 718 Teaneck Road, Teaneck, NJ 07666; tel: 201-837-0727; Internet: www.mscare.org). The CMSC is made up of numerous MS centers throughout the United States and Canada. The Consortium's mission is to disseminate information to clinicians, increase resources and opportunities for research, and advance the standard of care for multiple sclerosis. The CMSC is a multidisciplinary organization, bringing together health care professionals from many fields involved in MS patient care.

Department of Veterans Affairs (VA) (810 Vermont Avenue, N.W., Washington, D.C. 20420; tel: 202-273-5400; Internet: www.va.org). The VA provides a wide range of benefits and services to those who have served in the armed forces, their dependents, beneficiaries of deceased veterans, and dependent children of veterans with severe disabilities.

Equal Employment Opportunity Commission (EEOC) (Office of Communication and Legislative Affairs, 1801 L Street, N.W., 10th Floor, Washington, D.C. 20507; tel: 800-669-3362 (to order publications); 800-669-4000 (to speak to an investigator; 202-663-4900; Internet: www.eeoc.gov). The EEOC is responsible for monitoring the section of the ADA on employment regulations. Copies of the regulations are available.

Eastern Paralyzed Veterans Association (EPVA) (75-20 Astoria Boulevard, Jackson Heights, NY 11370; tel: 718-803-EPVA; Internet: www.epva.org). EPVA is a private, nonprofit organization dedicated to serving the needs of its members as well as other people with disabilities. While offering a wide range of benefits to member veterans with spinal cord dysfunction (including hospital liaison, sports and recreation, wheelchair repair, adaptive architectural consultations, research and educational services, communications, and library and information services, they will also provide brochures and information on a variety of subjects, free of charge to the general public (see Appendix D).

Handicapped Organized Women (HOW) (P.O. Box 35481, Charlotte, NC 28235; tel: 704-376-4735). HOW strives to build self-esteem and confidence among disabled women by encouraging volunteer community involvement. HOW seeks to train disabled women for leadership positions and works in conjunction with the National Organization of Women (NOW).

Multiple Sclerosis Society of Canada (250 Bloor Street East, Suite 1000, Toronto, Ontario M4W 3P9, Canada; tel: 416-922-6065; in Canada: 800-268-7582; Internet: www.mssoc.ca). A national organization that funds research, promotes public education, and produces publications in both English and French. They provide an "ASK MS Information System" database of articles on a wide variety of topics including treatment, research, and social services. Regional divisions and chapters are located throughout Canada.

Health Resource Center for Women with Disabilities (Rehabilitation Institute of Chicago, 345 East Superior Street, Chicago, IL 60611; tel: 312-908-7997; Internet: www.rehabchicago.org). The Center is a project run by and for women with disabilities. It publishes a free newsletter, "Resourceful Women," and offers support groups and educational seminars addressing issues from a disabled woman's perspective. Among its many educational resources, the Center has developed a video on mothering with a disability.

National Council on Disability (NCD) (1331 F Street, N.W., Suite 1050, Washington, D.C. 20004; tel: 202-272-2004; Internet: www.ncd.gov). The Council is an independent federal agency whose role is to study and make recommendations about public policy for people with disabilities. Publishes a free newsletter, "Focus."

National Family Caregivers Association (NFCA) (10605 Concord Street, Kensington, MD 20895; tel: 301-942-6430; Internet: www.nfcacares.org). NFCA is dedicated to improving the quality of life of America's 18,000,000 caregivers. It publishes a quarterly newsletter and has a resource guide, an information clearinghouse, and a toll-free hotline: 800-896-3650.

National Multiple Sclerosis Society (NMSS) (733 Third Avenue, New York, NY 10017; tel: 800-FIGHT MS; Internet: www.nmss.org). The NMSS is a nonprofit organization that supports national and international research into the prevention, cure, and treatment of MS. The Society's goals include provision of nationwide services to assist people with MS and their families, and provision of information to those with MS, their families, professionals, and the public. The programs and services of the Society promote knowledge, health, and independence while providing education and emotional support:

◇ Toll-free access to your local chapter by selecting the option one at 800-FIGHT MS.

◇ Internet web site with updated information about treatments, current research, and programs (http://www, nmss.org); local home page in many areas.

◇ Knowledge Is Power self-study program (serial mailings) for people *newly diagnosed* with MS and their families, available through most chapters.

◇ Living well with MS, a series of workbooks, written for, and by, people who have been living with MS for some time.

◇ Moving Forward, an on-line education series for people *newly diagnosed* with MS and their families, available on the NMSS website.

◇ Printed materials available on a variety of topics from your local chapter.

◇ Educational programs on various topics throughout the year, provided through your local chapter.

◇ Annual national teleconference at over 500 sites throughout the United States; call your chapter for the location nearest you.

◇ Swimming and other exercise programs sponsored or co-sponsored by some chapters, or referral to existing programs in the community.

◇ Wellness programs in some chapters.

National Park Service, U.S. Department of the Interior (P.O. Box 37127, Washington, D.C. 20013-7127; Internet: www.nps.gov). The service will provide you with a listing of national parks and numbers for you to call to obtain up-to-date accessibility information for the individual parks.

Office on the Americans with Disabilities Act (Department of Justice, Civil Rights Division, P.O. Box 66118, Washington, D.C. 20035; tel: 202-514-0301). This office is responsible for enforcing the ADA. To order copies of its regulations, call 202-514-6193.

Paralyzed Veterans of America (PVA) (801 Eighteenth Street N.W., Washington, D.C. 20006; tel: 800-424-8200; Internet: www.pva.org). PVA is a national information and advocacy agency working to restore function and quality of life for veterans with spinal cord dysfunction. It supports and funds education and research and has a national advocacy program that focuses on accessibility issues. PVA publishes brochures on many issues related to rehabilitation.

Social Security Administration (6401 Security Boulevard, Baltimore, MD 21235; tel: 800-772-1213; Internet: www.ssa.gov). To apply for social security benefits based on disability, call this office or visit your local social security branch office. The Office of Disability within the Social Security Administration publishes a free brochure entitled "Social Security Regulations: Rules for Determining Disability and Blindness."

Through the Looking Glass: National Research and Training Center on Families of Adults with Disabilities (2198 Sixth Street, Suite 100, Berkeley, CA 94710; tel: 510-848-4445; 800-644-2666; Internet: www.lookingglass.org).

Well Spouse Foundation (610 Lexington Avenue, New York, NY 10022-6005; tel: 212-644-1241; 800-838-0879). An emotional support network for people married to or living with a chronically ill partner. Advocacy for home health and long-term care and a newsletter are among the services offered.

Assistive Technology

Access to Recreation: Adaptive Recreation Equipment for the Physically Challenged (2509 E. Thousand Oaks Boulevard, Suite 430, Thousand Oaks, CA 91362; tel: 800-634-4351). Products include exercise equipment and assistive devices for sports, environmental access, games, crafts, and hobbies.

adaptABILITY (Department 2082, 75 Mill Street, Colchester, CT 06415; tel: 800-243-9232). A free catalog of assistive devices and self-care equipment designed to enhance independence.

Adaptive Parenting:Idea Book I (Though the Looking Glass, 2198 Sixth Street, Suite 100, Berkeley, CA 94710; tel: 510-848-1112; 800-644-2666).

American Automobile Association (1712 G Street N.W., Washington, D.C. 20015; Internet: www.AAA.com). The AAA will provide a list of automobile hand-control manufacturers.

American Medical Alert (3265 Lawson Blvd., Oceanside, NY 11572; tel: 516-536-5850 or 800-645-3244; Internet: www.amacalert.com). Personal emergency response system that links a person living alone with a 24-hour emergency response center, as well as other services.

Interim In-Touch (2050 Spectrum Blvd., Fort Lauderdale, FL 33309; tel: 800-900-8208). Personal emergency response system that links a person living alone with a 24-hour emergency response center as well as other services.

Lifeline Systems, Inc. (640 Memorial Drive, Cambridge, MA 02139; tel: 800-543-3546 or 617-679-1000; Internet: www.lifelinesys.com). Personal emergency response system that links a person living alone with a 24-hour emergency response center, as well as other services.

Life Enhancement Technologies, LLC (2682 Middlefield Road, Bldg. L, Redwood City, CA 94063; tel:800-779-6953; Internet: www.2bcool.com). The company manufactures a variety of cooling suits that can be used in management of heat-related symptoms in MS.

Medic Alert Foundation International (P.O. Box 1009, Turlock, CA 95380; tel: 800-344-3226; 209-668-3333; Internet: www.medicalert.org). A medical identification tag worn to identify a person's medical condition, medications, and any other important information that might be needed in case of an emergency. A file of the person's health data is maintained in a central database to be accessed by a physician or other emergency personnel who need to know the person's pertinent medical information.

National Rehabilitation Information Center (NARIC) (1010 Wayne Avenue, Suite 800, Silver Spring, MD 20910-5633; tel: 301-562-2400; fax: 301-562-2401; Internet: www.naric.com). NARIC is a library and information center on disability and rehabilitation, funded by the National Institute on Disability and Rehabilitation Research (NIDRR). NARIC operates two databases—ABLEDATA and REHABDATA. NARIC collects and disseminates the results of federally funded research projects and has a collection that includes commercially published books, journal articles, and audiovisual materials. NARIC is committed to serving both professionals and consumers who are interested in disability and rehabilitation. Information specialists can answer simple information requests and provide referrals immediately and at no cost. More complex database searches are available at nominal cost.

◇ ABLEDATA (8455 Colesville Road, Suite 935, Silver Spring, MD 20910; tel: 301-588-9284; 800-227-0216; fax: 301-589-3563; Internet: www.abledata.com/index.htm). ABLEDATA is a national database of information on assistive technology designed to enable persons with disabilities to identify and locate the devices that will assist them in their home, work, and leisure activities. Information specialists are available to answer questions during regular business hours. ABLE INFORM BBS is available twenty-four hours a day to customers with a computer, modem, and telecommunications software.

◇ REHABDATA (8455 Colesville Road, Suite 935, Silver Spring, MD 20910; tel: 301-588-9284; 800-346-2742; Internet: www.naric.com/naric/search/rhab/browse.html). REHABDATA is a database containing bibliographic records with abstracts and summaries of the materials contained in the NARIC (National Rehabilitation Information Information Center) library of disability rehabilitation materials. Information specialists are available to conduct a database search on any rehabilitation related topic.

RESNA: Rehabilitation, Engineering, and Assistive Technology Society of North America (1700 North Moore Street, Suite 1540, Arlington, VA 22209-1903; tel:703-524-6686, P.O. Box 969, Etobicoke Station U, Etobicoke, Ontario M82 5P9; Internet: www.resna.org). RESNA is an international association for the advancement of rehabilitation technology. Their objectives are to improve the quality of life for the disabled through the application of science and technology and to influence policy relating to the delivery of technology to disabled persons. They will respond by mail to specific questions about modifying existing equipment and designing new devices.

Sears Home Health Care Catalog (P.O. Box 3123, Naperville, IL 60566; tel: 800-326-1750). The catalog includes medical equipment such as hospital beds, commodes, and wheelchairs, as well as adaptive clothing.

SOS Wireless Communication (11 W. Cooke Road, Suite 8, Columbus, OH 43214; tel: 800-259-8327; Internet: www.sosphone.com). This mobile emergency response system operates on the existing national cellular network, providing 24-hour personalized service, nationwide roadside service, and free 911 calls.

Steele, Inc. (26112 Iowa Avenue, N.E., P.O. Box 7304, Kingston, WA 98346; tel: 360-297-4555). The company manufactures the Steele Vest® for cooling. It can be used for the management of heat-related symptoms in MS.

Environmental Adaptations

A Consumer's Guide to Home Adaptation (Adaptive Environments Center, 374 Congress Street, Suite 301, Boston, MA 02210; tel: 617-695-1225). A workbook for planning adaptive home modifications such as lowering kitchen countertops and widening doorways.

"Adapting the Home for the Physically Challenged" (A/V Health Services, P.O. Box 1622, West Sacramento, CA 95691; tel: 540-389-4339). A 22-minute videotape that describes home modifications for individuals who use walkers or wheelchairs. Ramp construction and room modification specifications are included.

American Institute of Architects (AIA) (1735 New York Avenue, N.W., Washington, D.C. 20006; tel: 202-626-7300; publications catalog and orders: 800-365-2724). This organization will make referrals to architects who are familiar with the design requirements of people with disabilities.

Financing Home Accessibility Modifications (Center for Universal Design, North Carolina State University, Box 8613, Raleigh, NC 27695; tel: 919-515-3082). This publication identifies state and local sources of financial assistance for homeowners (or tenants) who need to make modifications in their homes.

GE Answer Center (9500 Williamsburg Plaza, Louisville, KY 40222; tel: 800-626-2000). The Center, which is open twenty-four hours a day, seven days a week, offers assistance to individuals with disabilities as well as the general public. They offer two free brochures, "Appliance Help for Those with Special Needs," and "Basic Kitchen Planning for the Physically Handicapped."

National Association of Home Builders (NAHB) (NAHB Research Center, Economics and Policy Analysis Division, 400 Prince George's Boulevard, Upper Marlboro, MD 20774; tel: 301-249-4000; Internet: www.nahb.com). The Research Center produces publications and provides training on housing and special needs. A publication entitled "Homes for a Lifetime" includes an accessibility checklist, financing options, and recommendations for working with builders and remodelers.

National Kitchen and Bath Association (687 Willow Grove Street, Hackettstown, NJ 07840; tel: 908-852-0033; Internet: www.nkba.org). The Association produces a technical manual of barrier-free planning and has directories of certified designers and planners.

Travel

Accessible Journeys (tel: 800-846-4537 or 610-521-0339; Internet: www.disabilitytravel.com). A company that arranges travel for mobility-impaired travelers, and is affiliated with a network of offices in nine European countries.

Directory of Travel Agencies for the Disabled. (Written by Helen Hecker, published by Twin Peaks Press, P.O. Box 129, Vancouver, WA 98666-0129). This directory lists travel agents who specialize in arranging travel plans for people with disabilities.

The Disability Bookshop (P.O. Box 129, Vancouver, WA 98666; tel: 800-637-2256). The Disability Bookshop has an extensive list of books for disabled travelers, dealing with such topics as accessibility, travel agencies, accessible van rentals, medical resources, air travel, and guides to national parks.

Information for Handicapped Travelers (available free of charge from the National Library Service for the Blind and Physically Handicapped, 1291 Taylor Street, N.W., Washington, D.C. 20542; tel: 800-424-8567; 202-707-5100). A booklet providing information about travel agents, transportation, and information centers for individuals with disabilities.

Project Action (Internet: www.projectaction.org). Maintains a database on its website of information about the availability of accessible transportation anywhere in the United States. Users can highlight the state and city they plan to visit and view all transportation services available to them. The database also includes travel agencies specializing in travel arrangements for people with disabilities.

Society for the Advancement of Travel for the Handicapped (SATH) (347 Fifth Avenue, Suite 610, New York, NY 10016; tel: 212-447-7284; Internet: www.sath.org). SATH is a nonprofit organization that acts as a clearinghouse for accessible tourism information and is in contact with organizations in many countries to promote the development of facilities for disabled people. SATH publishes a quarterly magazine, "Access to Travel."

Travel for the Disabled: A Handbook of Travel Resources and 500 Worldwide Access Guides. (Written by Helen Hecker, published by Twin Peaks Press, P.O. Box 129, Vancouver, WA 98666; tel: 800-637-2256). The handbook provides information for disabled travelers about accessibility.

Travel Information Service (Moss Rehabilitation Hospital, 1200 West Tabor Road, Philadelphia, PA 19141; tel: 215-456-9900). The Service provides information and referrals for people with disabilities.

Travelin' Talk (P.O. Box 3534, Clarksville, TN 37043; tel: 615-552-6670). A network of more than one thousand people and organizations around the world who are willing to provide assistance to travelers with disabilities and share their knowledge about the areas in which they live. Travelin' Talk publishes a newsletter by the same name and has an extensive resource directory.

The Wheelchair Traveler (Accent on Living, P.O. Box 700, Bloomington, IL 61702; tel: 309-378-2961). A directory that provides ratings of hotels and motels in the United States.

Wilderness Inquiry (1313 5th Street, S.E., Box 84, Minneapolis, MN 55414; tel: 800-728-0719; 612-379-3858). Wilderness Inquiry sponsors trips into the wilderness for people with disabilities or chronic conditions.

Visual Impairment

Canadian National Institute for the Blind (CNIB) (1929 Bayview Avenue, Toronto, Ontario M4G 3E8, Canada; tel: 416-480-7580;

Internet: www.navnet.net/~mic/cnib/index.html). The Institute provides counseling and rehabilitation services for Canadians with any degree of functional visual impairment. They offer public information literature and operate resource and technology centers. The national office has a list of provincial and local CNIB offices.

The Lighthouse Low Vision Products Consumer Catalog (36-20 Northern Boulevard, Long Island City, NY 11101; tel: 800-829-0500). This large-print catalog offers a wide range of products designed to help people with impaired vision.

The Library of Congress, Division for the Blind and Physically Handicapped (1291 Taylor Street, N.W., Washington, D.C. 20542; tel: 800-424-8567; 800-424-9100; for application: 202-287-5100; Internet: lcweb.loc.gov/nls). The Library Service provides free talking book equipment on loan as well as a full range of recorded books for individuals with disabilities or visual impairment. It also provides a variety of free library services through one hundred forty cooperating libraries.

Publishing Companies Specializing in Health and Disability Issues

Demos Vermande (386 Park Avenue South, Suite 201, New York, NY 10016; tel: 800-532-8663).

Grey House Publishing (Pocket Knife Square, P.O. Box 1866, Lakeville, CT 06039; tel: 800-562-2139; fax: 860-435-3004; e-mail: www.greyhouse.com).

Resources for Rehabilitation (33 Bedford Street, Suite 19A, Lexington, MA 02173; tel: 617-862-6455; Internet: www.rfr.org).

Twin Peaks Press (P.O. Box 129, Vancouver, WA 98666; tel: 800-637-2256).

Woodbine House (Publishers of the Special-Needs Collection) (6510 Bells Mill Road, Bethesda, MD 20817; tel: 301-897-3570; 800-843-7323; Internet: www.woodbinehouse.com).

Appendix F

Professional Biographies of the Authors

Kathy Birk, M.D.

Kathy Birk, M.D., received her medical degree from the University of Missouri and completed her residency in obstetrics and gynecology. It was in 1984, during her first year of medical school, that Dr. Birk was diagnosed with MS. During her residency, Dr. Birk cared for two women with MS who were concerned that becoming pregnant might worsen their disease. Sharing these concerns, and finding there was little written about this topic in the medical literature, Dr. Birk decided to pursue the answer in her own research. While the study did not identify any hormone or protein in the blood of pregnant women that could explain why women with MS tend to have fewer exacerbations during pregnancy, Dr. Birk did conclude that having MS was not sufficient reason for women with MS to avoid becoming pregnant.

Following her residency, Dr. Birk practiced primary care office gynecology, delivered babies, and performed surgery. Beginning in 1994, she had a series of mild relapses, and intense fatigue forced her to restrict her practice to the office setting. She subsequently retired from her medical practice in 1997, following a significant seizure that left her unable to be kind of active and involved physician she had always been. After a year of retirement, Dr. Birk is once again very busy— serving on boards, speaking for charitable groups, writing for the professional and lay literature, and working at an Integrative Health center that offers complementary and alternative therapies.

Dr. Birk's interest and involvement in MS grew out of her own experience with the disease and that of her grandmother, who lived most of her life with the disease. Dr. Birk has dedicated this chapter to her grandmother's memory.

Angela Chan, B.P.T., M.H.Sc.

Angela Chan received her degree in physical therapy from McGill University in Montreal, Canada. Ms. Chan also received a Master of Health Sciences degree in Health Administration from the University of Toronto in 1998. Since 1981, Ms. Chan has been the specialist physical therapist for the Multiple Sclerosis Clinic at St. Michael's Hospital in Toronto, Canada, giving individuals with MS recommendations to improve their physical well-being and mobility.

In addition to providing clinical care to individuals with MS, Ms. Chan has extensive experience teaching about MS care to physical therapy students, health care practitioners, and various chapters of the MS Society of Canada. Ms. Chan holds the title of Lecturer of the Department of Physical Therapy at the University of Toronto.

Ms. Chan is an active member of the Consortium of Multiple Sclerosis Centers. She served as Co-Chair and subsequently Chairperson of the Consortium's Clinical Care Committee from 1992 to 1994. Ms. Chan was senior author of the paper entitled "Balance and Spasticity: What We Know and What We Believe," published in a special issue of the *Journal of Neurologic Rehabilitation* in 1994, devoted to the outcome of a two-year research project spearheaded by the Consortium. She also completed a research study to measure the effects of tilting the wheelchair seat position on individuals with advanced MS. The results of this study provided evidence of the positive impact from utilizing this device on breathing, posture and fatigue management of individuals with advanced MS. This evidence can be used to justify the prescription of this equipment to funding agencies.

Laura Cooper, Esq.

Laura Cooper graduated from the University Washington Law School in 1986. She has been a practicing attorney for the past 14 years, two as counsel to the Chairman of the Interstate Commerce Commission in Washington, D.C., and the latter eight focusing on disability rights and consumer-based health law on behalf of the National Multiple Sclerosis Society. She also serves the National MS Society as Life Planning and Legal Consultant, Special Consultant on Employment Initiatives, and a member of the Services Subcommittee on Independent Living.

Ms. Cooper has been a member of the National Advisory Board, National Center for Medical Rehabilitation & Research, National Institute of Child Health & Human Development, National Institutes of Health, U.S. Department of Health and Human Services, since 1995. She served as Chairperson of this committee from 1997-1998.

Ms. Cooper was teaching science on an Indian reservation when she first experienced gait problems, vertigo, numbness, and tingling. The severity of her MS forced her to leave her job at age 22. She enrolled in a couple of graduate school courses, paid her tuition with savings, and received support from the Department of Vocational Rehabilitation for wheelchair assistance. Her failing health put her in and out of hospitals and eventually, at age 23, into a nursing home. Three months later, Ms. Cooper found an ad in a newspaper for a wheelchair-accessible apartment complex. She negotiated for herself the space, some furniture, a hospital bed, and a commode, which she ordered on an old Visa card, and used her Social Security payment to help pay the rent. Her parents helped her by purchasing a lift-equipped van.

Ms. Cooper applied to law school and received a full tuition scholarship to Gonzaga University in Spokane, Washington. While in law school, she experienced several exacerbations that left her temporarily blind and quadriplegic. She transferred to the University of Washington to finish her degree, following which she was named one of the twenty outstanding young American lawyers "who make a difference" by the American Bar Association. During her search for employment, Ms. Cooper received more than 400 rejections, until one law firm was willing to look at her abilities instead of her disabilities.

Robert Enteen, Ph.D.

Robert Enteen is Director of Multimedia at Medscape, Inc., considered by many to be the leading medical website on the Internet. He is responsible for creating and hosting customized radio and webcast educational programs for physicians, allied health professionals, and consumers in the United States and internationally. These programs include web-based, accredited continuing medical education (CME) courses, as well as live, interactive medical symposia.

For twelve years, Dr. Enteen served as Director of Health Research and Policy Programs at the National Multiple Sclerosis Society. In this position, he conceived, designed, and oversaw the Society's grant, contract, and dissertation fellowship programs in health services, psychosocial, and policy research.

Since his introduction to the disability community and disability policy issues in 1976, Dr. Enteen has served as an advisor to numerous organizations, boards, and programs aimed at promoting optimal quality of life for people with disabilities and their families. He has been a guest speaker at over 400 professional and consumer conferences in the United States, Canada, and Europe.

In 1992, Dr. Enteen authored *Health Insurance: How to Get It, Keep It, or Improve What You Have.* A second edition of the book was published in 1996 by Demos Medical Publishing, and an update is planned for the year 2000. In 1998, this book was a finalist for the Kulp-Wright Book Award at the Wharton School, University of Pennsylvania, in the category "best book on insurance." It has also been identified as one of the 50 most popular health books on the Internet.

In 1994, Dr. Enteen initiated what later became the first nationally-syndicated radio show focusijng on disability, chronic disease, and aging. The show, entitled "Living Without Limits," is currently broadcast weekly on approximately 50 FM and AM stations throught the United States, as well as on several hundred Radio Reading Services (RRSs) for listeners who are blind, visually impaired, or "print-disabled."

Jill Fischer, Ph.D.

Jill Fischer, a clinical neuropsychologist, developed the Psychology Program at the Cleveland Clinic's interdisciplinary Mellen Center for MS Treatment and Research. Since receiving her doctorate in Clinical Psychology from the University of Wisconsin-Madison in 1985, she has maintained both an active clinical practice and an active research program, and has published numerous scientific articles and book chapters related to her work.

Dr. Fischer's interests include assessment of individuals whose cognitive function has changed as a result of MS, development of interventions for individuals with MS-related cognitive deficits, and refinement of methods for monitoring cognitive function over time. She was Principal Investigator on a four-year National Multiple Sclerosis Society (NMSS)-funded study of interventions for MS-related cognitive dysfunction, as well as Neuropsychology Principal Investigator on the National Institute of Neurologic Diseases and Stroke (NINDS)-funded multicenter trial of Avonex® for relapsing MS and on the NMSS-funded trial of oral methotrexate in chronic-progressive MS. Her interests extend to outcome assessment in MS in general, and toward that end, she participated in the development of the MS Quality of Life Inventory (MSQLI) and the MS Functional Composite (MSFC) measure, both funded by the NMSS.

Dr. Fischer is also active in national and international professional societies. She is a member of the NMSS Scientific Peer Review Committee C (Patient Management Technologies) and of the Board of Trustees of the Consortium of Multiple Sclerosis Centers (CMSC). She is also a past President of the CMSC (1992–1993) and has served on the Executive Committee of the American Psychological Association's Division 40-Clinical Neuropsychology (1994–1997).

Frederick W. Foley, Ph.D.

Frederick Foley is an Associate Professor in Clinical Health Psychology at Ferkauf Graduate School of Psychology and the Albert Einstein College of Medicine, of Yeshiva University, Bronx, New York. He is also a staff psychologist at the Bernard W. Gimbel Multiple Sclerosis Comprehensive Care Center of Holy Name Hospital in Teaneck, New Jersey. Dr. Foley has been actively involved in conducting research, training, and patient care for persons with MS and their families since 1978. He has published numerous scientific articles and book chapters related to psychological issues and outcomes in MS, and has received research grants from the National Institutes on Disability and

Rehabilitation Research, the Towbes Foundation, and the Multiple Sclerosis Society of Great Britain and Northern Ireland for his work. Dr. Foley has also served in a scientific advisory capacity for several MS research projects in the United States and Canada.

For his work in MS, Dr. Foley has received the Dorfman Award from the Academy of Psychosomatic Medicine and the Berlex Award for Patient Education from the Consortium of Multiple Sclerosis Centers. He has been on the Professional Advisory Committees of the New York City and Northern New Jersey Chapters of the National MS Society, and serves on the Intimacy and Sexuality Subcommittee of the Family Services Committee of the International Federation of Multiple Sclerosis Societies. Dr. Foley has recently been elected to serve as Secretary of the Board of Directors of the Consortium of MS Centers.

Debra Frankel, MS, OTR

Debra Frankel received a master's degree in occupational therapy from Boston University in 1977. After working in a rehabilitation setting for several years, Ms. Frankel joined the Massachusetts Chapter of the National Multiple Sclerosis Society as Director of Chapter Programs. In this capacity, she worked at developing a wide range of programs for people with MS, their families and the health care provider community. In 1981, she also became a consultant to the NMSS home office, where she worked with other chapters to strengthen their local programs. She also worked on several national program initiatives.

After almost 18 years with the chapter (now the Central New England Chapter), Ms. Frankel accepted a position as Senior Analyst with Abt Associates of Cambridge, Mass., a research and consulting firm. At Abt Associates she is working on an NMSS-funded contract to develop an MS longitudinal database. This project will follow almost 2000 people with MS over time to collect data about clinical and quality of life issues. The data will be used to address a number of research questions regarding access to health care, costs of care, the course and clinical characteristics of MS, the impact of MS on quality of life, health care utilization and more.

Ms. Frankel continues to serve as Senior Consultant to the Client Programs and Clinical Programs Departments of the NMSS. She is a member of the NMSS Long Term Care Advisory

Task Force, a member of the NMSS Education Committee, and is currently working on revising several NMSS client program manuals. She is the author of numerous publications and articles about multiple sclerosis, long term care and other health promotion issues.

June Halper, MSN, RN.CS, ANP, FAAN

June Halper is a certified adult nurse practitioner who has specialized in multiple sclerosis since 1978. She was a founder of the Gimbel MS Center in Teaneck, New Jersey, and has been the Executive Director since 1989. With the Multiple Sclerosis Research and Treatment Center of the University of Medicine and Dentistry of New Jersey (UMDNJ), the Gimbel Center established the Multiple Sclerosis Network of New Jersey in 1998. In 1993, the Gimbel MS Center was named the administrative seat of the Consortium of Multiple Sclerosis Centers (CMSC), the largest organization of MS healthcare professionals in the world. Ms. Halper was president of the CMSC from 1995-1997 has been Executive Director since 1997.

Ms Halper spearheaded the development of the national taskforce on disabled women's health issues that culminated in a nationally-attended conference in June, 1996 focusing on autoimmune diseases in women. She has published and lectured extensively on multiple sclerosis and its ramifications, and is the editor of *Comprehensive Nursing Care in Multiple Sclerosis* and co-editor of *Staying Well with Multiple Sclerosis: A Self-Care Guide*. Ms. Halper chaired the first Multiple Sclerosis Nurse Specialist Consensus Committee's development of a monograph on the nurse's role in adherence to complex protocols; the impact of cognitive impairment in nursing care; and the nurse's role in the patient's and family's quality of life.

Ms. Halper is a member of the American Academy of Nursing, the founding director of IOMSN, the International Organization of MS Nurses, and the recipient of the IOMSN's first June Halper Award for Excellence in Nursing in Multiple Sclerosis.

Robert M. Herndon, M.D.

Robert Herndon graduated from the University of Chicago in 1955 and from the University of Tennessee Medical School with honors in 1958. He did his internship and residency in Neurology at Wayne State University, followed by a fellowship in Neuropathology at the Montreal Neurological Institute. After two years in the Air Force, he did an additional year of fellowship in Anatomy at Harvard University Medical School.

Dr. Herndon joined the faculty at Stanford University Medical School as Assistant Professor of Neurology in 1966. There he began his research in MS, reporting the discovery of myelin fragments in the spinal fluid in 1968. In 1969 he became Associate Professor of Neurology at Johns Hopkins Medical School where he continued his research on spinal fluid and began studying myelin regeneration. Dr. Herndon became director of the MS clinic at Johns Hopkins in 1974. In 1977, he left Johns Hopkins to become Professor and director of the Center for Brain Research at the University of Rochester where he also directed the Rochester Area Multiple Sclerosis Society MS Clinic. After the Center for Brain Research was closed in 1977, he left to become Chief of Neurology at Good Samaritan Hospital in Portland Oregon, and Professor of Neurology at Oregon Health Sciences University, where he directed an MS clinic and was site principal investigator in the Phase III Avonex trial. After the University withdrew the training program from Good Samaritan Hospital he went into private practice for a short period, and then moved to the University of Mississippi and the Jackson VA Medical Center where he has continued his interest in MS.

Dr. Herndon is a past president of the Consortium of MS Centers and serves on the Medical Advisory Board of the National Multiple Sclerosis Society and the International Federation of Multiple Sclerosis Societies. He is the editor of the International Journal of MS Care.

Jean Hietpas, OTR, LCSW

Jean Hietpas is the Coordinator of Clinical Research at the University of California, San Francisco Multiple Sclerosis Center. In this role, she directs clinical trials of disease modifying therapies and symptomatic treatments.

Previously, Ms. Hietpas provided occupational therapy services to MS patients in her position as Clinical Specialist with the Department of Rehabilitation at the University of California in San Francisco.

Following her training at the University of Wisconsin, Milwaukee in both Occupational Therapy and Clinical Social Work,

Ms. Hietpas remained at the University to teach courses in occupational therapy. She served as Program Director of the Mental Health and Alcohol and Drug Abuse Clinic at dePaul Rehabilitation Hospital in Milwaukee from 1986 to 1987, and then became Clinical Director of Drug and Alcohol Programs at Elmbrook Memorial Hospital in Milwaukee.

Ms. Hietpas is a contributing author of several publications including a chapter on multiple sclerosis in *Occupational Therapy Practice Skills for Physical Dysfunction (4th edition)*.

Jean is a member of the Professional Advisory Committee for the Northern California Chapter of the National Multiple Sclerosis Society, and a task force member for professional education on the disease and its treatment.

Nancy J. Holland, Ed.D., R.N.

Nancy Holland is Vice President of Clinical Programs at the National Multiple Sclerosis Society in New York. She directs the Society's activities to improve access to healthcare, and the quality of that healthcare, for people with MS. Dr. Holland earned a doctorate in higher and adult education from Teachers College, Columbia University, and holds undergraduate and graduate degrees in nursing. Her career in the field of MS began in 1974 at the first comprehensive care center for people with MS in the country. Her roles in this setting included clinician, clinical coordinator, director of training, co-therapist for MS support groups, and research associate. Dr. Holland was also recipient of a Career Development Award from the National Institute on Disability and Rehabilitation Research.

Dr. Holland is the author/editor of more than 60 MS-related articles and books, including: *Multiple Sclerosis: A Guide for Patients and Their Families; Multiple Sclerosis: A Guide for the Newly Diagnosed; Comprehensive Nursing Care in Multiple Sclerosis; and Multiple Sclerosis: A Self-Care Guide to Wellness.*

Rosalind C. Kalb, Ph.D.

Rosalind Kalb is a clinical psychologist at the MS Care Center at St. Agnes Hospital in White Plains, New York, and Clinical Assistant Professor of Neurology at New York Medical College. She is also Director of Information Resources for the National Multiple Sclerosis Society, developing educational materials for professional and lay audiences. In her private clinical practice, she specializes in the needs of individuals and families living with chronic illness and disability.

After receiving her doctorate from Fordham University, she began her career in MS, providing individual, group, and family therapy at the MS Care Center at the Albert Einstein College of Medicine. Following the Center's relocation to New York Medical College, Dr. Kalb added a variety of other clinical and research activities to her work in MS, including groups for well spouses and couples living with MS, and neuropsychological evaluation and cognitive rehabilitation for research and treatment purposes.

Dr. Kalb has authored or edited a number of publications about multiple sclerosis. She is the author of *Families Affected by Multiple Sclerosis: Disease Impacts and Coping Strategies*, a monograph published in 1995 by the National MS Society. She also wrote, with Marla Shawaryn, M.A., the *Knowledge is Power* series for individuals newly diagnosed with MS, published by the National MS Society in 1998. In addition to *Multiple Sclerosis: The Questions You Have, The Answers You Need*, first published in 1996, she is the editor of *Multiple Sclerosis: A Guide for Families, published in 1998.*

With funding from the National MS Society, Dr. Kalb investigated "The Impact of Multiple Sclerosis in Childhood and Adolescence." The study evaluated the effects of early-onset MS on intellectual function and academic performance, as well as a variety of psychosocial variables. Dr. Kalb also collaborated with Drs. Nicholas LaRocca and Charles Smith on a study, funded by the National Institute on Disability and Rehabilitation Research, entitled The Psychosocial Impact of Parental Multiple Sclerosis on Children and Adolescents.

Nicholas G. LaRocca, Ph.D.

Nicholas LaRocca, who received his doctorate in Clinical Psychology from Fordham University, has been the Director of Health Care Delivery and Policy Research at the National Multiple Sclerosis Society in New York City since 1997. Before coming to the Society, Dr. LaRocca was the Director of Research at the Medical Rehabilitation Research and Training Center for MS at St. Agnes Hospital, White Plains, New York, and Associate Professor of Neurology and Medicine at New York Medical College.

Dr. LaRocca has extensive experience in both psychosocial research and psychological treatment in multiple sclerosis. He has designed, administered, and analyzed a number of clinical studies in MS, including neurogenic bladder dysfunction, comparisons of inpatient and outpatient rehabilitation, and the role of stressful life events in MS. Dr. LaRocca was Principal Investigator of a project funded by the National Institute on Disability and Rehabilitation Research entitled "The Comprehensive Rehabilitation of Cognitive Dysfunction in Multiple Sclerosis." He also served as Principal Investigator of a National MS Society-funded "Program to Facilitate Retention of Employment Among Persons with Multiple Sclerosis," and as Co-Principal Investigator for the National MS Society-funded project entitled "Development of a Multiple Sclerosis Quality of Life Measurement."

Dr. LaRocca has led support groups for persons with MS and their spouses, and has given innumerable workshops and presentations for both lay and professional audiences. In 1992, Dr. LaRocca was the invited speaker for the National MS Society audioteleconference entitled "Multiple Sclerosis: Understanding Your Mind and Emotions." He is the author of a number of scientific papers and book chapters, and wrote a monograph entitled "Employment and Multiple Sclerosis" that was published by the National MS Society in 1995. He also serves on the editorial boards of *Neurorehabilitation and Neural Repair*, *MS Quarterly Report*, and *Real Living with MS*.

Jeri Logemann, Ph.D.

Jeri Logemann is the Ralph and Jean Sundin Professor of Communication Sciences and Disorders at Northwestern University, Evanston, Illinois, and Professor of Otolaryngology and Maxillofacial Surgery and Neurology at Northwestern University Medical School in Chicago.

For over twenty years, Dr. Logemann has received funding from the National Institutes of Health for her work in the area of normal swallowing physiology and evaluation and treatment of swallowing disorders. She has a particular interest in the assessment and treatment of speech and swallowing dysfunction in people with cancer and those with neurological impairments. She has completed several studies of swallowing disorders resulting from multiple sclerosis, and has worked with other speech-language pathologists to identify research priorities for

MS-related speech and swallowing problems. She is currently Principal Investigator of the Communication Sciences and Disorders Clinical Trials Research Group.

Dr. Logemann is co-author of the *Fisher-Logemann Test of Articulation Competence*, author of *Evaluation and Treatment of Swallowing Disorders* and *Manual for the Videofluorographic Study of Swallowing*. In 1994, she served as President of the American Speech-Language-Hearing Association (ASHA).

Deborah M. Miller, Ph.D., LISW

Deborah M. Miller, Ph.D., LISW, is Director of Comprehensive Care at the Mellen Center for MS Treatment and Research of the Cleveland Clinic. In this capacity, her responsibilities include program development and outcomes research, providing clinical care, conducting psychosocial research, and assuring integration of the Center's clinical, research, and operational activities. She obtained her MSSA and Ph.D. from the School of Applied Social Sciences, Case Western Reserve University. She is Chair of the Consortium of Multiple Sclerosis Centers' (CMSC) Clinical Care Committee and the MS Council for Clinical Practice Guidelines.

A social worker with 18 years experience in the area of chronic disability, Dr. Miller has been a member of the Mellen Center's interdisciplinary care team since 1985. Her practice interests focus on marital and family adjustment to the consequences of MS. Her research interests include developing disease-specific quality of life measures, assessing impact of clinical interventions on health status, and identifying predictors of service utilization.

Using her clinical experience, Dr. Miller has developed and facilitated group treatment programs for school age children and teenagers whose parents have MS and for adults who have parenting concerns because of MS. She has lectured nationally on these subjects.

Dr. Miller has numerous affiliations with the National Multiple Sclerosis Society, including consultant to the Office of Client and Community Services, Chair of the National Panel of Professional Advisors, and member of the committee to establish guidelines for known and suspected abuse. She is a member of the Northeast Ohio Chapter's Patient Services Committee and won that Chapter's "Health Care Professional" Award in 1991. In addition, Dr. Miller is a President of the Board of Trustees of the Long Term Care Ombuds Program.

Aaron Miller, M.D.

Aaron Miller, M.D., Director of the Division of Neurology and of the Multiple Sclerosis Center at Maimonides Medical Center in Brooklyn, New York, and Professor of Clinical Neurology at the State University of New York—Health Sciences Center at Brooklyn, graduated from New York University School of Medicine in 1968. Following his residency in neurology at the Albert Einstein College of Medicine, he received additional postdoctoral training in neurovirology and immunology at the Johns Hopkins University School of Hygiene and Public Health and at Albert Einstein. During this time, he was the recipient of a fellowship from the National Multiple Sclerosis Society (NMSS).

Dr. Miller currently serves as the Chairman of the Professional Education Committee of the NMSS, chairman of the Professional Advisory Committee of the New York City Chapter of the NMSS, and is a past president of the Consortium of MS Centers. He has participated in numerous clinical trials of new treatments for MS and is the author of many articles and chapters on MS and other neurologic subjects.

Dr. Miller is also very active with the American Academy of Neurology. He was the first chairman of the Multiple Sclerosis section of the Academy. He currently serves as Co-chairman of the Education Committee and Chairman of the Annual Meeting Subcommittee. Prior to assuming this position, he served as chairman of the Program Accreditation and Development Subcommittee. Dr. Miller has developed, and for many years directed, a popular seminar at the annual meeting of the American Academy of Neurology entitled *MS: Patient Management.*

Phillip D. Rumrill, Jr., Ph.D., CRC

Phillip Rumrill is an Associate Professor and Coordinator of the graduate Rehabilitation Counseling Program at Kent State University. He received his Masters Degree in Educational Counseling in 1991 and his Ph.D. in Rehabilitation Counseling in 1993. Currently, Dr. Rumrill teaches courses in the psychosocial, medical, and vocational aspects of disability, and serves as Director of Kent State's Center for Disability Studies, an institute for training, demonstration, and research projects concerning disability issues across the life span.

Dr. Rumrill has extensive experience conducting applied research on the career development implications of chronic illnesses and other disabling conditions. He was involved with the Career Possibilities Project and the Progressive Request Model Intervention, both funded by the National MS Society, as well as Project Alliance, funded by the Rehabilitation Services Administration of the U.S. Department of Education. His research interests include job placement and retention for people with disabilities, disability policy, and psychological adjustment to disability. Dr. Rumrill also serves as Special Project Consultant on Employment Issues for the National Multiple Sclerosis Society.

Dr. Rumrill has authored more than 100 professional publications, including books entitled *Employment Issues and Multiple Sclerosis*, *Research in Rehabilitation Counseling*, and *Research in Special Education*.

Dr. Rumrill has received numerous honors for his research and program development efforts, including the 1998 Distinguished Scholar Award from the Arla Institute in Finland, the 1996 Innovative Program Award from the National Association of Student Personnel Administrators, and the 1993 National TRIO Achiever Award.

Charles R. Smith, M.D.

Charles Smith has been Director of the Multiple Sclerosis Comprehensive Care Center at St. Agnes Hospital and New York Medical College since 1992. He has served as Director of the Departments of Neurology, since 1991, and Rehabilitation Medicine, since 1994, at the Bronx Lebanon Hospital Center, Bronx, New York. Following his training in internal medicine and neurology at the University of Toronto, he came to the Albert Einstein College of Medicine, Bronx, New York, to study mechanisms of viral persistence in tissue culture as a grantee of the National Multiple Sclerosis Society of Canada.

From 1989 to 1998, Dr. Smith was the Principal Investigator of the Medical Rehabilitation Research and Training Center for Multiple Sclerosis at Albert Einstein and, later, at New York Medical College. His particular interests have included clinical evaluation of fatigue and tremor in MS and the management of spasticity. He has been awarded research grants from the Social Security Administration and the National MS Society. He enjoys clinical management of patients with MS and frequently lectures to lay and professional groups about the illness. He has many published articles in both the professional and lay press on various aspects of the disease.

Pamela M. Sorensen, M.A., C.C.C.-S.L.P.

Pamela Sorensen, M.A., C.C.C.-S.L.P. earned her master's degree from the University of Denver and has provided evaluation and treatment for the speech, swallowing and cognitive-language problems of neurologically impaired adults since 1976. She served as Director of Speech/Language Pathology and Co-ordinator of the Comprehensive Outpatient Program for Evaluation (COPE) at the Rocky Mountain Multiple Sclerosis Center from 1988 to 1996, and has been a consulting Speech-Language Pathologist for the Jimmie Heuga Center medical programs since 1992.

Ms. Sorensen has been active with the Consortium of Multiple Sclerosis Centers (CMSC) since 1990. She directed the speech-language pathology segment of the Consortium's 1993 conference entitled *What Do We Know About MS*. She has served on the Clinical Care, Research, and Nominating Committees of the CMSC as well as the steering committees for MS Management Strategies, the North American Research Consortium on Multiple Sclerosis (NARCOMS) and the Paralyzed Veteran's of America (PVA)-sponsored MS Council for the development of Clinical Practice Guidelines (serving as an American Speech-Language and Hearing Association liaison). Ms. Sorensen was elected to the Executive Committee of the CMSC Board in 1996 as Vice President. She subsequently served as President-Elect in 1997, and President in 1999-2000.

Ms. Sorensen serves on the Employment Committee for the National MS Society and on the Editorial Advisory Board for the monthly publication Real Living with MS. In addition, she has published several articles and chapters on MS patient care, including "Communication Disorders and Dysphagia" in the *Journal of Neurologic Rehabilitation* (1994) and "Dysarthria in Multiple Sclerosis" in *The Diagnosis and Treatment of Symptoms and Signs in Multiple Sclerosis* (1999).

Michael A Werner, M.D.

Michael Werner is on the faculty of the New York Medical College in the Department of Urology, and serves as Regional Medical Advisor for New York and Connecticut for the Impotence Institute of America.

Following his residency in urology at Mount Sinai Medical Center in New York, Dr. Werner received his specialized fellowship training in male infertility and male sexual dysfunction at Boston University Medical Center. Dr. Werner has authored many chapters and articles for professional journals on male infertility and sexual dysfunction. One of his areas of particular interest is ejaculatory dysfunction. Dr. Werner works with men with MS to maximize their fertility and sexual function.

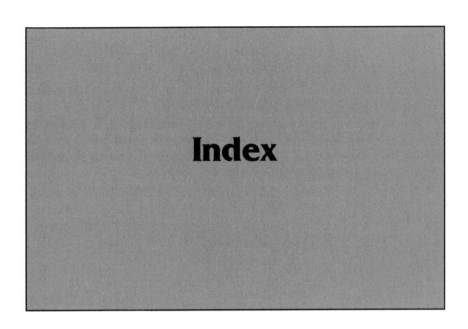

Index

Note: Boldface numbers indicate illustrations.

Demos Medical Publishing, Inc. publishes numerous books on multiple sclerosis. These include:

Alternative Medicine and Multiple Sclerosis
Allen C. Bowling, M.D.

Meeting the Challenge of Progressive Multiple Sclerosis
Patricia K. Coyle and June Halper

Multiple Sclerosis: A Guide for Families
Rosalind C. Kalb

Multiple Sclerosis: A Wellness Approach
George H. Kraft and Marci Catanzaro

300 Tips for Making Life with Multiple Sclerosis Easier
Shelley Peterman Schwarz

Symptom Management in Multiple Sclerosis, 3rd ed.
Randall T. Schapiro

Multiple Sclerosis: Your Legal Rights
Lanny Perkins and Sara Perkins

Insurance Solutions: Plan Well, Live Better
Laura Cooper